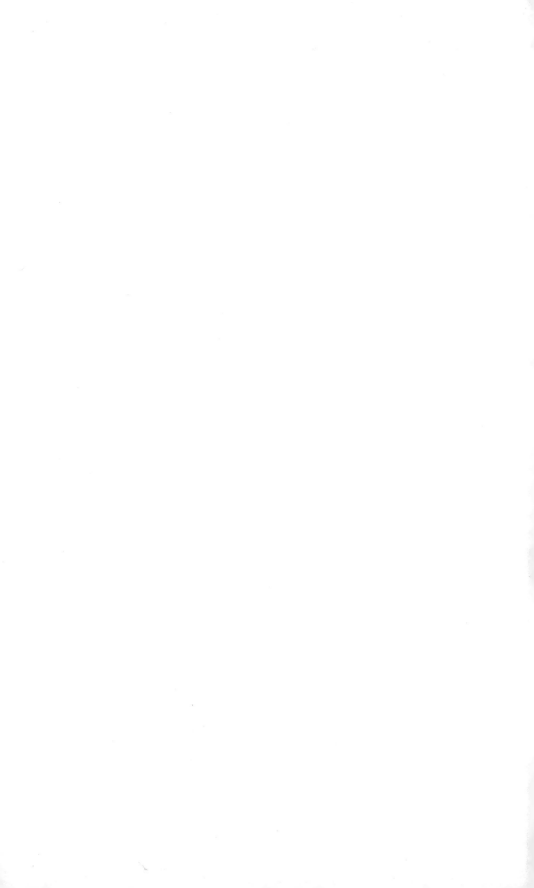

David E. Wazer · Douglas W. Arthur · Frank A. Vicini (Eds.)

Accelerated Partial Breast Irradiation

David E. Wazer · Douglas W. Arthur · Frank A. Vicini (Eds.)

Accelerated Partial Breast Irradiation

Techniques and Clinical Implementation

With 125 Figures and 42 Tables

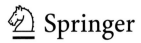 Springer

David E. Wazer
Department of Radiation Oncology
Tufts-New England Medical Center
Tufts University School of Medicine
750 Washington Street
Boston, MA 02111
USA

Frank A. Vicini
Department of Radiation Oncology
William Beaumont Hospital
3577 W. Thirteen Mile Road, Ste. 210
Royal Oak, MI 48073
USA

Douglas W. Arthur
Department of Radiation Oncology
Virginia Commonwealth University Medical
Center
Medical College Virginia Campus
401 College St
Richmond, VA 23298-0058
USA

Library of Congress Control Number: 2005937527

ISBN-10 3-540-28202-5 Springer Berlin Heidelberg New York
ISBN-13 978-3-540-28202-0 Springer Berlin Heidelberg New York

Springer is a part of Springer Science + Business Media
springer.com
© Springer-Verlag Berlin Heidelberg 2006
Printed in Germany

The use of general descriptive names, registered names, trademarks, etc. in this publication does not imply, even in the absence of a specific statement, that such names are exempt from the relevant protective laws and regulations and therefore free for general use.

Product liability: The publishers cannot guarantee the accuracy of any information about dosage and application contained in this book. In every individual case the user must check such information by consulting the relevant literature.

Editor: Dr. Ute Heilmann
Desk Editor: Meike Stoeck
Production & Typesetting: LE-TeX Jelonek, Schmidt & Vöckler GbR, Leipzig
Cover: Frido Steinen-Broo, Estudio Calamar, Spain

Printed on acid-free paper   21/3100/YL   5 4 3 2 1 0

Contents

List of Contributors

Douglas W. Arthur
Department of Radiation Oncology,
Virginia Commonwealth University
Medical Center,
Medical College Virginia Campus,
401 College Street
Richmond, VA 23298 USA

Thomas A. Buchholz
Department of Radiation Oncology,
The University of Texas
M. D. Anderson Cancer Center,
1515 Holcombe Blvd., Unit 1202,
Houston, TX 77030, USA

Peter Y. Chen
Department of Radiation Oncology,
William Beaumont Hospital,
3601 W. 13 Mile Road,
Royal Oak, MI 48073, USA

Laurie W. Cuttino
Department of Radiation Oncology,
Virginia Commonwealth University,
Richmond, VA 23298, USA

Rupak Das
Department of Human Oncology,
University of Wisconsin,
K4/B100 Clinical Sciences Center,
Madison, WI 53792, USA

Gregory K. Edmundson
Cytyc Surgical Products,
P.O. Box 944, Rough and Ready,
CA 95975, USA

Neal S. Goldstein
Department of Anatomic Pathology,
William Beaumont Hospital,
3601 West Thirteen Mile Road,
Royal Oak, MI 48073, USA

Yasmin Hasan
William Beaumont Hospital,
3601 West Thirteen Mile Road,
Royal Oak, MI 48073-6769, USA

Shruti Jolly
Department of Radiation Oncology,
William Beaumont Hospital,
3601 West Thirteen Mile Road,
Royal Oak, MI 48073, USA

Martin E. Keisch
Mt. Sinai Medical Center,
4300 Alton Road, Blum Bldg,
Miami Beach, FL 33140, USA

Joseph R. Kelley
Department of Radiation Oncology,
Virginia Commonwealth University
Medical Center,
Medical College Virginia Campus,
401 College Street
Richmond, VA 23298 USA

Larry L. Kestin
Department of Radiation Oncology,
William Beaumont Hospital,
3601 West Thirteen Mile Road,
Royal Oak, MI 48073, USA

Henry M. Kuerer
Department of Surgical Oncology,
The University of Texas,
M. D. Anderson Cancer Center,
Box 444, 1515 Holcombe Boulevard,
Houston, TX 77030, USA

Robert R. Kuske Jr.
Arizona Oncology Services,
8994 E Desert Cove Avenue, Ste. 100,
Scottsdale, AZ 85260, USA

Tibor Major
Department of Radiotherapy,
National Institute of Oncology,
Ráth Gy. u. 7-9.,
Budapest 1122, Hungary

Peter Niehoff
Department of Radiation Oncology,
University Hospital Schleswig-Holstein
Campus Kiel, Arnold-Heller Str. 9,
24105 Kiel, Germany

Oliver J. Ott
Department of Radiation Oncology,
University Hospital Erlangen,
Universitätsstr. 27,
91054 Erlangen, Germany

Rakesh R. Patel
Department of Human Oncology,
University of Wisconsin,
600 Highland Avenue K4/B100,
Madison, WI 53792, USA

Csaba Polgár
Department of Radiotherapy,
National Institute of Oncology,
Ráth Gy. u. 7-9.,
Budapest 1122, Hungary

Simon N. Powell
Department of Radiation Oncology,
Washington University School of Medicine,
4511 Forest Park,
St. Louis, MO 63108, USA

Mark J. Rivard
Department of Radiation Oncology,
Tufts-New England Medical Center,
750 Washington Street,
Boston, MA 02111, USA

Vratislav Strnad
Department of Radiation Oncology,
University Hospital Erlangen,
Universitätsstr. 27,
91054 Erlangen, Germany

Eric A. Strom
Department of Radiation Oncology,
The University of Texas
M. D. Anderson Cancer Center,
1515 Holcombe Blvd.,
Houston, TX 77030, USA

Alphonse G. Taghian
Department of Radiation Oncology,
Massachusetts General Hospital,
Harvard Medical School,
55 Fruit Street,
Boston, MA 02114, USA

Bruce Thomadsen
Departments of Medical Physics and
Human Oncology,
University of Wisconsin,
1530 Medical Sciences Center,
Madison, WI 53706, USA

Jayant S. Vaidya
Department of Surgery and Molecular
Oncology,
University of Dundee, Level 6,
Ninewells Hospital and Medical School,
Dundee DD1 9SY, UK

Frank A. Vicini
Department of Radiation Oncology,
William Beaumont Hospital,
3577 W. Thirteen Mile Road, Ste. 210,
Royal Oak, MI 48073, USA

David E. Wazer
Department of Radiation Oncology,
Tufts-New England Medical Center,
Tufts University School of Medicine,
750 Washington Street,
Boston, MA 02111, USA

Accelerated Partial Breast Irradiation: History, Rationale, and Controversies

1

Thomas A. Buchholz
and Eric A. Strom

Contents

1.1 Introduction

Results from two decades of study have conclusively shown that radiation therapy has an important role in ensuring local control for patients with early-stage breast cancer who are treated with breast-conserving surgery. When breast-conservation therapy was first explored as an alternative to mastectomy, many trials investigated whether surgical resection of the tumor-bearing region of the breast was sufficient, or whether adjuvant irradiation of the entire breast would be required to improve patient outcome. These trials showed that whole-breast irradiation significantly reduced the risk of ipsilateral tumor recurrence after resection of the tumor and the tissue immediately surrounding the tumor (Fisher et al. 2002a; Veronesi et al. 2001; Vinh-Hung and Verschraegen 2004).

On the basis of the results of these phase III trials, whole-breast irradiation became a standard component of breast-conservation therapy. Subsequently, two randomized trials investigated whether the addition of a tumor-bed boost following whole-breast irradiation offered further benefit (Bartelink et al. 2002; Romestaing et al. 1997). Both of these studies demonstrated a small but statistically significant reduction in ipsilateral breast tumor recurrence. Correspondingly, the available medical evidence to date suggests that the optimal radiation treatment schedule should include 5 weeks of daily therapy directed to the ipsilateral breast followed by 1 to 1.5 weeks of additional daily therapy directed to the tumor-bed region. A single randomized study has suggested that a 16-fraction course of whole-breast irradiation might also be considered for selected elderly patients with stage I disease (Whelan et al. 2002).

The studies investigating radiation and breast-conservation therapy proved to be one of the more significant advances in the local–regional management of breast cancer. It is now accepted that whole-breast irradiation after breast-conserving surgery decreases the risk of local recurrence to very low levels that are comparable to those achieved with mastectomy. Correspondingly, there is consensus that nearly all patients with early-stage breast cancer should be offered the option of being treated with a breast-conserving approach. An equally positive finding of these studies is that the radiation component of breast-conservation therapy is associated with a very low rate of toxicity to normal tissue and that modern local–regional treatment has little impact on the long-term quality of life for breast cancer survivors. Finally, with optimal surgical and radiation treatment the long-term aesthetic outcomes associated with this approach are excellent (Taylor et al. 1995; Wazer et al. 1992).

However, despite its many positive benefits, radiation therapy is also associated with some disadvantages, the foremost of which is perhaps the fact that it is a relatively complex and expensive treatment. Radiation treatments require physical resources, such as linear accelerators, simulators, and treatment planning systems, in addition to significant personnel resources, such as specialty-trained physicians, physicists, dosimetrists, and therapists. This level of expertise is not available in every city and the level varies from country to country. A second major downside of radiation therapy is that the treatments are inconvenient. As mentioned, standard whole-breast irradiation in the United States is typically administered over 6–7 weeks and treatments are preceded by 2 or 3 days of treatment planning. The 5-day-a-week treatment schedule may require patients to miss work and can lead to other significant life-style disruptions. These factors are particularly relevant for patients who do not live in close proximity to a radiation treatment facility. Standard whole-breast treatment may require such individuals to temporarily relocate, which might cause financial burdens such as temporary lodging expenses and the costs of missing work. Furthermore, such relocation may mean separating patients from their family, friends, and other supporters.

These downsides of radiation have been proven to have consequences. First, some women elect to forgo breast-conservation therapy and to be treated with mastectomy in order to avoid the need for radiation treatments. In fact, a number of studies have found an inverse relationship between the use of breast-conservation therapy and the distance from a patient's home to the nearest radiation facility (Athas et al. 2000). Furthermore, the regions of the country with the lowest density of radiation treatment facilities have the lowest rates of breast-conserving treatments (Farrow et al. 1992). An even more serious consequence that can result from the inconvenience of the radiation treatment schedule is that some patients treated with breast-conservation therapy elect to forgo the radiation component of their treatment. Recent pattern-of-care studies have indicated that approximately 20% of patients with early-stage invasive breast cancer treated in the United States do not receive radiation as a component of breast-conservation therapy (Nattinger et al. 2000). This option has been proven to place these patients at higher risk of tumor recurrence and possibly a higher risk of death.

The magnitude of the problem posed by the time required to administer radiation treatments is much greater outside the United States. The shortage of radiation treatment facilities in many countries makes the traditional scheduling of breast treatments impractical. In these countries, there can be extended delays in starting radiation therapy due to patient backlogs, and in other countries, the scheduling of radiation and the shortage of facilities have hindered the use of breast-conservation therapy.

One strategy to overcome some of these issues is to accelerate the course of radiation treatments. Although this may seem an intuitive solution, there are biological reasons why the 5- to 6-week treatment course for whole-breast radiation was originally developed. In brief, this schedule was thought to optimize the therapeutic ratio (defined as the probability of achieving tumor control versus the probability of causing normal-tissue injury). Decreasing the radiation treatment schedule to less than 5 weeks would require increasing the daily dose per fraction, and this increase, unfortunately, has a greater effect on the probability of normal-tissue injury than tumor control. A second important determinant of normal-tissue injury in addition to fraction size is the volume of normal tissue that is irradiated. Therefore, it was rational to hypothesize that an optimal therapeutic ratio could be maintained with an accelerated radiation schedule if the volume of normal tissue included in the irradiated volume was minimized.

This rationale, along with the clinical desire to shorten the radiation course, led to the investigation of accelerated partial breast irradiation (APBI). In this strategy, radiation is delivered only to the tumor bed region of the breast plus an arbitrarily defined margin. To date, APBI has been delivered with a variety of techniques, including single-fraction intraoperative electron or orthovoltage treatment, low-dose-rate interstitial brachytherapy (temporary implantation of radioactive sources), high-dose-rate interstitial brachytherapy, high-dose-rate brachytherapy delivered with a balloon catheter system (MammoSite; Proxima Therapeutics, Alpharetta, GA), and three-dimensional conformal external beam radiation treatment. Although these strategies differ with respect to many key variables, such as the dose of radiation delivered and the volume of breast tissue treated, they all share the common characteristic of attempting to shorten the treatment schedule from 6 to 7 weeks to a course that lasts 1 week or less.

1.2 History of APBI

Over the past 5 years, APBI has generated a great degree of enthusiasm among both cancer care providers and breast cancer patients. However, the first investigations of APBI as an alternative to conventional whole-breast irradiation began some time ago and were abandoned because of lack of efficacy. The first two trials investigating APBI were conducted in the United Kingdom in the early 1990s. Investigators at Guy's Hospital, London, conducted a relatively small phase I/II trial in which a low-dose-rate brachytherapy implant directed to the tumor bed region was used as the sole radiation component of breast-conservation therapy (Fentiman et al. 1996). After a median follow-up of 6 years, local in-breast relapse had developed in ten patients (37%). This rate is similar to that predicted for treatment with lumpectomy without any radiation. A much larger phase III clinical trial comparing whole-breast external beam irradiation to APBI was conducted at the Christie Hospital (Manchester, UK) during this same period (Magee et al. 1998). The APBI approach used in this trial was a fractionated external beam approach that utilized a single electron field. It should be recognized that the targeting of the APBI to the region at greatest risk in this trial was relatively crude by today's standards. Since this study, a number of improvements in imagining and treatment planning have been developed. In the Christie Hospital trial, APBI proved to be an inferior treatment to whole-breast irradiation. The 8-year actuarial local recurrence rate was 25% for those treated with partial-breast therapy and 13% for those receiving whole-breast treatment (Magee et al. 1998). These discouraging results led to a reluctance to pursue further the concept of APBI for some time.

In the late 1990s, interest in APBI was renewed. Investigators hoped that the high local recurrence rates noted in the early studies could be avoided with more stringent patient selection criteria, more uniform definitions of target volumes, a greater ability to define the target due to improved imaging and treatment planning, and more uniform dose prescriptions. In addition, in the first APBI trials, many important pathological factors that were subsequently found to be associated with local–regional recurrence were not evaluated systematically. Specifically, these studies included patients with unassessed or positive surgical margins and patients who did not undergo axillary lymph node evaluation. Finally, the presence or absence of invasion of the lymphovascular space and/or an extensive intraductal component were not analyzed.

In the United States, the first studies of APBI investigated treatment delivered with an interstitial implant (usually a double-plane implant) with the targeted region typically being the tumor bed plus a margin of 2.0–2.5 cm. Eligibility was limited to patients with tumors less than 4 cm in size with no more than three positive lymph nodes who were treated with a breast-conserving surgery that achieved negative surgical margins. Unlike previous experiences, these initial studies showed 3- to 5-year breast recurrence rates ranging from 1% to 5% (King et al. 2000; Vicini et al. 2003a). The short-term efficacy of the interstitial implant approach was also confirmed in many European centers. One of the leading European centers investigating APBI has been the National Institute of Oncology in Hungary. Investigators from this institution completed a phase I/II trial with encouraging results and have begun a follow-up phase III trial (Polgar et al. 2004). On the basis of the initial favorable data from approaches utilizing multicatheter implants, the Radiation Therapy Oncology Group (RTOG) conducted a multicenter phase II trial investigating a double-plane brachytherapy approach to APBI. Again, after a relatively short median follow-up period, the short-term in-breast recurrence rate and the normal-tissue toxicity rate were both excellent (Kuske et al. 2004).

The double-plane interstitial breast brachytherapy approach to APBI, however, has not been widely adopted in the United States. The treatment technique requires a specialized skill set, and the procedure and its planning require a significant amount of time. More recent technological advances, such as the use of template-guided approaches, have improved the reproducibility and convenience of interstitial brachytherapy, but even with these improvements brachytherapy remains a less popular option for APBI in the United States.

The initial therapeutic success of interstitial brachytherapy, coupled with its lack of widespread adoption, led to the development of a number of other methods of delivering APBI. In Italy and the United Kingdom, single-fraction intraoperative electron-beam or orthovoltage treatments have been studied in phase II trials, and both of these approaches are now being tested in phase III studies (Vaidya et al. 2004; Veronesi et al. 2003). In the United States, alternatives to double-plane interstitial implants have also been developed. At William Beaumont University (Vicini et al. 2003b) and New York University (Formenti et al. 2004) a conformal three-dimensional external-beam approach to APBI has been studied in pilot trials that were followed by a phase II RTOG study, which proved the feasibility of this approach in a multicenter setting. Another approach developed in the United States that has proven to be the most popular method of APBI has been the use of the MammoSite delivery device to deliver fractionated high-dose rate brachytherapy. The MammoSite is a balloon catheter that can be inserted into the tumor bed in a relatively straightforward fashion. After initial studies, the Food and Drug Administration approved the MammoSite applicator as a treatment-delivery device. It has been estimated that this device has been used in over 3000 patients.

Arguably, the use of APBI has outpaced the clinical data proving that it is an appropriate alternative to whole-breast treatment. The most mature data to date concerning the safety and efficacy of APBI have been derived from studies investigating the double-plane brachytherapy approach; however, as mentioned, this approach represents a relatively small percentage of the current APBI practice pattern. Brachytherapy treatment using the MammoSite device is different from that using a double-plane interstitial implant in many ways, and although the early results of a registry trial appear promising, there are no 5-year data available concerning the safety and efficacy of treatments using the MammoSite device. Despite this, the majority of MammoSite treatments are currently being given outside of a protocol setting.

Whether APBI should be considered an investigational treatment or be accepted as an alternative to whole-breast irradiation is a controversial issue. Table 1.1 lists some reasons for and against considering APBI to be an accepted standard of care. In 2003, the American Brachytherapy Society issued a report suggesting that APBI could be considered an appropriate treatment option for selected patients provided there was an ad-

Table 1.1 Should APBI be considered investigational or an accepted standard of care?

Reasons to consider APBI as an investigational treatment	Reasons to consider APBI an acceptable standard of care for selected patients
There have been no completed phase III trials comparing more recent APBI approaches to whole-breast treatment. The only APBI phase III study completed to date showed this approach to be inferior	Mature results from a comparative phase III trial will likely not be available for a decade
	Whole-breast irradiation is not an option for some breast cancer patients because of its protracted treatment schedule
The long-term efficacy of APBI with modern techniques remains unknown	
	Initial institutional and phase II multicenter trials investigating APBI have shown excellent local control rates and low rates of serious normal-tissue injury
The appropriate patient selection criteria for APBI treatment are unknown	
The late normal-tissue effects of APBI are unknown. The majority of long-term quality-of-life complications associated with hypofractionated radiation treatments develop years after completion of treatment and are not necessarily related to the absence of short-term side effects	

equate quality-assurance program in place (Arthur et al. 2003). However, we and others have contended that whole-breast irradiation should continue to be the standard of care until longer term safety and efficacy data are available from well-designed clinical trials of APBI (Buchholz 2003; McCormick 2003). This is particularly true for patients who are able to undergo whole-breast treatment with only minor inconvenience. For those who are truly unable to receive a 6- to 7-week course of therapy and who do not have the option of conventional treatment, APBI should be considered as an unproven alternative that would likely be better than complete omission of radiation therapy.

1.3 Controversies Regarding the Use of APBI

The major question concerning the use of APBI as an alternative to whole-breast irradiation is whether APBI will prove to be as safe and effective. Breast cancer therapy has achieved considerable success over the past two decades. Since 1990, there has been a consistent 7% annual decrease in the breast cancer death rate in the United States (Wingo et al. 2003). Advances in public education, screening programs, diagnostic imaging, surgery, systemic treatments, and radiation therapy have all contributed towards this improved outcome. Specific examples of such advances in the field of medical oncology are the use of anthracyclines, taxanes, specific dose schedules, and new classes of compounds such as aromatase inhibitors and molecular specific therapies such as trastuzumab. There have also been advances in radiation therapy. Because of advances in radiation delivery techniques, important potentially life-threatening injuries can be overcome and treatment efficacy has been improved.

The benefits derived from radiation therapy as a component of breast-conservation are very significant. A meta-analysis of trials investigating radiation therapy after breast-conservation surgery has shown that radiation not only reduces the recurrence rate but also improves overall survival (Vinh-Hung and Verschraegen 2004). These considerations are particularly important in that other studies have indicated that the majority of patients are willing to accept the toxicity and inconvenience of treatments if they perceive there to be even a 1% decrease in the risk of recurrence (Ravdin et al. 1998).

Whether whole-breast irradiation offers an advantage over APBI in decreasing the risk of ipsilateral breast tumor recurrence will only be determined by a comparative phase III trial. The degree of difference between the two approaches will likely be dependent on patient selection criteria. It should be appreciated that patients with favorable disease characteristics achieve an excellent rate of success with conventional approaches, providing a high benchmark against which APBI needs to be compared. For example, for patients with lymph node-negative disease who are treated with surgery that achieves a negative margin, whole-breast irradiation, tumor bed boost irradiation, and some form of systemic therapy, the estimated annual risk of local recurrence is approximately 0.5% (Buchholz et al. 2001; Fisher et al. 2002b). It is highly unlikely that APBI will improve upon this excellent result, but when the risk of recurrence is so low, it may be appropriate to consider accepting a slightly higher risk for the convenience benefits.

1.3.1 Does APBI Treat an Adequate Volume of Breast Tissue?

An important rationale for considering less than whole-breast treatment concerns the patterns of breast tumor recurrence in patients treated with breast conservation without adjuvant radiation therapy. Data from clinical trials suggest that of the 30% of patients who experience breast tumor recurrence when radiation therapy is not delivered, the vast majority (approximately 80%) will have the recurrence develop at the site of the original disease (Clark et al. 1992; Liljegren et al. 1999; Veronesi et al. 2001). In addition, the absolute percentage of recurrences that develop in a location far away from the tumor bed is low, ranging from 3% to 5% (Clark et al. 1992; Liljegren et al. 1999; Veronesi et al. 2001). From these data, many researchers have hypothesized that treatment directed solely to the site of the primary tumor may be adequate.

It is important to recognize that there is an inherent limitation in using data from studies that have investigated patterns of recurrence in patients treated with surgery alone to support the concept of treating only a small volume of breast tissue around the tumor bed. Most breast cancer recurrences develop from residual disease that was a component of the original primary tumor and therefore is in part adjacent to the surgical cavity. In fact, for patients with residual disease, it is likely that the greatest disease burden will be located next to the tumor bed cavity and that the density will diminish as a function of distance from the cavity. However, this does not mean that the area around the cavity will be the only site of residual disease. In fact, clinical evidence suggests that residual disease may also extend into volumes not included within APBI-targeted regions. A representation of this important concept is shown in Fig. 1.1. If a patient with such extent of disease did not receive any additional treatment, the regions closest to the tumor bed would be identified as the first sites of tumor recurrence. As effective treatment was given to an extended volume around the tumor bed, recurrences within that treatment volume may be avoided, but there would continue to be a risk that some volume of disease would be left untreated. In such a scenario, the first site of recurrence would again be at the margin of the treatment. If the margin were extended, the most common site of first recurrence would then be at the new margin of treatment.

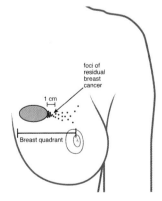

Fig. 1.1 Illustration of a medial tumor bed with residual disease extending from the tumor bed into the upper lateral quadrant. If no radiation was given in this situation, it is likely that the tumor would recur first at the tumor bed site. However, it is clear that giving radiation only to a volume of radius 1 cm around the tumor site would also be an ineffective strategy (reprinted with permission from Buchholz et al. 2005)

The concept described above is supported by studies of the distribution of disease in mastectomy specimens, which suggest that residual disease may extend beyond a margin of 1–2.5 cm around the tumor excision cavity. One of the first pieces of evidence for this came from the work of Holland et al. in 1985, in which mastectomy specimens from 282 women with localized T1 and T2 tumors were carefully examined (Holland et al. 1985). In this study, 28% of the cases of index tumors measuring 2 cm or smaller where found to have a focus of residual in situ or invasive carcinoma more than 2 cm from the primary tumor. Later, Faverly et al. (2001) mapped the disease extent in 135 patients with tumors smaller than 4 cm and again found that a large percentage of patients had disease that extended beyond the margins around the primary tumor that are typically included in APBI treatment. Finally, Vaidya et al. also performed a careful three-dimensional pathological analysis of whole-mount mastectomy specimens and reconstructed the residual tumor volume present after an initial lumpectomy (Vaidya et al. 1996). Residual disease was detected in 63% of the patients, and in 79% of these patients, the disease extended beyond 25% of the breast volume surrounding the lumpectomy cavity. It is important to recognize that if such patients were treated with breast-conserving surgery without radiation, the most common site of recurrence would be the primary tumor site. However, these data indicate that this pattern of failure does not provide a scientific rationale for directing therapies to a tissue margin of 1–2 cm around the tumor bed.

Data from studies investigating the value of magnetic resonance imaging (MRI) in patients with early-stage breast cancer also raise questions as to whether APBI treatment covers the appropriate volume of tissue at risk of residual disease. For example, in a study of 267 patients who were undergoing breast-conservation surgery, MRI scans showed that 18% of patients had foci of disease outside the index tumor bed (Bedrosian et al. 2003). Furthermore, in an international collaborative study of 417 patients with early-stage breast cancer, MRI scans showed incidental lesions away from the index site of disease in 24% of patients (Bluemke et al. 2004). Of these lesions, 71% were histologically confirmed to be cancer, and only 8% of these incidental lesions were detected by mammography. As MRI scans are not routinely performed prior to APBI, these studies suggest that a percentage of patients treated with APBI will have disease that extends beyond the treatment volume.

In addition to the pathological and radiological rationale for the use of whole-breast treatment, the clinical data available to date suggest that APBI approaches may not include all areas at risk of residual disease. Attempts have been made to avoid whole-breast irradiation by treating the tumor bed plus a wider margin with surgery, but these approaches have been unsuccessful. Specifically, the Milan III trial compared results using very wide excision (quadrantectomy) with and without whole-breast radiation (Veronesi et al. 2001). The 10-year rate of breast tumor recurrence in the quadrantectomy-only group was 24% versus 6% in the surgery plus whole-breast irradiation arm. The trial was not powered to analyze effects in particular subgroups, but a particularly high recurrence rate was noted in younger patients and those with tumors had an extensive intraductal component in the surgery-only arm. Another important finding was that patients with positive lymph nodes who were randomized to not receive radiation therapy had a poorer survival (P=0.038), again suggesting that the prevention of local recurrences by radiation is of paramount importance.

These data suggest that the volume of breast irradiated and the patient selection criteria will in part determine the success of APBI. It should be recognized that the volume of breast treatment is determined both by the extent of surgical resection and by the type of APBI approach used. Ideally, the surgical resection should provide widely negative margins, and the APBI approach should treat as large a volume of tissue around the surgical cavity as possible. Indeed, some of the early data concerning outcomes after APBI treatment suggest that larger volumes are associated with lower rates of recurrence. For example, Vicini et al. at William Beaumont Hospital reported their single-institution experience. They achieved excellent 5-year tumor control rates in highly selected patients treated with a large-volume implant that included the tumor bed with 2-cm margins (Vicini et al. 2003a). However, Perera et al. at the London (Ontario) Regional Cancer Center used implants that treated only the tumor bed as delineated by surgical clips, and reported a 5-year breast tumor recurrence rate of 16%. Two-thirds of these recurrences developed outside of the implanted volume (Perera et al. 2003).

As these data indicate, one of the limitations to current APBI approaches is the uncertainty of what constitutes the most appropriate target volume. APBI is often considered to be a single therapeutic strategy, but it is important to recognize that different APBI approaches target different volumes of peritumoral tissue. In addition, the necessary volume of tissue to be included in APBI treatments is also dependent on the completeness of the surgical procedure. Currently, there is no consensus on the optimal volume of breast tissue that should be treated with APBI and the language used to describe treatment volumes is inconsistent. These factors make comparisons between institutional experiences difficult. There continues to be a need to standardize APBI treatments in order to provide a better understanding of benefits and shortcomings. A major advance in this area has been the development of standards for a national phase III APBI trial that recently began enrolling patients in the United States.

1.3.2 Which Patients May Be The Most Appropriate for APBI?

Patient selection is a critical determinant of whether APBI treatments will likely include the region at risk of residual disease. Randomized trials that have investigated radiation omission have helped define the factors that are associated with a lower risk of residual disease after surgery. These factors include older age (particularly over 70 years), wide negative surgical margins, T1 primary disease, lack of an extensive intraductal component, lack of lobular histology, estrogen receptor-positive disease, treatment with sys-

Table 1.2 Patient selection criteria for APBI

	ASBC[a]	ABS[b]	NSABP/RTOG
Age (years)	>50	≥45	>45
Histology	IDC, DCIS	Unifocal IDC	DCIS or any histology
Size (cm)	≤2	≤3	≤3
Margins	≥2 mm	No tumor on ink	No tumor on ink
Lymph nodes	Negative	Negative	<4 positive LN

[a] American Society of Breast Surgeons (2005)
[b] Arthur et al. (2003)

temic therapy, and pathological N0 disease (Veronesi et al. 2001). These factors are all associated with a lower risk of recurrence when patients are treated with surgery alone, so it is likely that those with residual disease after surgery will have a lower disease burden that is more often localized near the tumor bed. There is no uniform consensus on the patient and disease characteristics that are appropriate for consideration of APBI. Table 1.2 provides details about statements concerning patient selection that have been issued by the American Society of Breast Surgeons and the American Brachytherapy Society (American Society of Breast Surgeons 2005; Arthur et al. 2003). Also included is the eligibility criteria for an ongoing National Surgical Adjuvant Breast and Bowel Project (NSABP)/RTOG phase III trial that is comparing APBI to whole-breast treatment

1.3.3 Does APBI Deliver an Adequate Radiation Dose?

A final issue of importance when considering whether APBI will prove to be as effective as whole-breast treatment concerns the dose of radiation. In general, whole-breast irradiation plus a tumor-bed boost provides a significantly higher biologically effective dose to the peritumoral area. Although a variety of dose schedules have been used in APBI treatments, the most common prescription dose (and the dose selected for the planned American phase III clinical trial) is 34 Gy delivered in ten fractions, with fractions given twice daily over a period of 5 days. Rosenstein et al. recently estimated the biological equivalent dose (BED) of this schedule for tumors and late-responding normal tissues compared to standard whole-breast treatment plus a tumor-bed boost (Rosenstein et al. 2004). The BED for the tumor was 1.7 times higher for the whole-breast plus boost schedule compared to the 34-Gy in ten fraction schedule (assuming an alpha/beta ratio for tumor of 10 Gy) and 1.4 times higher for late effects in normal tissue (alpha/beta ratio of 2 Gy). These data indicate that the dose to the area at greatest risk of disease is less with APBI. This is an important consideration given that trials investigating use versus omission of a tumor-bed boost after whole-breast treatment suggest that dose escalation minimizes the risk of recurrence (Bartelink et al. 2002; Romestaing et al. 1997).

Estimating the success of APBI through calculations of BED significantly oversimplifies a very complex process. Most APBI techniques, particularly MammoSite, have significant dose inhomogeneity within the treated volume. For example, the treatment dose with a MammoSite device is almost twice as high at the surface of the balloon as it is at the prescription dose point located 1 cm from the balloon. Therefore, regions within the target volume may receive significantly higher BEDs if they are close to the applicator surface. In addition, the effectiveness of radiation is also dependent on treatment time and the shortened treatment course associated with APBI may reduce the risk of tumor cell repopulation during treatment. Finally, the biological properties of breast cancers vary; correspondingly, the alpha/beta ratios and proliferation rates are also likely to vary from case to case. Therefore, dose comparisons between the two treatment schedules are difficult.

1.3.4 Can APBI Increase Rates of Normal Tissue Injury?

Data from phase II trials and institutional reports suggest that APBI approaches are associated with low rates of acute injury to normal tissue (Keisch et al. 2003; Vicini et al. 2003a). However, the more important question that has yet to be fully answered is whether late normal-tissue complications may be increased. As highlighted above, dosages of 34 Gy in ten fractions provide a lower BED to late-responding normal tissues compared to 66 Gy in 33 fractions and, therefore, would be predicted to carry less risk of injury (Rosenstein et al. 2004). Furthermore, the decreased volume of irradiated tissue will also be an important factor in decreasing the risk of injury with APBI, and this component is not considered in BED calculations. One possible concern, however, is that, as previously noted, many APBI techniques have significant dose inhomogeneity within the treatment volume. For example, a MammoSite catheter placed against the chest wall may give a significantly higher BED to this important normal tissue than conventional therapy. Therefore, it is important that these promising APBI techniques be investigated in protocols that carefully track and record late radiation injuries. Late injuries to normal tissue resulting from radiation are difficult to study in that they may occur many years after treatment. For example, in a study of breast cancer patients who were treated with a hypofractionated radiation regimen, Bentzen et al. found that it took 15 years of follow-up after treatment to detect 90% of the ultimate incidence of late grade 3 complications (Bentzen et al. 1990).

1.4 Convenience Benefits of APBI

It is clear that APBI offers a convenience advantage over whole-breast irradiation. Five-day APBI treatment approaches are potentially 85% shorter than conventional whole-breast plus tumor-bed boost therapy. However, for patients treated with surgery and chemotherapy, the shortened course of radiation would lead to only a 10–15% decrease in the overall length of the breast cancer treatment. In addition, it should be recognized that there is an alternative to APBI for patients for whom treatment time is a major issue. A Canadian phase III trial found equivalent 5-year control and toxicity rates for a 3-week hypofractionated whole-breast irradiation schedule (42.5 Gy in 16 fractions) compared to a 5-week irradiation schedule for carefully selected patients (Whelan et al. 2002). When compared to this whole-breast treatment approach, most APBI schedules require only six fewer treatment visits, making the convenience benefits of APBI less relevant. Finally, some patients may find the twice-daily treatment required by most APBI schemes to cause a greater disruption to their lives than once-daily treatment.

1.4.1 Will APBI Increase Access to Medical Facilities and Reduce Costs?

One potential advantage of APBI would be to improve access to radiation therapy facilities. However, unlike in other countries, few patients in the United States endure long delays before starting radiation therapy because of limited access to treatment machines. In the Unites States, more common rate-limiting steps in getting patients onto treatment is limited physician time and treatment planning resources. Most APBI approaches require significantly greater treatment planning and quality assurance and, therefore, require significantly more physician and physicist time than conventional external beam whole-breast treatments. Therefore, the total impact of APBI in improving access to care may not be significant in the United States.

With respect to treatment cost, there is currently no evidence that treatment with either MammoSite or a double-plane interstitial implant costs less than conventional whole-breast irradiation followed by a boost. In fact, in a recent study, Suh et al. calculated direct medical costs and Medicare fee schedules and modeled treatment costs to the patients and society (Suh et al. 2003). These authors found that APBI using either of these brachytherapy techniques was significantly more expensive than conventional whole-breast plus tumor-bed boost therapy.

1.5 Conclusions

APBI has the potential to be an exciting improvement in radiation treatment for patients with early-stage breast cancer. However, new advances in breast cancer treatment should be carefully evaluated in clinical trials that are appropriately designed to assess safety and efficacy end-points. Premature adoption of initially promising therapies can lead to long-term setbacks. A perfect example of this in breast cancer was the premature adoption of high-dose chemotherapy with bone marrow transplant. Widespread adoption of this approach after favorable short-term phase II trials impaired the completion of phase III studies. As most of the phase III trials were eventually negative, it became apparent that thousands of patients received a treatment that was later proven to be less than optimal.

Studying APBI as an alternative to whole-breast treatment is difficult because it requires long-term follow-up. Furthermore, depending on the patient selection criteria used, differences between these two approaches may be subtle, and detecting such a difference in comparative trials would require thousands of patients. To date, such trials have not been completed. The only relatively mature studies available concerning efficacy and safety of APBI have been from institutional studies using double-plane interstitial brachytherapy as the APBI technique. No 5-year follow-up data are available from the external beam or MammoSite APBI approaches.

It is imperative to recognize that short-term success may not translate into a long-term satisfactory result, with respect to both efficacy and toxicity. As previously indicated, the complications of a hypofractionated APBI scheme may not appear for many years. An example of the necessity for long-term follow-up is found in the unsuccessful phase II trial at Guy's Hospital that investigated APBI with an interstitial brachytherapy technique. The original publication of the Guy's Hospital experience reported "encouraging" results in 1991 (Fentiman et al. 1991); however, in 1996, as the data matured, the authors concluded that this approach was inadequate (Magee et al. 1998).

Modern conventional whole-breast irradiation provides excellent outcomes for patients treated with breast conservation, providing a high benchmark against which new treatments must be compared. It is highly unlikely that APBI will improve upon these excellent results, because it is a less intensive approach, both with respect to volume of treatment and the dose delivered to the targeted treatment volume. Whereas some patients may accept a small increase in probability of recurrence for the added convenience of APBI, most breast cancer patients report that they wish to do everything possible to minimize this risk. To study whether APBI will be equally efficacious, a comparative phase III trial is needed. Recently, such a trial opened in the United States, allowing the entire oncology community the option of contributing to the resolution of these important questions.

References

1. American Society of Breast Surgeons (2005) Consensus statement for accelerated partial breast irradiation. http://www.breastsurgeons.org/apbi.shtml

2. Arthur D, Vicini F, Kuske RR, et al (2003) Accelerated partial breast irradiation: an updated report from the American Brachytherapy Society. Brachytherapy 2:124–130

3. Athas WF, Adams-Cameron M, Hunt WC, et al (2000) Travel distance to radiation therapy and receipt of radiotherapy following breast-conserving surgery. J Natl Cancer Inst 92(3):269–271

4. Bartelink H, Horiot JC, Poortmans, et al (2002) Recurrence rates after treatment of breast cancer with standard radiotherapy with or without additional radiation. J Clin Oncol 20:4141–4149

5. Bedrosian I, Mick R, Orel SG, et al (2003) Changes in the surgical management of patients with breast carcinoma based on preoperative magnetic resonance imaging. Cancer 98:468–473

6. Bentzen SM, Turesson I, Thames HD (1990) Fractionation sensitivity and latency of telangiectasia after postmastectomy radiotherapy: a graded-response analysis. Radiother Oncol 18:95–106

7. Bluemke D, Gatsonis CA, Chen MH, et al (2004) Magnetic resonance imaging of the breast prior to biopsy. JAMA 292(22):2735–2742

8. Buchholz TA (2003) Partial breast irradiation: is it ready for prime time? Int J Radiat Oncol Biol Phys 57(5):1214–1216

9. Buchholz TA, Tucker SL, Mathur D, et al (2001) Impact of systemic treatment on local control for lymph-node negative breast cancer patients treated with breast-conservation therapy. J Clin Oncol 19:2240–2246

10. Buchholz TA, Kuerer HM, Strom EA (2005) Is partial breast irradiation a step forward or backward? Semin Radiat Oncol 15(2):69–75

11. Clark RM, McCulloch PB, Levine MN, et al (1992) Randomized clinical trial to assess the effectiveness of breast irradiation following lumpectomy and axillary dissection for node-negative breast cancer. J Natl Cancer Inst 84:683–689

12. Farrow DC, Hunt WC, Samet JM (1992) Geographic variation in the treatment of localized breast cancer. N Engl J Med 326:1097–1101

13. Faverly DR, Hendriks JH, Holland R (2001) Breast carcinomas of limited extent: frequency, radiologic–pathologic characteristics, and surgical margin requirements. Cancer 91:647–659

14. Fentiman IS, Poole C, Tong D, et al (1991) Iridium implant treatment without external radiotherapy for operable breast cancer: a pilot study. Eur J Cancer 27(4):447–450

15. Fentiman IS, Poole C, Tong D, et al (1996) Inadequacy of iridium implant as sole radiation treatment for operable breast cancer. Eur J Cancer 32A:608–611

16. Fisher B, Anderson S, Bryant J, et al (2002a) Twenty-year follow-up of a randomized trial comparing total mastectomy, lumpectomy, and lumpectomy plus irradiation for the treatment of invasive breast cancer. N Engl J Med 347:1233–1241

17. Fisher B, Bryant J, Dignam JJ, et al; National Surgical Adjuvant Breast and Bowel Project (2002b) Tamoxifen, radiation therapy, or both for prevention of ipsilateral breast tumor recurrence after lumpectomy in women with invasive breast cancers of one centimeter or less. J Clin Oncol 20:4141–4149

18. Formenti SC, Truong MT, Goldberg JD, et al (2004) Prone accelerated partial breast irradiation after breast-conserving surgery: preliminary clinical results and dose-volume histogram analysis. Int J Radiat Oncol Biol Phys 60:493–504

19. Holland R, Veling SH, Mravunac M, et al (1985) Histologic multifocality of Tis, T1-2 breast carcinomas. Implications for clinical trials of breast-conserving surgery. Cancer 56(5):979–990

20. Keisch M, Vicini F, Kuske RR, et al (2003) Initial clinical experience with the MammoSite breast brachytherapy applicator in women with early-stage breast cancer treated with breast-conserving therapy. Int J Radiat Oncol Biol Phys 55:289–293

21. King TA, Bolton JS, Kuske RR, et al (2000) Long-term results of wide-field brachytherapy as the sole method of radiation therapy after segmental mastectomy for T(is,1,2) breast cancer. Am J Surg 180(4):299–304

22. Kuske RR, Winter K, Arthur DW, et al (2004) A phase II trial of brachytherapy alone following lumpectomy for stage I or II breast cancer: initial outcomes of RTOG 9517 (abstract). Proc Am Soc Clin Oncol 23:18

23. Liljegren G, Holmberg L, Bergh J, et al (1999) 10-Year results after sector resection with or without postoperative radiotherapy for stage I breast cancer: a randomized trial. J Clin Oncol 17:2326–2333

24. Magee B, Young EA, Swindell R (1998) Patterns of breast relapse following breast conserving surgery and radiotherapy (abstract O69). Br J Cancer 78 [Suppl 2]:24

25. McCormick B (2003) The politics and the ethics of breast cancer. Brachytherapy 2(2):119–120

26. Nattinger AB, Hoffmann RG, Kneusel RT, et al (2000) Relation between appropriateness of primary therapy for early-stage breast carcinoma and increased use of breast-conserving surgery. Lancet 356:1148–1153

27. Perera F, Yu E, Engel J, et al (2003) Patterns of breast recurrence in a pilot study of brachytherapy confined to the lumpectomy site for early breast cancer with six years' minimum follow-up. Int J Radiat Oncol Biol Phys 57:1239–1246

28. Polgar C, Major T, Fodor J, et al (2004) High-dose-rate brachytherapy alone versus whole-breast radiotherapy with or without tumor bed boost after breast-conserving surgery: seven-year results of a comparative study. Int J Radiat Oncol Biol Phys 60(4):1173–1181

29. Ravdin PM, Siminoff IA, Harvey JA (1998) Survey of breast cancer patients concerning their knowledge and expectations of adjuvant therapy. J Clin Oncol 16:515–521

30. Romestaing P, Lehingue Y, Carrie C, et al (1997) Role of a 10-Gy boost in the conservative treatment of early breast cancer: results of a randomized clinical trial in Lyon, France. J Clin Oncol 15(3):963–968

31. Rosenstein BS, Lymberis SC, Formenti SC (2004) Biologic comparison of partial breast irradiation protocols. Int J Radiat Oncol Biol Phys 60(5):1393–1404

32. Suh WW, Pierce LJ, Vicini FA, et al (2003) Comparing the cost of partial versus whole-breast irradiation following breast conserving surgery for early-stage breast cancer (abstract). Breast Cancer Res Treat 82:S181

33. Taylor ME, Perez CA, Halverson KJ, et al (1995) Factors influencing cosmetic results after conservation therapy for breast cancer. Int J Radiat Oncol Biol Phys 4(31):753–764

34. Vaidya JS, Vyas JJ, Chinoy RF, et al (1996) Multicentricity of breast cancer: whole-organ analysis and clinical implications. Br J Cancer 74:820–824

35. Vaidya JS, Tobias JS, Baum M, et al (2004) Intraoperative radiotherapy for breast cancer. Lancet Oncol 5:165–173

36. Veronesi U, Marubini E, Mariani L, et al (2001) Radiotherapy after breast-conserving surgery in small breast carcinoma: long-term results of a randomized trial. Ann Oncol 12:997–1003

37. Veronesi U, Gatti G, Luini A, et al (2003) Full-dose intraoperative radiotherapy with electrons during breast-conserving surgery. Arch Surg 138:1253–1256

38. Vicini FA, Kestin L, Chen P, et al (2003a) Limited-field radiation therapy in the management of early-stage breast cancer. J Natl Cancer Inst 95:1205–1210

39. Vicini FA, Remouchamps V, Wallace M, et al (2003b) Ongoing clinical experience utilizing 3D conformal external beam radiotherapy to deliver partial-breast irradiation in patients with early-stage breast cancer treated with breast-conserving therapy. Int J Radiat Oncol Biol Phys 57:1247–1253

40. Vinh-Hung V, Verschraegen C (2004) Breast-conserving surgery with or without radiotherapy: pooled-analysis for risks of ipsilateral breast tumor recurrence and mortality. J Natl Cancer Inst 96:115–121

41. Wazer DE, DiPetrillo T, Schmidt-Ullrich R, et al (1992) Factors influencing cosmetic outcome and complication risk after conservative surgery and radiotherapy for early-stage breast carcinoma. J Clin Oncol 10(3):356–363

42. Whelan T, McKenzie R, Julian J, et al (2002) Randomized trial of breast irradiation schedules after lumpectomy for women with node-negative breast cancer .J Natl Cancer Inst 94:1143–1150

43. Wingo PA, Cardinez CJ, Landis SH, et al (2003) Long-term trends in cancer mortality in the United States, 1930-1998. Cancer 97:3133–3275

Who is a Candidate for Accelerated Partial Breast Irradiation?

Douglas W. Arthur, Frank A. Vicini
and David E. Wazer

2

Contents

2.1 Introduction

There are many aspects to consider when determining whether a woman is an appropriate candidate for accelerated partial breast irradiation (APBI). First, however, it is necessary to have a full appreciation of the challenge that this new approach presents to the conventional treatment paradigm for early-stage breast cancer. Until recently, the accepted local management of breast cancer has always stressed the importance of treatment directed to the entire breast. Over the past three decades the management of early breast cancer has evolved from radical en bloc regional resection to breast-conserving surgery followed by radiotherapy, but the minimal target tissue requirement has always included the entire breast. Prior to screening mammograms, breast cancer went undetected until clinically evident and often presented in a locally advanced stage. However, as public awareness has increased regarding the role of mammographic screening, breast cancer is increasingly detected earlier in the disease process and frequently presents as a small, non-palpable tumor. In view of this changed clinical presentation, it is appropriate to ask the question as to whether there should be a parallel reduction in the extent of local treatment.

The concept that the extent of treatment to the breast could be safely reduced was first tested by moving from mastectomy to lumpectomy. When introduced, the concept of breast preservation was initially considered to be extreme and dangerous. Many felt that to compromise the radical extent of the surgical resection would result in a diminished ability to cure the cancer. It was the carefully measured steps of a handful of pioneering surgeons and radiation oncologists that ultimately led to the widespread acceptance that breast conservation was both safe and practical. This profound shift in treatment paradigm nonetheless held fast to the philosophy of treating the entire breast with the addition of adjuvant radiotherapy—a practice that was ultimately embraced with remarkable speed as the requisite radiation therapy technology was widely available and easily applied.

Despite initial controversy, many years of rigorous investigation led to breast conservation becoming established as an appropriate alternative to mastectomy in properly selected early-stage breast cancer. In 1990, based upon early but compelling clinical trial results, the National Institutes of Health published a consensus statement on early-stage breast cancer supporting breast conservation surgery followed by radiotherapy as an appropriate method of primary therapy for women with stage I–II breast cancer (NIH Consensus Development Conference 1990). More recently, survival data after a 20-year follow-up of large prospectively randomized studies have become available that definitively establish the equivalence of lumpectomy followed by whole-breast radiotherapy as compared to mastectomy (Fisher et al. 2002; Veronesi et al. 2002). However, despite this overwhelming evidence, many women who are eligible for breast conservation therapy continue to lose their breasts to mastectomy (Athas et al. 2000; Du et al. 1999; Hahn et al. 2003; Hebert-Croteau et al. 1999). This phenomenon is likely due to many factors, but the logistical barriers of treatment duration and travel distance encountered with the standard 5–7 weeks of daily whole-breast radiotherapy can be a hardship for many women and can play a role in treatment decisions. These factors may push a number of women towards mastectomy (when they would rather preserve the breast) or towards lumpectomy only (where they face an increased risk of in-breast failure). The desire to avoid conventional whole-breast radiotherapy, as a result of either patient preference or physician bias, has been documented through data from the National Cancer Institute Surveillance, Epidemiology, and End Results registry which finds a steady increase in the rate of breast-conserving surgery without radiotherapy (Nattinger et al. 2000).

Local treatment options for breast cancer depend upon the definition of the tissue at risk. If the target tissue following lumpectomy is indeed the whole breast, then the constraints of normal tissue tolerance dictate that radiation treatment be delivered daily over several weeks to achieve the dose necessary to eradicate microscopic residual disease. However, if the volume of the target can be substantially reduced to include only a portion of the breast, then dose–volume relationships strongly suggest that the radiation treatment course can be safely accelerated and completed in a matter of days. As such, APBI could potentially overcome the barriers presented by conventional whole-breast irradiation, and provide more patients with the option of breast-conservation treatment. Additionally, APBI may open the option of breast preservation for patients who are not currently considered as candidates. For example, in patients who have experienced a local recurrence following breast conservation with whole-breast irradiation and those diagnosed with breast cancer after having previously received mantle irradiation for Hodgkin's disease (Kuerer et al. 2004).

As previously noted, the change in focus from a treatment target that encompasses the entire breast to one that encompasses only part of the breast represents a shift of the treatment paradigm that is as profound, and likely as controversial, as the step from mastectomy to breast conservation. For a new treatment paradigm of this nature to be broadly accepted, four components are necessary: (1) supporting data with respect to both the pathologic anatomy of breast cancer and in-breast failure patterns, (2) appropriate patient selection criteria, (3) partial breast treatment techniques that can be safely and widely performed, and (4) solid clinical data that demonstrate that APBI can offer equivalent local control, complication rates, and cosmetic outcomes to those achieved with conventional whole-breast radiotherapy. This chapter focuses on a review of the supporting background data and appropriate patient selection criteria. In subsequent chapters treatment techniques and outcome data are reviewed.

2.2 Pathologic Data

There are no data that unequivocally demonstrate that radiotherapy to the *entire* breast is required to achieve local control in patients with early-stage breast cancer. In fact, the literature regarding the pathologic anatomy of breast cancer offers limited guidance. Prior to 1990, most papers on this subject suggested that breast cancer was a diffuse, multicentric process that extended well beyond the confines of the clinically obvious tumor mass (Holland et al. 1985). Extrapolation of the findings of these older, methodologically limited studies to contemporary early-stage breast cancer patients is of questionable utility. Patients in these early studies presented with clinically advanced, palpable cancers that were subjected to mastectomy. These mastectomy specimens were then histologically examined for residual tumor after a "simulated" gross tumor excision meant to estimate the "lumpectomy" that would have been performed were breast conservation pursued. While of historical interest, such studies have little or no relevance to current breast cancer management. In this era of meticulous mammographic, surgical, and pathologic assessment techniques, patients present more commonly with small, non-palpable tumors that are completely resected with carefully evaluated microscopically negative margins. In contemporary studies of patients managed in accordance with such modern practice, limited pathologic data are available that detail the extent of microscopic residual disease within the breast after "lumpectomy"—information that would have direct relevance for defining the remaining target tissue. In the contemporary studies that have addressed this question, extensive microscopic evaluation of both mastectomy and quadrantectomy specimens has consistently found that residual disease beyond the clinically evident primary tumor mass is most likely ductal carcinoma in situ (DCIS) (Faverly et al. 1992, 1994; Imamura et al. 2000; Ohtake et al. 1995). These studies have consistently provided evidence that suggests that the extension of tumor in most patients is limited to less than 1 cm from the primary lesion.

2.3 Anatomic Patterns of In-Breast Failure after Breast-Conserving Treatment

The strongest support for partial breast treatment as an appropriate option for early-stage breast cancer is the anatomic location of in-breast failures following lumpectomy. Three prospective randomized studies of lumpectomy only versus lumpectomy plus whole-breast radiotherapy have documented the specific location in the breast of local recurrences (Clark et al. 1992; Fisher and Anderson 1994; Holli et al. 2001; Uppsala-Orebro Breast Cancer Study Group 1990; Veronesi et al. 2001a). The location of in-breast failure was categorized as either adjacent to the lumpectomy cavity (true recurrence) or far removed from the lumpectomy cavity ("elsewhere failure") (Clark et al. 1992; Uppsala-

Orebro Breast Cancer Study Group 1990; Veronesi et al. 2001a). Each of these studies found that the primary location of treatment failure is at the site of lumpectomy and "elsewhere failures" occur at a rate of less than 4%. Of particular note, "elsewhere failures" occurred with equal frequency in both the group of patients receiving whole-breast radiotherapy and the group treated with lumpectomy alone (Table 2.1). The conclusion drawn from these data is that "elsewhere failures" likely represent a new primary tumor and that the primary benefit of whole-breast radiotherapy is to prevent breast cancer recurrence in the lumpectomy bed (Morrow 2002). This is compelling evidence to support the view that equivalent rates of local control may be achieved if radiotherapy is directed to the lumpectomy cavity plus a 1–2 cm margin.

If a partial breast target can be appropriately defined, a direct follow-on question would ask if comparable local control could be achieved with a wider local excision and no radiotherapy. The answer to this is complex but, under most circumstances, appears to be "no" as prospective clinical trials of partial mastectomy alone have been associated with high rates of local recurrence. For example, in a study reported by Veronesi et al., quadrantectomy was compared to quadrantectomy plus whole-breast radiotherapy (Veronesi et al. 2001a) and local failure was observed in 23.5% vs. 5.8%, respectively. The local failure rate was found to be independent of the extent of partial breast resection which indicates that radiotherapy is required in addition to conservative surgery. The inability to remove all microscopic disease is not necessarily due to an inadequacy of surgery, but rather to unrecognized multifocality, unrecognized extent of microscopic disease, and/or the inadequacy of microscopic margin assessment (Fisher et al. 1999).

Table 2.1 Location of in-breast failure reported in prospective randomized trials investigating breast-conservation therapy (*WBI* post-lumpectomy whole-breast radiotherapy)

reference	No. of patients	Median follow-up (months)	In-breast failures (%)		True recurrence[a] (%)		Elsewhere failures[b] (%)	
			No WBI	WBI	No WBI	WBI	No WBI	WBI
Veronesi et al. 2001a	579	109	20.5	5.4	17.6	3.7	2.9	0.7
Clark et al. 1992	837	43	25.7	5.5	22.1	4.5	3.5	1.0
Uppsala-Orebro Breast Cancer Study Group 1990	381	33	5.7	2.2	4.1	1.6	1.5	0.5

[a] Recurrence at the site of lumpectomy.
[b] Recurrence beyond the site of lumpectomy.
Reproduced with permission from Arthur 2003

2.4 Proper Selection Criteria

The importance of proper patient selection for APBI cannot be overstated. A comprehensive evaluation must be performed to include patient and tumor characteristics as well as technical feasibility. Further, patients must be informed participants in the treatment decision process with a balanced educational approach when obtaining informed consent.

The formation of selection criteria for APBI has to date been a careful exercise of choosing specific patient and tumor characteristics to minimize the risk of tumor recurrence or complications. The goals of current criteria are to identify patients in whom the tissue at risk after lumpectomy is most likely to be in immediate proximity to the excision cavity and the risk of harboring residual microscopic disease at remote locations "elsewhere" within the breast is limited (Recht and Houlihan 1995).

All selection criteria must include patients who, first and foremost, are appropriate candidates for breast-conservation therapy. Patients with documented multicentric tumor and at increased risk of complications (pregnancy, connective tissue disorders) are excluded. Small primary tumor size, older age, no evidence of axillary nodal metastases, histology limited to invasive ductal carcinoma, and negative microscopic margins of excision are the primary criteria currently applied. However, a comparison of different institutional experiences shows that, despite their common cautious theme, there is some variability in the criteria chosen (Table 2.2). The presence of an extensive intraductal component (EIC), up to three positive axillary nodes, infiltrating lobular histology, pure DCIS, and young age have been allowed in some series (Arthur et al. 2003; King et al. 2000; Krishnan et al. 2001; Kuske and Bolton 1995; Kuske et al. 2002, 2004; Lawenda et al. 2003; Polgar et al. 2002, 2005; Strnad et al. 2004; Vicini et al. 2002, 2003b; Wazer et al. 2001, 2002). Most authors currently advocate the position that the presence of any of these features should exclude patients from consideration for APBI (American Society of Breast Surgeons 2005; Arthur et al. 2002; Vicini et al. 2003a).

In addition to clinical patient selection criteria, the one additional aspect that is crucial to the implementation of APBI is a quality assurance program that ensures that a treatment target is appropriately defined and dosimetrically covered within the intended prescription dose.

Examples of improper patient selection criteria and inadequate quality assurance methods for partial breast irradiation are presented in Table 2.3. These trials represent early partial breast irradiation studies from Europe and convincingly demonstrate that poor selection and poor technique will lead to poor results (Fentiman et al. 1996; Magee et al. 1996; Ribeiro et al. 1993). Microscopic margin assessment was not employed in two of the studies and it is unclear as to how many of the accrued patients would have been eligible for breast-conservation treatment by modern standards. Further, the authors acknowledge problems in the quality assurance of the treatments including poorly defined methods for target delineation and the inability to confirm dosimetric coverage of the target.

An additional treatment experience with a high rate of local failure that used interstitial brachytherapy for APBI has been reported from Canada (Perera et al. 2003). The patient cohort in this trial comprised 39 patients with T1 or T2 breast cancers and treated to 37.2 Gy in ten fractions (given twice daily) over 1 week. The 5-year actuarial rate of ipsilateral breast recurrence was 16%, comprising six ipsilateral recurrences, of which

Table 2.2 Selection criteria and quality assurance methods in successful partial breast irradiation experiences (<5% in-breast failure rate) (? unknown/not reported)

Series	Reference	No. of patients	Tumor size, median (range)	EIC+[a]	IDC only[b]	N+c	Age limit (years)	Negative margins required	Quality assurance method[d]
William Beaumont Hospital	Vicini et al. 2003b	199	11 mm	No	Yes	Yes[e] (13%)	>45	Yes (≥2 mm)	Postimplant CT
Virginia Commonwealth University	Arthur et al. 2003	44	11 mm (3–40 mm)	No	No (9%)	Yes (18%)	>45f	Yes	Postimplant CT
Oschner Clinic	King et al. 2000	51	14 mm (mean)	Yes (14%)	No	Yes (18%)	>45	Yes	Postimplant CT
Tufts/Brown Universities	Wazer et al. 2001, 2002	33	1.3 mm (0.5–2.0 mm)	Yes (55%)	Yes	Yes (9%)	None	Yes	Direct visualization or orthogonal pair
Massachusetts General Hospital	Lawenda et al. 2003	48	? (<20 mm)	No	?	No	None	Yes	Direct visualization or orthogonal pair
University of Kansas	Krishnan et al. 2001	25	10 mm (mean)	No	No (12% ILC)	No	>45	No[g]	Orthogonal pair
RTOG 95-17	Kuske and Bolton 1995; Kuske et al. 2002, 2004	99	? (<3 cm)	No	Yes	Yes	None	Yes	Orthogonal pair
Budapest, Hungary	Polgar et al. 2002, 2005; Vicini et al. 2002	81	13 mm (1–20 mm)	No	Yes	Yes (Micro-mets)	No	Yes (≥2 mm)	Variable angle orthogonal pair
German–Austrian phase II trial	Strnad et al. 2004	251	? (<3 cm)	No	?	Micro only	<35	Yes	Postimplant CT

a Included patients whose tumors contained an extensive intraductal component. In parentheses: proportion of patients in study with such findings.
b Patients with infiltrating ductal carcinomas only. If no, then in parentheses: proportion of patients in study non-IDC.
c Included patients with histologically positive axillary lymph nodes. In parentheses: proportion of patients in study with such findings.
d Methods of assuring target received prescription dose.
e Patients with positive axillary nodes were excluded beginning in 1995.
f Early experience allowed four patients <45 years old.
g Having a focus of microscopic disease at margin allowed.

Table 2.3 Selection criteria and quality assurance methods in unsuccessful partial breast irradiation experiences (>15% in-breast failure rate) (? unknown/not reported)

Institution	Reference	No. of patients	Tumor size	EIC+[a]	ILC[b]	N+c	Age limit (years)	Negative margins required	Quality assurance method[d]
Guy's Hospital London, England	Fentiman et al. 1996	27	<4 cm clinically (three were >4 cm)	Yes (30%)	No (16%)	Yes (32%)	<70	No, gross resection only	No
Christie Hospital Manchester, England	Magee et al. 1996	353	<4 cm (75% were 2–4 cm)	Yes (3%)	No (15%)	? No dissection	<70	No, gross resection only	No
London Regional Cancer Center	Perera et al. 2003; Ribeiro et al. 1993	39	Mean 15.6 cm, range 0.4–45 cm	Yes (8%)	No	Yes[e] (21%)	None	Yes	Orthogonal pair, clip coverage

[a] Included patients whose tumors contained an extensive intraductal component. In parentheses: proportion of patients in study with such findings.
[b] Included patients with infiltrating lobular carcinomas. In parentheses: proportion of patients in study with such findings.
[c] Included patients with histologically positive axillary lymph nodes. In parentheses: proportion of patients in study with such findings.
[d] Methods of assuring target received prescription dose.
[e] Includes two patients with unknown nodal status.

two occurred within the lumpectomy site and four were categorized as new primaries located at a distance from the initial lesion. The local failure rate was higher then most institutional APBI experiences reported to date and prompted a careful evaluation of the selection criteria and treatment technique employed. Nineteen percent of patients had infiltrating lobular carcinomas and the minimum tumor-free margin width was 2 mm or less in 31% of patients. Of particular note, the median implant volume in this study was 30 cm³ (range 10–111 cm³), which is significantly smaller than the implant volumes reported in any other single-institution study (60–215 cm³) (Vicini et al. 2003a). The high rate of local failure observed in this study was most likely due to an inadequately defined target volume which included only tissue encompassed within the confines of surgical clips. As surgical clips are placed to define just the lumpectomy cavity, this would exclude immediately adjacent tissue-at-risk from the prescribed radiation dose.

Physician and patient interest in APBI has continued to increase. In response to this interest, two professional societies have issued recommendations regarding patient selection criteria. Both societies seek to incorporate the lessons learned from accumulated clinical experience and to provide the broader medical community with guidance in the selection of potentially eligible patients. The American Brachytherapy Society (ABS) and the American Society of Breast Surgeons (ASBS) have independently developed patient selection criteria that are generally viewed as both cautious and reasonable (American Society of Breast Surgeons 2005; Arthur et al. 2002). Both societies based their criteria on previously published data and focus on five characteristics felt to best define risk: patient age, tumor size, histologic type, axillary nodal status, and microscopic margin assessment. These criteria are detailed in Table 2.4. The ABS criteria include: patients ≥45 years of age, invasive ductal carcinoma only, tumor size of ≤3 cm, negative resection margins (defined as "no tumor on ink"), and a negative axillary nodal status. Similar in concept to those promulgated by the ABS, the ASBS patient selection criteria includes: patients ≥50 years of age, invasive ductal carcinoma or DCIS, tumor size of ≤2 cm, negative resection margins (defined as at least 2 mm in all directions), and a negative axillary nodal status.

Table 2.4 Patient selection criteria

	American Brachytherapy Society[a]	American Society of Breast Surgeons[b]
Age (years)	≥45	≥50
Diagnosis	Invasive ductal carcinoma	Invasive ductal carcinoma or ductal carcinoma in situ
Size (cm)	≤3	≤2
Margin status	Negative; no tumor involving inked margin	Negative; at least 2 mm in all directions
Nodal status	Negative; axillary lymph node dissection or sentinel lymph node evaluation	Negative; axillary lymph node dissection or sentinel lymph node evaluation

[a] Arthur 2003; Arthur et al. 2002
[b] American Society of Breast Surgeons 2005; Arthur 2003

Interestingly, there is a notable discrepancy between the two sets of criteria in that the ASBS includes the treatment of DCIS whereas the ABS does not. This difference of opinion reflects a surgical perspective largely influenced by research work on the conservative management of DCIS by Silverstein et al. (American Society of Breast Surgeons 2005; Silverstein 2000). These authors have claimed that when unifocal DCIS is resected with a pathologically confirmed circumferentially clear margin of >1 cm, then the addition of postoperative whole-breast irradiation is of no benefit. These findings are neither universally accepted nor supported by prospective clinical trial data, but they are nonetheless embraced by many in the surgical community and have led some to manage selected cases of DCIS with wide resection only. Therefore, there has been a greater willingness amongst surgeons to include those with DCIS as candidates for APBI.

Currently, there are four principal methods of APBI: (1) multicatheter brachytherapy, (2) balloon-based brachytherapy (MammoSite radiation therapy system, RTS), (3) external beam three-dimensional conformal radiotherapy (3D-CRT), and (4) intraoperative radiotherapy with electrons or 50-kV photons. The experience with intraoperative treatment was initiated in United Kingdom (50-kV photons) and Milan, Italy (electrons) (Vaidya et al. 2001a, 2001b, 2004; Veronesi et al. 2001b, 2003). The former is recruiting patients in an international randomised trial (Targit trial) in several centres in the UK, USA, Germany, Italy and Australia. Most long-term clinical experience with APBI has been accumulated with multicatheter brachytherapy, MammoSite RTS, and 3D-CRT. The first technique employed for APBI was by multicatheter interstitial brachytherapy and this method is currently being tested in phase III trials in both Europe and North America. The newer techniques of MammoSite RTS and 3D-CRT are being tested as part of a phase III trial in North America.

Each APBI technique offers a unique treatment approach with advantages and disadvantages depending upon the individual patient and treatment anatomy. As such, a technical feasibility assessment for each technique must be included as part of the evaluation of each patient. An important technical requirement is the ability to definitively identify the target. This is followed by an evaluation of which technique will best optimize target coverage and limit the risk of toxicity. If APBI is to be performed intraoperatively such that lumpectomy is immediately followed with the placement of brachytherapy catheters or the MammoSite RTS, then the target geometry at the time of wound closure will need to be anticipated. However, there is an increasing preference to perform APBI only in the postoperative setting when pathologic review is complete and patient eligibility can be fully assessed. In the postlumpectomy setting, CT or ultrasound imaging is necessary to define the excision cavity as well to evaluate for technical feasibility. Both imaging information and physical examination are essential to determine the feasibility of APBI and to guide the choice of the method of delivery. Often, more than one approach can be successfully employed at which point patient preference can be considered.

Multicatheter interstitial brachytherapy was the originally employed APBI technique and as a consequence has generated clinical experience with the longest follow-up duration. This APBI technique requires the highest level of skill but also offers the most flexible and adaptable technique of the three now commonly used. With this approach, an implant can be constructed to encompass each individual target regardless of size, location, or proximity to skin and/or chest wall. Multicatheter brachytherapy allows the physician to be less concerned with whether or not the target can be covered, and focus instead on how to optimize the construction of the implant. Factors such as catheter number and the direction and location of catheter exit and entrance sites need to be considered as this may affect the degree of patient discomfort and the ultimate cosmetic result (punctate scarring) (Cuttino et al. 2005; Kuske 1999). Many treatment centers have mastered the ability to deliver multicatheter brachytherapy. However, an integral part of proper patient selection for this technique is the anticipation of a patient's ability to tolerate additional breast trauma and whether the size of the implant and number of catheters needed to cover the target is excessive.

The MammoSite RTS is an innovative treatment device designed to simplify brachytherapy treatment delivery for both the physician and the patient (Arthur and Vicini 2004; Keisch et al. 2003a, 2003b). Although its design goals have been largely achieved, additional technical aspects need to be considered in its clinical implementation. In contrast to a multicatheter implant where the catheters are placed to conform to the target, the MammoSite RTS is placed so that the target conforms to the balloon surface. Appropriate patient selection is critically dependent upon the geometry and location of the lumpectomy cavity and these are dependent upon the characteristics of the breast, size of the tumor, and the communication between the surgeon and the radiation oncologist. When selecting a patient for MammoSite RTS, additional technical factors to consider include the achievable volume after balloon inflation, balloon symmetry, cavity conformance to the applicator, and balloon-to-skin distance. Preplacement assessment must anticipate whether the balloon can be inflated properly and the treatment dose delivered successfully. The size and shape of the cavity and the anticipated distance from the balloon surface and skin need to be carefully evaluated by either intraoperative visual inspection or postoperative imaging. Currently there are three different balloon designs: small and large spherical shapes and a single-sized ellipsoid shape. In order to minimize the risk of a wasted unused catheter, complete cavity imaging and geometry assessment will help to determine whether the patient is an appropriate candidate for balloon brachytherapy, whether a balloon can be successfully placed, which balloon size/shape is optimal, and where on the surface of the breast would be the best entry point for the catheter.

The use of 3D-CRT has added a non-invasive option to techniques for APBI (Baglan et al. 2003; Formenti et al. 2002, 2004; Vicini et al. 2003c). With external beam treatment, beam configurations can be adjusted to achieve dosimetric goals set by the treating physicians. However, as with other APBI techniques, proper patient selection for 3D-CRT is critical. In contrast to brachytherapy, 3D-CRT results in a markedly increased integral dose, the degree of which is dependent upon the field arrangement. Because of the necessity to account for both beam entry and exit, dose limits to surrounding normal tissues need to be carefully considered. To accomplish this, patient selection for this technique must include a thorough assessment of the size, shape and location of the target with respect to patient anatomy. Two characteristics of the excision cavity have been identified that make 3D-CRT APBI difficult to apply. The first relates to the size of the defined target as breathing motion and patient set-up error must be compensated for by further increasing the field size. This results in an increased dose to the surrounding structures such that normal tissues receive doses that exceed currently prescribed limits. In general, it appears that when the excision cavity volume exceeds 20% of the ipsilateral breast volume, 3D-CRT will exceed acceptable normal tissue dose-volume constraints. The second limiting factor for 3D-CRT APBI is the location of the excision cavity within the breast. When the cavity is located in the lower, inner aspect of the left breast, the resultant dose to the heart may exceed acceptable limits. In the upper portions of the breast, cavity location may limit the choice of beam arrangements that result in excessive radiation doses to normal ipsilateral breast tissue. Finally, more subjective limiting factors are the reproducibility of the patient set-up position, the position of the breast, and the positional reproducibility of the partial breast target. A fidgety patient and/or a patient with large pendulous breasts represent examples of poor patient selection for this technique.

The appeal of completing postoperative radiation treatment in a short time period must not overshadow the need for the eligible patient to thoroughly understand the risks and benefits of this new adjuvant treatment approach. A central part of the patient selection process for APBI, as for any treatment, must be thorough informed consent. As physician and patient enthusiasm for APBI expands, we must remember—and our patients should know—that there is a marked difference in the scope and follow-up of clinical trial data support between standard breast-conservation treatment with whole-breast irradiation and APBI. Conventional whole-breast irradiation is supported by large robust randomized trials and decades of common clinical practice. In comparison, there are only several hundred women treated with APBI who have been followed for more than 5 years. This underscores the need to support phase III clinical trials that compare APBI to whole-breast irradiation. In the interim, though, if APBI is to be offered to patients, the clinician must carefully acknowledge the controversy as to the role of APBI in the management of early breast cancer and thoroughly educate the patient as to the justification for treating a partial breast target and the extent of clinical trial data currently available to support such an approach.

In summary, patient selection for APBI incorporates patient and tumor characteristics, technical considerations and thorough informed consent. A cautious and highly selective approach is recommended with the goal of maintaining in-breast control rates that approach 95–100% and acceptable cosmetic results equivalent to those achieved with whole-breast irradiation. Ongoing studies will not only help further define the potential of APBI, but also better define appropriate selection criteria so that as many women as possible will have the opportunity to pursue this innovative treatment approach.

References

1. American Society of Breast Surgeons (2005) Consensus Statement for Accelerated Partial Breast Irradiation. http://www.breastsurgeons.org/apbi.shtml
2. Arthur D (2003) Accelerated partial breast irradiation: a change in treatment paradigm for early stage breast cancer. J Surg Oncol 84:185–191
3. Arthur DW, Vicini FA (2004) MammoSite RTS: the reporting of initial experiences and how to interpret. Ann Surg Oncol 11:723–724
4. Arthur DW, Vicini FA, Kuske RR, et al (2002) Accelerated partial breast irradiation: an updated report from the American Brachytherapy Society. Brachytherapy 1:184–190
5. Arthur DW, Koo D, Zwicker RD, et al (2003) Partial breast brachytherapy after lumpectomy: low-dose-rate and high-dose-rate experience. Int J Radiat Oncol Biol Phys 56:681–689

6. Athas WF, Adams-Cameron M, Hunt WC, et al (2000) Travel distance to radiation therapy and receipt of radiotherapy following breast-conserving surgery. J Natl Cancer Inst 92:269–271

7. Baglan KL, Sharpe MB, Jaffray D, et al (2003) Accelerated partial breast irradiation using 3D conformal radiation therapy (3D-CRT). Int J Radiat Oncol Biol Phys 55:302–311

8. Clark RM, McCulloch PB, Levine MN, et al (1992) Randomized clinical trial to assess the effectiveness of breast irradiation following lumpectomy and axillary dissection for node-negative breast cancer. J Natl Cancer Inst 84:683–689

9. Cuttino LW, Todor D, Arthur DW (2005) CT-guided multi-catheter insertion technique for partial breast brachytherapy: reliable target coverage and dose homogeneity. Brachytherapy 4:10–17

10. Du X, Freeman JL, Freeman DH, et al (1999) Temporal and regional variation in the use of breast-conserving surgery and radiotherapy for older women with early-stage breast cancer from 1983 to 1995. J Gerontol A Biol Sci Med Sci 54:M474–478

11. Faverly D, Holland R, Burgers L (1992) An original stereomicroscopic analysis of the mammary glandular tree. Virchows Arch A Pathol Anat Histopathol 421:115–119

12. Faverly DR, Burgers L, Bult P, et al (1994) Three dimensional imaging of mammary ductal carcinoma in situ: clinical implications. Semin Diagn Pathol 11:193–198

13. Fentiman IS, Poole C, Tong D, et al (1996) Inadequacy of iridium implant as sole radiation treatment for operable breast cancer. Eur J Cancer 32A:608–611

14. Fisher B, Anderson S (1994) Conservative surgery for the management of invasive and non-invasive carcinoma of the breast: NSABP trials. National Surgical Adjuvant Breast and Bowel Project. World J Surg 18:63–69

15. Fisher B, Anderson S, Bryant J, et al (2002) Twenty-year follow-up of a randomized trial comparing total mastectomy, lumpectomy, and lumpectomy plus irradiation for the treatment of invasive breast cancer. N Engl J Med 347:1233–1241

16. Fisher ER, Dignam J, Tan-Chiu E, et al (1999) Pathologic findings from the National Surgical Adjuvant Breast Project (NSABP) eight-year update of Protocol B-17: intraductal carcinoma. Cancer 86:429–438

17. Formenti SC, Rosenstein B, Skinner KA, et al (2002) T1 stage breast cancer: adjuvant hypofractionated conformal radiation therapy to tumor bed in selected postmenopausal breast cancer patients – pilot feasibility study. Radiology 222:171–178

18. Formenti SC, Truong MT, Goldberg JD, et al (2004) Prone accelerated partial breast irradiation after breast-conserving surgery: preliminary clinical results and dose-volume histogram analysis. Int J Radiat Oncol Biol Phys 60:493–504

19. Hahn CA, Marks LB, Chen DY, et al (2003) Breast conservation rates-barriers between tertiary care and community practice. Int J Radiat Oncol Biol Phys 55:1196–1199

20. Hebert-Croteau N, Brisson J, Latreille J, et al (1999) Compliance with consensus recommendations for the treatment of early stage breast carcinoma in elderly women. Cancer 85:1104–1113

21. Holland R, Veling SH, Mravunac M, et al (1985) Histologic multifocality of Tis, T1-2 breast carcinomas. Implications for clinical trials of breast-conserving surgery. Cancer 56:979–990

22. Holli K, Saaristo R, Isola J, et al (2001) Lumpectomy with or without postoperative radiotherapy for breast cancer with favourable prognostic features: results of a randomized study. Br J Cancer 84:164–169

23. Imamura H, Haga S, Shimizu T, et al (2000) Relationship between the morphological and biological characteristics of intraductal components accompanying invasive ductal breast carcinoma and patient age. Breast Cancer Res Treat 62:177–184

24. Keisch M, Vicini F, Kuske RR (2003a) Two-year outcome with the MammoSite breast brachytherapy applicator: factors associated with optimal cosmetic results when performing partial breast irradiation. Int J Radiat Oncol Biol Phys 60 [Suppl 1]:s315

25. Keisch M, Vicini F, Kuske RR, et al (2003b) Initial clinical experience with the MammoSite breast brachytherapy applicator in women with early-stage breast cancer treated with breast-conserving therapy. Int J Radiat Oncol Biol Phys 55:289–293

26. King TA, Bolton JS, Kuske RR, et al (2000) Long-term results of wide-field brachytherapy as the sole method of radiation therapy after segmental mastectomy for T(is,1,2) breast cancer. Am J Surg 180:299–304

27. Krishnan L, Jewell WR, Tawfik OW, et al (2001) Breast conservation therapy with tumor bed irradiation alone in a selected group of patients with stage I breast cancer. Breast J 7:91–96

28. Kuerer HM, Arthur DW, Haffty BG (2004) Repeat breast-conserving surgery for in-breast local breast carcinoma recurrence: the potential role of partial breast irradiation. Cancer 100:2269–2280

29. Kuske RR Jr (1999) Breast brachytherapy. Hematol Oncol Clin North Am 13:543–558, vi–vii

30. Kuske RR, Bolton JS (1995) A phase I/II trial to evaluate brachytherapy as the sole method of radiation therapy for stage I and II breast carcinoma (publication no. 1055). Radiation Therapy Oncology Group

31. Kuske RR, Winter K, Arthur D, et al (2002) A phase I/II trial of brachytherapy alone following lumpectomy for select breast cancer: toxicity analysis of Radiation Therapy Oncology Group 95-17 (abstract). Int J Radiat Oncol Biol Phys 54 (2 Suppl)

32. Kuske RR, Winter K, Arthur DW, et al (2004) A phase II trial of brachytherapy alone following lumpectomy for stage I or II breast cancer: initial outcomes of RTOG 9517 (abstract 565). Proc Am Soc Clin Oncol 23

33. Lawenda BD, Taghian AG, Kachnic LA, et al (2003) Dose-volume analysis of radiotherapy for T1N0 invasive breast cancer treated by local excision and partial breast irradiation by low-dose-rate interstitial implant. Int J Radiat Oncol Biol Phys 56:671–680

34. Magee B, Swindell R, Harris M, et al (1996) Prognostic factors for breast recurrence after conservative breast surgery and radiotherapy: results from a randomised trial. Radiother Oncol 39:223–227

35. Morrow M (2002) Rational local therapy for breast cancer. N Engl J Med 347:1270–1271

36. Nattinger AB, Hoffmann RG, Kneusel RT, et al (2000) Relation between appropriateness of primary therapy for early-stage breast carcinoma and increased use of breast-conserving surgery. Lancet 356:1148–1153

37. NIH Consensus Development Conference (1990) Treatment of early-stage breast cancer. Consensus statement. Vol 8. June 18–21. Bethesda, MD, pp 1–9

38. Ohtake T, Abe R, Kimijima I, et al (1995) Intraductal extension of primary invasive breast carcinoma treated by breast-conservative surgery. Computer graphic three-dimensional reconstruction of the mammary duct-lobular systems. Cancer 76:32–45

39. Perera F, Yu E, Engel J, et al (2003) Patterns of breast recurrence in a pilot study of brachytherapy confined to the lumpectomy site for early breast cancer with six years' minimum follow-up. Int J Radiat Oncol Biol Phys 57:1239–1246

40. Polgar C, Sulyok Z, Fodor J, et al (2002) Sole brachytherapy of the tumor bed after conservative surgery for T1 breast cancer: five-year results of a phase I-II study and initial findings of a randomized phase III trial. J Surg Oncol 80:121–128; discussion 129

41. Polgar C, Strnad V, Major T (2005) Brachytherapy for partial breast irradiation: the European experience. Semin Radiat Oncol 15:116–122

42. Recht A, Houlihan MJ (1995) Conservative surgery without radiotherapy in the treatment of patients with early-stage invasive breast cancer. A review. Ann Surg 222:9–18

43. Ribeiro GG, Magee B, Swindell R, et al (1993) The Christie Hospital breast conservation trial: an update at 8 years from inception. Clin Oncol (R Coll Radiol) 5:278–283

44. Silverstein MJ (2000) Current management of noninvasive (in situ) breast cancer. Adv Surg 34:17–41

45. Strnad V, Ott O, Potter R, et al (2004) Interstitial brachytherapy alone after breast conserving surgery: interim results of a German-Austrian multicenter phase II trial. Brachytherapy 3:115–119

46. Uppsala-Orebro Breast Cancer Study Group (1990) Sector resection with or without postoperative radiotherapy for stage I breast cancer: a randomized trial. J Natl Cancer Inst 82:277–282

47. Vaidya JS, Baum M, Tobias JS, et al (2001a) Targeted intra-operative radiotherapy (Targit): an innovative method of treatment for early breast cancer. Ann Oncol 12:1075–1080

48. Vaidya JS, Tobias JS, Baum M, et al (2001b) Targeted intra-operative radiotherapy (Targit) for breast cancer: a randomized trial. Radiology [Suppl] 221:234

49. Vaidya JS, Tobias JS, Baum M, et al (2004) Intraoperative radiotherapy for breast cancer. Lancet Oncol 5:165–173

50. Veronesi U, Marubini E, Mariani L, et al (2001a) Radiotherapy after breast-conserving surgery in small breast carcinoma: long-term results of a randomized trial. Ann Oncol 12:997–1003

51. Veronesi U, Orecchia R, Luini A, et al (2001b) A preliminary report of intraoperative radiotherapy (IORT) in limited-stage breast cancers that are conservatively treated. Eur J Cancer 37:2178–2183

52. Veronesi U, Cascinelli N, Mariani L, et al (2002) Twenty-year follow-up of a randomized study comparing breast-conserving surgery with radical mastectomy for early breast cancer. N Engl J Med 347:1227–1232

53. Veronesi U, Gatti G, Luini A, et al (2003) Full-dose intraoperative radiotherapy with electrons during breast-conserving surgery. Arch Surg 138:1253–1256

54. Vicini FA, Arthur DW, Wazer DE (2002) Inconsistency, perspective, double talk, and false virtue. Brachytherapy 1:181–183

55. Vicini F, Arthur D, Polgar C, et al (2003a) Defining the efficacy of accelerated partial breast irradiation: the importance of proper patient selection, optimal quality assurance, and common sense. Int J Radiat Oncol Biol Phys 57:1210–1213

56. Vicini FA, Kestin L, Chen P, et al (2003b) Limited-field radiation therapy in the management of early-stage breast cancer. J Natl Cancer Inst 95:1205–1210

57. Vicini FA, Remouchamps V, Wallace M, et al (2003c) Ongoing clinical experience utilizing 3D conformal external beam radiotherapy to deliver partial-breast irradiation in patients with early-stage breast cancer treated with breast-conserving therapy. Int J Radiat Oncol Biol Phys 57:1247–1253

58. Wazer DE, Lowther D, Boyle T, et al (2001) Clinically evident fat necrosis in women treated with high-dose-rate brachytherapy alone for early-stage breast cancer. Int J Radiat Oncol Biol Phys 50:107–111

59. Wazer D, Berle L, Graham R, et al (2002) Preliminary results of a phase I/II study of HDR brachytherapy alone for T1/T2 breast cancer. Int J Radiat Oncol Biol Phys 53:889–897

Pathologic Anatomy of Early-Stage Breast Cancer and its Relevance to Accelerated Partial Breast Irradiation: Defining the Target

3

Shruti Jolly, Larry L. Kestin,
Neal S. Goldstein and Frank A. Vicini

Contents

3.1 Determining the Extent of Disease Beyond the Lumpectomy Cavity

While several recent studies have demonstrated excellent 5-year results using accelerated partial breast irradiation (APBI), the optimal clinical target volume (CTV) to be used in these patients has not been clearly defined (Vicini et al. 2003; Wallner et al. 2004). The CTV, which refers to the volume of breast tissue around the lumpectomy cavity requiring radiotherapy (RT), is crucial in determining the efficacy of adjuvant PBI in comparison to whole-breast RT. It is important to consider whether PBI treats the appropriate volume of breast tissue at risk of harboring residual disease.

There are three bodies of data that can be used to help define the optimal CTV for APBI. These data include (1) mastectomy studies in which the distribution of cancer in the breast is correlated with the site of the initial tumor, (2) re-excision studies in which the presence, amount, and distance of residual disease is correlated with the initial tumor, and (3) published results with APBI in which the actual CTV used is correlated with the local recurrence rates.

3.1.1 Mastectomy Studies

The classic pathologic evaluation of mastectomy specimens performed by Holland et al. suggested that microscopic disease was present in a multicentric pattern with relatively high frequency. Breast cancer multifocality was studied in mastectomy specimens by correlated specimen radiography and histologic techniques. It was found that up to 40% of patients undergoing breast conservation therapy (BCT) might have residual tumor within the breast. This analysis justified the concept that whole-breast treatment, either with surgery or RT, was necessary to achieve local control. It was also one of the main sources of pathologic information that supported the use of whole-breast RT as a component of standard BCT in the 1980s (Faverly et al. 1992; Holland et al. 1985).

However, since the publication of these data, there have been significant advances in the detection, selection, and management process of patients receiving BCT, and it is uncertain how many of the patients included in the study of Holland et al. would have been eligible for BCT by modern standards. In addition, this study suggested that residual disease could be found in the breast after simulated gross excisions >2 cm from the primary tumor in >29% of patients (with no extensive intraductal component). However, a review of the study details shows that in the majority of patients tumor was clinically detected (>80%) with a median size of almost 4 cm. Additionally, the extensive mapping procedure that was used was described as having an error of "less than 15 mm", which is significant when considering the possibility of performing PBI. The most important aspect to consider is that it is impossible to extrapolate the data generated from the "gross simulated excision" used in this study to a lumpectomy with negative microscopic margins routinely achieved in the clinic today. For example, in the analysis from William Beaumont Hospital, disease extended more than 10 mm into the breast in approximately 26% of patients after an initial lumpectomy with positive margins vs. only 10% in patients with initial negative margins (Goldstein et al. 2003). As a result, it is difficult to know whether the findings of Holland et al. can be applied to patients selected for BCT with modern mammographic evaluation and rigorous pathologic evaluation.

Contrary to the data of Holland et al., recent studies applying thorough pathologic processing of quadrantectomy and mastectomy specimens from women considered appropriate for BCT by modern standards reveal that the microscopic extension of malignant cells is much less likely to be beyond 1 cm. For example, Ohtake et al. used a subgross and stereomicroscopic technique to examine the extent of residual ductal carcinoma in situ (DCIS) remaining in the breast after *actual* quadrantectomies in 20 patients with invasive cancer. Using a computer graphic three-dimensional reconstruction of the mammary duct–lobular system, the average *maximum* distance of extension was 11.9 mm. Patients >50 years of age had a maximum extension of <8 mm. In contrast to the study of Holland et al., the mean tumor size in this contemporary study was 1.7 cm (Ohtake et al. 1995).

In a related study, Imamura et al. measured the maximal DCIS extension in 253 mastectomy specimens in women with invasive breast cancer. The authors found that the median DCIS extension was only 9 mm and was related to patient age. The maximum disease extension was measured in relation to the edge of the invasive tumor. In patients ≥40 years of age, the maximum extension was <9 mm in all cases (Imamura et al. 2000).

Table 3.1 Factors in initial excision specimens and the presence of ≥1 cm extension of carcinoma in re-excision specimens (combining margin status with invasive carcinoma/specimen dimension ratio)

Initial excision specimen margin group	Percentage of re-excision specimens with >1 cm maximum extension (no. of patients)			
	Initial excision specimen invasive carcinoma:specimen dimension ratio			Totals
	<0.3	0.3–<0.6	≥0.6	
Negative	0% (0/13)	0% (0/3)	100% (2/2)	28% (2/18)
Near:least amount	0% (0/40)	0% (0/13)	40% (2/5)	3% (2/58)
Near:intermediate amount	0% (0/10)	5% (1/20)	0% (0/4)	3% (1/34)
Near:greatest amount	36% (4/11)	57% (4/7)	0% (0/5)	35% (8/23)
Totals (>1.0 cm extension)	5% (4/74)	12% (5/43)	25% (4/16)	9.7% (13/133)

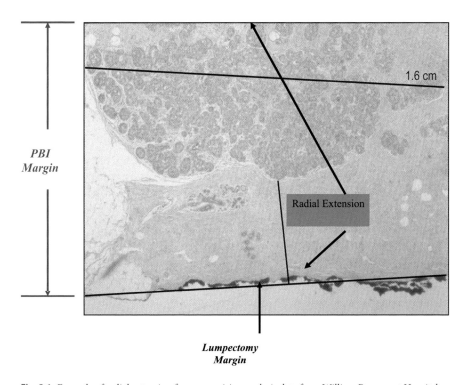

Fig. 3.1 Example of radial extension from re-excision analysis data from William Beaumont Hospital

The results of these studies point out two key issues. First, it is unlikely that the distribution of cancer in a breast in contemporary cases detected through screening mammography is similar to the findings in clinically detected cases from the early 1980s reported by Holland et al. Second, selection criteria for PBI clearly identify patients with smaller tumors and negative margins whose patterns of disease distribution in the breast are more likely to mirror those described in the studies of Imamura et al. and Ohtake et al., and current studies. Hopefully, additional pathologic analyses using contemporary patients will help to further clarify these issues.

3.1.2 Re-Excision Pathologic Studies

One primary re-excision study of patients treated at William Beaumont Hospital, Royal Oak, Michigan, was conducted to help define the CTV for APBI. The study population comprised 441 patients derived from a dataset of 607 consecutive patients (reviewed by one pathologist) who underwent re-excision before RT (as part of their standard BCT). The surgical treatment in all patients included an initial excisional resection with a rim of normal breast parenchyma around the clinically apparent tumor or the tissue around the tip of the needle localization wire. Patients underwent a re-excision of the primary tumor site for inadequate margin distances or questionable post-surgical mammography results at the discretion of the surgeon or radiation oncologist. The re-excision specimens were reviewed for presence, type, amount, and linear (radial) extension of cancer cells from the edge of the original margin (see Fig. 3.1) (Goldstein et al. 2003; Vicini et al. 2004).

In the specimens from 333 of these 441 patients, it was possible to measure the greatest perpendicular extension of any residual disease (DCIS or invasive cancer) from the edge of the original lumpectomy specimen. Because no PBI protocols allow patients with positive margins to be enrolled, only 134 patients with initial negative margins (per NSABP criteria) were studied (199 patients had initial positive margins). In more than 90% of these 134 patients, if any residual disease was present (38% of patients) it was limited to <10 mm from the edge of the original lumpectomy margin. If more restrictive criteria were used (e.g., initial excision specimens with margins that were negative, near: least-amount, or near:intermediate-amount with invasive carcinoma:specimen maximum dimension ratios of <0.3 or margins that are negative or near:least-amount with invasive carcinoma:specimen maximum dimension ratios of <0.6), it was possible to accurately identify all 13 patients (9.7%) with disease extending ≥10 mm from the edge of the margin (Table 3.1).

These results suggest that using NSABP criteria for negative margins (no tumor on ink), a margin of 10 mm beyond the tumor bed is adequate to cover any residual disease remaining in the breast in >90% of patients treated with PBI. In addition, it is possible to accurately identify all patients with disease extending beyond 10 mm using more restrictive pathologic criteria.

3.1.2.1 Concerns Regarding Re-Excision Analysis

Although the results in the current re-excision analysis suggest that a 1.0-cm margin beyond the lumpectomy cavity provides an adequate CTV for PBI (with negative margins per NSABP criteria), they are by no means conclusive. Clearly, it is not certain if the assumption that the maximal, perpendicular extension distance of invasive carcinoma or DCIS measured from the inner edge of the granulation tissue reaction in the re-excision specimen provides an accurate representation of residual cancer distribution in the breast. Because a variable amount of breast tissue is removed (or destroyed) around the lumpectomy edges through electrocautery or tissue processing, the actual extension of disease in some patients may be underestimated. However, the results obtained were from numerous surgeons using various surgical techniques. Despite obvious inconsistencies, the range and standard deviation of the maximal extension in all 333 patients were very small. Combined with the clinical results obtained with PBI, this pathologic analysis does provide some assurance that a 1.0-cm margin beyond the lumpectomy cavity may be sufficient for most patients treated with PBI. Additional similar pathologic studies and long-term clinical PBI data are needed to help clarify this issue.

3.1.3 Recurrence Patterns in PBI

The only clinical treatment data that can be used to correlate the volume of tissue irradiated (e.g., CTV) with local recurrence after PBI has been reported by Vicini et al. (Vicini et al. 1999; Kestin et al. 2000). In their analysis, 21 patients treated with PBI using high-dose-rate (HDR) brachytherapy who had surgical clips outlining the lumpectomy cavity and underwent computed tomography (CT) scanning after implant placement were analyzed. For each patient, the postimplant CT dataset was transferred to a three-dimensional treatment planning system. The lumpectomy cavity, target volume (lumpectomy cavity plus a 1-cm margin), and entire breast were outlined. The programmed HDR brachytherapy source positions and dwell times were then imported into the three-dimensional planning system. The implant dataset was then registered to the visible implant template in the CT dataset. The distribution of the implant dose was analyzed with respect to defined volumes via dose–volume histograms. Despite visual verification by the treating physician that surgical clips (with an appropriate margin) were within the boundaries of the implant needles, the median proportion of the lumpectomy cavity that received the prescribed dose was only 87% (range 73–98%). With respect to the CTV, a median of only 68% (range 56–81%) of this volume received 100% of the prescribed dose.

The minimum follow-up for the 21 patients in the analysis was 62 months, and the 5-year actuarial rate of local recurrence was 0.5%. The overall experience in 199 patients treated with PBI using the same CTV margins from the same group has recently been published. With a median follow-up of 5.4 years for all patients, the 5-year actuarial rate of local recurrence reported was 1.2%. Although no direct relationship between the precise volume of breast tissue receiving full-dose RT and outcome in all patients can be obtained, these findings suggest that a CTV of only the lumpectomy cavity plus 1.0 cm should be adequate in most patients and supports the conclusions from this re-excision analysis.

3.1.4 Composite Disease Extension

Using the above studies to delineate the target volume for partial breast irradiation, the composite maximum intraductal extension can be estimated. Imamura et al. and Ohtake et al. concluded the average maximum intraductal extension was 9 mm and 11.9 mm, respectively. The William Beaumont Hospital data using re-excision analysis revealed a maximum radial extension of <10 mm in 90% of patients. Therefore, if the radiation dose of PBI is prescribed to 1 cm around the lumpectomy cavity, the pathologic area of risk should be covered.

3.2 Impact of Radiation on Elsewhere Failures

The rationale for giving adjuvant whole-breast RT after lumpectomy in patients receiving BCT is that even after tumor excision with negative margins, many patients may harbor significant areas of occult, residual microscopic disease in the breast (see Table 3.2). Therefore, whole-breast radiation must be delivered to the lumpectomy cavity and the entire breast in an effort to "sterilize" any residual foci of cancer. There are multiple randomized trials comparing breast-conserving surgery alone versus breast-conserving surgery plus RT (see Table 3.3). The percentage of patients with elsewhere failures is not impacted by the addition of RT. In the study by Veronesi et al. (Veronesi et al. 2002), with 20 years of follow-up, the overall rate of ipsilateral breast recurrence was nearly identical to the rate of contralateral carcinomas in women who received postoperative whole-breast RT. Patterns of failure after standard BCT and after excision alone (without adjuvant radiation) show that the large majority of recurrences are in the immediate vicinity of the tumor bed. This suggests that the major value of post-lumpectomy RT is to eradicate residual disease in the region of the tumor bed and that areas of occult disease in the remainder of the breast may be of little practical significance in many patients.

A study from Yale (Smith et al. 2000) analyzed true recurrences vs. new primary ipsilateral breast tumor relapses. It was found that in 1152 patients treated with standard breast-conserving therapy utilizing whole-breast RT, at 15 years the elsewhere failure and contralateral failure rates were 13.1% and 10%, respectively. It was shown that a significant proportion of patients who experienced ipsilateral breast tumor relapses following conservative surgery and RT may have new primary tumors as opposed to true local recurrences.

Krauss et al. studied the rates and patterns of tumor recurrence following BCT. Their analysis showed that after 5 years the ipsilateral breast tumor recurrence rates approach the rates of development of a contralateral breast cancer. While elsewhere failures were less frequent than true recurrences, they more often contributed to the ipsilateral breast tumor recurrence rate (Krauss et al. 2004). This further emphasizes that elsewhere failures may increasingly represent new primary tumors rather than recurrences.

There are inherent inconsistencies in reporting recurrences following BCT. The rates of elsewhere failures vs. true recurrences vary depending on the classification scheme employed. The use of molecular techniques to identify markers, such as deletion/loss of heterozygosity analysis, may provide additional insight in determining whether genetically the ipsilateral tumor bed recurrences noted are secondary to new primary tumors

Table 3.2 Prospective randomized trials of lumpectomy with/without RT (*CS* conserving surgery)

Trial	Reference	No. of patients	Tumor size (cm)	Surgery	Patients with recurrence (%)		Reduction in recurrence, CS vs. CS + RT (%)
					CS alone	CS + RT	
NSABP B06	Fisher et al. 2002	1265	<4.0	Wide excision	36	12	67
Milan III	Veronesi et al. 1993	601	<2.5	Quadran-tectomy	24	6	75
Scottish	Forrest et al. 1996	584	<4.0	Wide excision	5	6	75
Sweden	Liljegren et al. 1994	381	<2.0	Quadran-tectomy	24	9	63
Ontario	Clark et al. 1996	837	<4.0	Wide excision	35	11	69
British	Renton et al. 1996	399	<5.0	Wide excision	35	13	63

Table 3.3 The impact of whole-breast radiation therapy on elsewhere failures (*CS* conserving surgery)

Trial	Reference	Elsewhere failures (%)	
		CS alone	CS + RT
NSABP B06	Fisher et al. 2002	2.7 (17/636)	3.8 (24/629)
Ontario	Clark et al. 1992	3.5 (15/421)	0.9 (4/416)
Milan	Veronesi et al. 2002	2.8 (8/280)	0.6 (2/299)
Sweden	Liljegren et al. 1994	1.5 (3/194)	0.5 (1/187)
Range		1.5–3.5	0.5–3.8

or an actual recurrence (Tsuda et al. 1999). Nonetheless, the above data suggest that there is a rate of developing new disease within the breast that whole-breast RT may not be able to prevent. The key benefit of whole-breast RT seems to be reduction of failures in the breast tissue immediately surrounding the lumpectomy cavity.

3.3 Conclusions

The optimal margin of tissue requiring RT after lumpectomy in patients treated with PBI remains controversial. However, recent radiographic and pathologic data suggest that a margin of 10 mm around the tumor bed appears adequate for coverage of any disease remaining in the breast after lumpectomy in most (>90%) patients treated with PBI, provided the final negative margins are negative using the NSABP criteria. More restrictive pathologic criteria can be used to identify patients with disease beyond 10 mm. Additional pathologic analysis as well as long-term clinical data on patients treated with PBI are required to provide stricter guidelines in establishing the optimal CTV for PBI.

References

1. Clark RM, McCulloch PB, Levine MN, et al (1992) Randomized clinical trial to assess the effectiveness of breast irradiation following lumpectomy and axillary dissection for node-negative breast cancer. J Natl Cancer Inst 84(9):683–689

2. Clark RM, Whelan T, Levine M, et al (1996) Randomized clinical trial of breast irradiation following lumpectomy and axillary dissection for node-negative breast cancer: an update. Ontario Clinical Oncology Group. J Natl Cancer Inst 88(22):1659–1664

3. Faverly D, Holland R, Burgers L (1992) An original stereomicroscopic analysis of the mammary glandular tree. Virchows Arch A Pathol Anat Histopathol 421(2):115–119

4. Fisher B, Anderson S, Bryant J, et al (2002) Twenty-year follow-up of a randomized trial comparing total mastectomy, lumpectomy, and lumpectomy plus irradiation for the treatment of invasive breast cancer. N Engl J Med 347(16):1233–1241

5. Forrest AP, Stewart HJ, Everington D, et al (1996) Randomised controlled trial of conservation therapy for breast cancer: 6-year analysis of the Scottish trial. Scottish Cancer Trials Breast Group. Lancet 348(9029):708–713

6. Goldstein NS, Kestin L, Vicini F (2003) Factors associated with ipsilateral breast failure and distant metastases in patients with invasive breast carcinoma treated with breast-conserving therapy. A clinicopathologic study of 607 neoplasms from 583 patients. Am J Clin Pathol 120(4):500–527

7. Holland R, Veling SH, Mravunac M, et al (1985) Histologic multifocality of Tis, T1-2 breast carcinomas. Implications for clinical trials of breast-conserving surgery. Cancer 56(5):979–990

8. Imamura H, Haga S, Shimizu T, et al (2000) Relationship between the morphological and biological characteristics of intraductal components accompanying invasive ductal breast carcinoma and patient age. Breast Cancer Res Treat 62(3):177–184

9. Kestin LL, Jaffray DA, Edmundson GK, et al (2000) Improving the dosimetric coverage of interstitial high-dose-rate breast implants. Int J Radiat Oncol Biol Phys 46(1):35–43

10. Krauss DJ, Kestin LL, Mitchell C, et al (2004) Changes in temporal patterns of local failure after breast-conserving therapy and their prognostic implications. Int J Radiat Oncol Biol Phys 60(3):731–740

11. Liljegren G, Holmberg L, Adami HO, et al (1994) Sector resection with or without postoperative radiotherapy for stage I breast cancer: five-year results of a randomized trial. Uppsala-Orebro Breast Cancer Study Group. J Natl Cancer Inst 86(9):717–722

12. Ohtake T, Abe R, Kimijima I, et al (1995) Intraductal extension of primary invasive breast carcinoma treated by breast-conservative surgery. Computer graphic three-dimensional reconstruction of the mammary duct-lobular systems. Cancer 76(1):32–45

13. Renton SC, Gazet JC, Ford HT, et al (1996) The importance of the resection margin in conservative surgery for breast cancer. Eur J Surg Oncol 22(1):17–22

14. Smith TE, Lee D, Turner BC, et al (2000) True recurrence vs. new primary ipsilateral breast tumor relapse: an analysis of clinical and pathologic differences and their implications in natural history, prognoses, and therapeutic management. Int J Radiat Oncol Biol Phys 48(5):1281–1289

15. Tsuda H, Takarabe T, Hirohashi S (1999) Correlation of numerical and structural status of chromosome 16 with histological type and grade of non-invasive and invasive breast carcinomas. Int J Cancer 84(4):381–387

16. Veronesi U, Luini A, Del Vecchio M, et al (1993) Radiotherapy after breast-preserving surgery in women with localized cancer of the breast. N Engl J Med 328(22):1587–1591

17. Veronesi U, Cascinelli N, Mariani L, et al (2002) Twenty-year follow-up of a randomized study comparing breast-conserving surgery with radical mastectomy for early breast cancer. N Engl J Med 347(16):1227–1232

18. Vicini FA, Kestin LL, Edmundson GK, et al (1999) Dose-volume analysis for quality assurance of interstitial brachytherapy for breast cancer. Int J Radiat Oncol Biol Phys 45(3):803–810

19. Vicini FA, Kestin L, Chen P, et al (2003) Limited-field radiation therapy in the management of early-stage breast cancer. J Natl Cancer Inst 95(16):1205–1210

20. Vicini FA, Kestin LL, Goldstein NS (2004) Defining the clinical target volume for patients with early-stage breast cancer treated with lumpectomy and accelerated partial breast irradiation: a pathologic analysis. Int J Radiat Oncol Biol Phys 60(3):722–730

21. Wallner P, Arthur D, Bartelink H, et al (2004) Workshop on partial breast irradiation: state of the art and the science, Bethesda, MD, December 8-10, 2002. J Natl Cancer Inst 96(3):175–184

Physics of Partial Breast Irradiation: Coping with the New Requirements of the NSABP B39/RTOG 0413 Protocol

4

Gregory K. Edmundson

Contents

4.1 Introduction

The National Surgical Adjuvant Breast and Bowel Project (NSABP) and the Radiation Therapy Oncology Group (RTOG) opened a randomized trial of partial breast irradiation (PBI) versus conventional whole-breast irradiation in March 2005. This trial is designated NSABP B-39/RTOG 0413. While PBI has been undertaken since 1992, this trial will be the first exposure of many users to PBI. In addition, it is destined to become the benchmark by which all PBI will be measured for some time to come. Accordingly, this chapter has three purposes: (1) to help users understand the requirements so that they may place patients into the trial, (2) to elucidate the background of some of the requirements which may be novel to some practitioners, and (3) to serve as a reference in future years for physicians interpreting the lessons of this important trial.

For each PBI modality, the following areas are covered:
- Required imaging studies
- Structures needing to be contoured
- Regions of interest (ROI) to be defined
- Evaluation parameters for ROIs
- Dose prescription and delivery
- Treatment verification

4.1.1 Imaging

For all modalities, the imaging (CT scan) requirements are identical:
- Supine position
- Superior border at or above the mandible
- Inferior border below the inframammary fold
- Include entire lung
- Include chin, shoulders, entire ipsilateral breast
- Include contralateral breast for external beam techniques
- Scan thickness ≤0.5 cm

These requirements make sense in the context of a trial, but go considerably beyond what is needed in typical clinical practice. This is an area where the protocol requirements will not likely extend beyond the scope of the trial itself. Especially for the brachytherapy procedures, smaller volumes may safely be imaged in routine practice. The implication of the requirements listed above is that many slices will generally be needed (over 100 in many cases). This presents issues for many current CT scanners in terms of throughput and Heat Unit considerations. The datasets themselves will be large, typically 0.5 MB per slice. This is an issue in radiation oncology in general, however, and something for which all departments should be preparing.

4.1.2 Breast Reference Volume

It is difficult to delineate the extent of actual breast tissue on CT. As a result, physicians outlining the breast by hand are expected to have poor reproducibility. For purposes of the study only, the 'whole breast reference volume' has been defined as that tissue, excluding lung, which would be irradiated using normal tangential external beams. Of note is that this will include chest wall. It is defined identically for all modalities except MammoSite, in which the volume occupied by the applicator is excluded. The breast reference volume is used in the definition of a number of normal tissue constraints, listed below.

4.2 Interstitial Multicatheter Technique

These structures must be outlined on all CT slices in which they appear:
- Excision cavity
- Ipsilateral breast reference volume

The excision cavity is usually visible on CT scan, especially if the surgery has been quite recent, which is a general requirement of the protocol. If it is not directly visualized, surgical clips may be left to mark the boundaries of the cavity. If the cavity cannot be visualized by one or the other of these techniques, the patient is not eligible for study participation.

4.2.2 Volumes of Interest

4.2.2.1 PTV_EVAL
For dosimetric evaluation of coverage, a new ROI is defined specifically for the study: the planning target volume (PTV) for evaluation (PTV_EVAL). Based upon the International Commission on Radiation Units and Measurements (ICRU) target definitions (ICRU 1993), it is defined for interstitial irradiation to be identical to the clinical target volume (CTV) and PTV. It is formed by placing a uniform 15 mm expansion around the excision cavity, with the exceptions that chest wall and pectoralis muscles are to be excluded, as is any portion which would extend outside the patient, or any portion within 5 mm of the skin surface. This latter restriction makes the evaluation comparable to that for external beam, where dose calculations in the build-up region are uncertain. It also is consistent with the practice of some (but not all) prior users of limiting the target volume near the skin, for optimization purposes. One of the problems with this definition is that not all currently available planning software can identify the 5-mm margin in three dimensions. In regions where the closest distance from the cavity to the skin lies oblique to the axial CT images, it is not possible to make this determination manually either. Note that this volume *includes* the excision cavity.

4.2.2.2 Breast Reference Volume
See above for definition. Note that the excision cavity and chest wall are included.

4.2.3 Appropriateness for Treatment: Evaluation of Dosimetric Parameters

For interstitial multicatheter implants, there are six criteria, one based on point dose and five based on dose–volume histogram (DVH) (see Table 4.1).

Table 4.1 Evaluation parameters for interstitial multicatheter brachytherapy

Parameter	Allowed value	Evaluation of
Skin dose	≤100% of the prescription dose	Maximum point dose
V90[a]	≥90% of PTV_EVAL	DVH of PTV_EVAL
V150[a]	≤70 cm^3	DVH of whole breast
V200[a]	≤20 cm^3	DVH of whole breast
V50[a]	<60%	DVH of whole breast
DHI[b]	≥0.75	

[a] Vn is the volume of tissue treated to at least n% of the prescribed dose
[b] DHI=(V100–V150)/V100 (Wu et al. 1988)

Skin dose is to be restricted to no more than the prescription dose of 340 cGy per fraction, evaluated at the skin–air interface. This criterion is easily achieved if care is taken to avoid placing dwell positions closer than 5 mm to the skin. Skin dose has rarely been a problem in the experiences of the early adopters. One important caveat to this is that the planning imaging shows the state of the breast at an early time following placement. There is frequently edema of the breast at this time, which usually resolves over a period of several days. It is prudent to carefully check for changes in the size of the breast at each fraction.

The parameter listed as V90 is a coverage indication, and is therefore to be evaluated on the histogram of the PTV_EVAL.

The parameters V150 and V200 represent the absolute tissue volumes exposed to doses of 150% (510 cGy per fraction) and 200% (680 cGy per fraction) of the prescribed dose. They are based upon the observation that large volumes at these doses are significantly correlated with the development of symptomatic fat necrosis (Wazer et al. 2001).

As a practical matter, it is helpful to consider the V90, V150 and V200 together as constraints which determine the lower and upper bounds for adjustment of the normalization. We have found it convenient to export the two histograms on which these parameters are calculated, and use them in a spreadsheet to show the DVHs and constraints together. If adjustment of the normalization is needed (usually to accommodate V90), the trade-off can be readily visualized.

The parameter listed here as V50 is not so identified in the protocol proper. This is the major normal breast tissue constraint. It would be equivalent to use D60 (minimum dose to 60% of the breast), with a limit of 50% of prescription dose (i.e. 170 cGy per fraction). This normal tissue constraint was originally derived in a retrospective review at William Beaumont Hospital (Baglan et al. 2003). In this review of 23 interstitial brachytherapy patients, the maximum breast volume treated to 20 Gy in eight fractions was

57% of the breast reference volume. The presumption is that, since toxicity was low in these patients, this volume–dose relationship should also predict low toxicity in other modalities intended to be equivalent. The same constraint, with the same value, is used in the protocol for all modes of accelerated treatment.

The dose homogeneity index (DHI) is defined in current terms as:

DHI=(V100–V150)/V100   (1)

DHI was first described in a time when true ROI DVHs were not commonly available for brachytherapy (Wu et al. 1988). As such, it should strictly be evaluated on the entire dose matrix. In practice, evaluating it on the breast reference volume is functionally equivalent. It is not strictly correct to evaluate it using the DVH of the PTV_EVAL, as interstitial implants are generally designed to encompass more than the PTV in order to achieve acceptable homogeneity within the PTV. DHI is a simple metric to calculate, but has not been shown to correlate with toxicity in the treatment of the breast (Wazer et al. 2001). It is, nonetheless, a useful index for implant quality. The value achieved will vary significantly depending on the implant method used.

4.2.4 Dose Prescription and Delivery

The prescribed dose is to be 3.4 Gy per fraction for ten fractions, delivered twice daily with a minimum 6-hour interval. What is not stated is how that prescription is to be defined, i.e. whether to a point, a series of points (as per the Paris system), or with respect to the DVH of the PTV. Any of these are allowed, and there may be some variability between participating centers. Care should therefore be taken in interpreting results. Overall treatment duration is explicitly stated as 5–10 days, meaning that breaks for weekends or slightly longer are specifically allowed. Once-per-day treatment is not explicitly addressed, but is not specifically excluded by this description. Treatment must begin within 3 weeks of the prerandomization CT scan.

4.2.5 Treatment Verification

Verification is via a written treatment verification record to be submitted to the Radiologic Physics Center (RPC) at M.D. Anderson Hospital in Houston. Two recommended items which are not part of the protocol documentation but should be part of the treatment record are (1) the calculated source strength-total dwell time product for each fraction (some afterloaders report this as total reference air kerma, or TRAK) and (2) some indication that the effect of breast edema has been measured. The source-strength may be indicated as activity or air kerma strength (i.e. Ci-sec or U-sec), and should be almost constant from one fraction to the next. It will also be similar from one patient to the next, given similar treatment volumes. Learning what product to expect for a given size implant will give confidence that the program is being implemented in a consistent way. The breast edema portion can be any measurement capable of detecting whether dwell positions are closer to the skin than they were at the time of planning (e.g. button-to-skin distances for each end of each catheter).

4.3 MammoSite

These structures must be outlined on all CT slices in which they appear:
- Balloon surface
- Trapped air/fluid outside of the balloon
- Ipsilateral breast reference volume

The balloon surface has two uses in this context. The first is that the applicator itself is subsequently removed from the evaluated regions of interest, as dose delivered to the balloon is of no consequence. The second is that this surface is a convenient proxy for the original excision margin. While it is recognized that the excision margin does not always precisely conform to this surface, the actual excision margin may at times be difficult to evaluate. At any rate, there is little one can do to compensate for the irregular shape of the cavity when it is not in contact. For that reason, a simple, reliable basis for the PTV is the balloon surface, with the caveat that if the conformity is not within defined limits, the treatment is not allowed to proceed.

Air, seroma or hematoma contiguous with the balloon surface are all considered to be equivalent, representing non-contact of the excision margin with the balloon surface ('non-conformance'). The total volume of this region is used in the calculation of conformance (see below). Note that some planning systems do not provide for structures which are not contiguous on every slice (e.g. separated air bubbles). In such cases, multiple ROIs must be constructed, and their volumes added. Any region of non-conformance is to be considered in its entirety, specifically to include any portion which extends beyond the 1.0-cm boundary of the PTV. It is the potential displacement of the excision margin away from the applicator which is the important concept. It is conservatively assumed that all such regions represent radial displacement of breast tissue away from the applicator. This will not always be the case, but it is not possible to distinguish circumferential spread (i.e. fracturing of tissue) from radial displacement.

Air trapped inside the balloon, on the other hand, must be considered part of the applicator. No accounting is made for the dosimetric effects of air either inside or outside of the balloon. The effects appear to be minor (Cheng et al. 2005), and are not represented in current planning systems.

4.3.1 Volumes of Interest

4.3.1.1 CTV=PTV=PTV_EVAL
Note that the PTV_EVAL is defined in a different manner from the equivalent ROI described above for the interstitial technique. It encompasses a uniform 10 mm expansion about the balloon, with the same exclusions as above, namely lung, chest wall, and the first 5 mm of tissue beneath the skin. The balloon proper is also excluded. This produces some difficulty for planning systems which do not support complex structures (i.e. noncontiguous as listed above for air, or having an inner surface which is not contiguous with the outer surface, as here). In such cases, there are several work-arounds. The first method is to make the contours contiguous by excluding a small strip of tissue on each slice (Fig. 4.1). If care is taken with this procedure, the resulting volume will produce DVH results closely approximating the true values. Care must be taken that not too much tissue is excluded in the 'bridge', and especially that the contours do not cross.

The second method is to create two volumes, one for the balloon proper and the other the balloon plus the 10-mm margin. The volumes of the dose levels of interest can be extracted from each, and subtracted. The third method is to create the two volumes of interest as above, taking care that the bin width and number are identical in the DVH calculations. The histograms are then exported to a spreadsheet, and subtracted bin-for-bin. The resulting histogram will correctly depict the dose-volume characteristics of the intended PTV_EVAL.

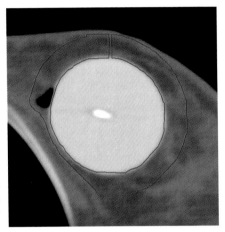

Fig. 4.1 Preparing a complex contour using the bridge technique. The contour has been 'broken' at the top. Note also that care must be taken for the contour not to cross at the chest wall

4.3.1.2 Volume of Nonconformity
Use of the MammoSite assumes that the tissues of interest conform to the applicator, rather than have the treatment conform to the pre-existing geometry of the tissue volume. It is possible that this conformity is not perfect, due to inclusions between the balloon applicator and the breast tissue. Air can be trapped in the cavity at the time the applicator is placed. In addition, accumulation of seroma or hematoma between the applicator and breast tissue has an identical effect. All of these nonconformance regions are contoured as one ROI as outlined above, to be compared to the volume of the PTV_EVAL (see evaluation, below).

4.3.1.3 Breast Reference Volume
See above for definition. Note that the chest wall is included, but the balloon volume is excluded, as it does not represent tissue. For planning systems not supporting complex ROIs the comments from the paragraph describing the PTV_EVAL definition apply.

4.3.2 Appropriateness for Treatment

For MammoSite, there are geometric parameters to be evaluated in addition to dosimetric parameters (Table 4.2).

The minimum distance from the balloon surface to the skin surface is 7 mm. This

Table 4.2 Evaluation parameters for MammoSite

Parameter	Allowed value	Evaluation of
Skin to balloon distance	≥7 mm (no dose eval) ≥5 mm (+ dose, below)	3D distance
Skin dose	≤145% of the prescription dose	Maximum point dose
Nonconformity[a]	≤10%	Volume of nonconformance/ volume of PTV_EVAL ×100%
V90[b]	≥90% of PTV_EVAL + percent nonconformity	DVH of PTV_EVAL
V150[b]	≤50 cm^3	DVH of whole breast
V200[b]	≤10 cm^3	DVH of whole breast
V50[b]	<60%	DVH of whole breast

[a] Nonconformity is the percentage of the PTV_EVAL displaced by air or seroma (see text)
[b] Vn is the volume of tissue treated to at least n% of the prescribed dose

may be decreased to 5 mm *provided* the dose to the skin is evaluated and remains below 145% of the prescribed dose (i.e. 493 cGy). It is recognized that the calculation of surface dose is subject to error due to the loss of backscatter, which is not accounted for in commercial planning systems (Pantelis et al. 2005). The protocol dose value is derived from considerable clinical experience, in which the loss of backscatter is also not accounted for. When more sophisticated planning is available in the future, this value will be adjusted downward for those systems.

There are several ways to make this measurement in practice. For planning systems having true 3D margining capability, it is straightforward to incrementally place a margin on the balloon surface and expanding the margin until it emerges through the skin surface (Fig 4.2). This process will determine not only what the minimum distance is, but where the closest approach is located. We have generally defined a special ROI for this purpose, which can be named something like 'skin distance'. Once the required margin to bring this ROI to the skin surface is determined, we rename the ROI to include this measurement as part of the structure name. The reason for this is that no current planning systems actually record the margin used to create the ROI. Embedding this information into the ROI name assures that this critical piece of information is properly and permanently recorded.

It is important to note also that this minimum distance represents the shortest distance in any arbitrary direction, not merely measured in axial CT planes. When the applicator is located low in the breast, this minimum distance is not evaluable from the axial slices alone, and to do so will systematically overestimate the distance. This will put the patient at risk of unexpected skin toxicity. In Fig. 4.3a, the skin distance is determined using the true 3D method above, and the true distance in this case was determined to be 12 mm. If the distance from the balloon to the skin were measured naively in the slices as in Fig. 4.3b, the minimum distance found would be 15 mm.

The nonconformity is calculated as the ratio of the volume of the nonconformance region to the volume of the PTV_EVAL, expressed as a percentage. If the percentage of the PTV_EVAL is greater than 10%, the patient is not considered suitable for treatment

Fig. 4.2 Iterative expansion to find skin distance. After the balloon is contoured, an expansion is performed with increasing margin until the new ROI emerges through the skin. If a skin rendering is available in the planning system, this is useful, as it gives the user an intuitive understanding as to where the highest skin dose will occur

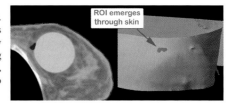

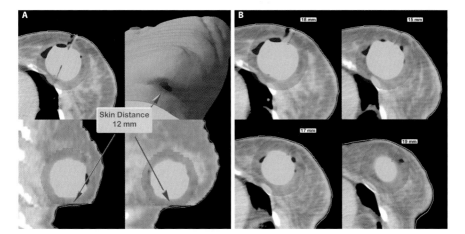

Fig. 4.3 **A** Clockwise from lower right: sagittal, coronal, axial and 3D rendered views of skin distance determined using the technique of shown in Fig. 4.2. The skin distance is 1.2 cm, and is directed in this case caudally. **B** Four axial views of the same case with the in-plane distance to skin illustrated. The apparent distance from these measurements is 1.5 cm, an over-estimation

(unless a way is found to physically reduce the nonconformity). Although the dose in the displaced portion of the PTV does not go to zero, this portion is considered 'lost' to the PTV for prescription purposes. For this reason, the coverage index (V90) requirement is adjusted upward in such cases.

The V90 parameter has the same meaning as for the interstitial technique, that is that it is a description of the coverage of the PTV_EVAL. For treatments with perfect conformance, 90% of the PTV_EVAL must be covered by the 90% dose. For increasing nonconformance, this volume is adjusted upward, i.e. for 3% nonconformance, 93% of the PTV_EVAL must be covered by the same dose level. When nonconformance exceeds 10%, it is no longer physically possible to achieve this, and the patient is excluded.

The V150 and V200 parameters are defined in the same way as for the interstitial technique (they represent absolute volumes of breast tissue), but the acceptable values are lower. In theory, they need to be evaluated on the whole breast volume, although the values will not be different if they are evaluated on the PTV_EVAL, unless a significant portion of this has a thickness of less than 1.0 cm (e.g. balloon is against the chest wall).

Similar to the interstitial case, the V90, V150 and V200 parameters can be considered simultaneously (see Fig. 4.4). The DVHs can be exported to a spreadsheet, and plotted together with the constraint values. The toxicity constraints have fixed absolute values (these are smaller than the values associated with interstitial). The coverage parameter must be calculated after determining the conformity. In the example shown, the PTV_ EVAL is 120 cm³, and the volume of the nonconformity region is 2.2 cm³, leading to a nonconformity percentage of 1.5%. The required value then is 90% + 1.5% = 91.5%, or 109.8 cm³ in this case.

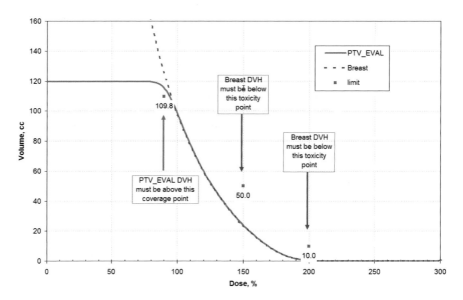

Fig. 4.4 Composite DVH of PTV_EVAL (*green*) and whole breast (*red*). Toxicity constraints have fixed values; coverage constraint is calculated (see text)

The V50 parameter has the same meaning and acceptable value as for both interstitial and 3D. It would be very unusual to see this constraint violated for MammoSite.

4.3.3 Dose Prescription and Delivery

Dose prescription and delivery requirements for MammoSite are identical to those for the interstitial technique above.

4.3.4 Treatment Verification

Proper balloon inflation is documented via the treatment verification sheet submitted to the RPC. Note that this implies that some form of imaging will be performed for every fraction. The primary concerns here are balloon leakage or deflation. Acceptable forms of imaging would include simulator x-rays, c-arm x-rays, ultrasound or CT scan. For users without x-ray projection imaging, note that CT is acceptable, but for this purpose it need not be a complete scan. A single slice through the balloon center is sufficient. For patients with iodine allergy, instillation of contrast medium into the balloon is contraindicated. In such cases, either CT or ultrasound work well. If balloon deflation occurs, a new balloon may be inserted, and the course of treatment completed.

4.4 3D Conformal External Beam

Intensity-modulated radiation therapy (IMRT) is *not* allowed. For protocol purposes, this means that any form of segmented fields with weights determined via inverse planning would not be acceptable. Simple segmented fields, used in the manner of wedged fields may be acceptable. The primary reasons for these exclusions are that IMRT methodologies are not entirely standardized at this time, and providing oversight for the technical aspects of delivery is inordinately time-consuming with current tools. It is to be expected that once this form of treatment becomes routine, off-protocol treatments will frequently make use of IMRT.

Tissue inhomogeneity correction must be used for all external beam calculations.

4.4.1 Contouring

These structures must be outlined on all CT slices in which they appear:
- Excision/lumpectomy cavity
- Skin
- Ipsilateral breast
- Contralateral breast
- Thyroid
- Heart

4.4.2 Volumes of Interest

The CTV is defined as the contoured excision cavity plus a 15 mm uniform margin. Pectoralis muscles are excluded, as well as any breast tissue within 5 mm of the skin surface. If the excision cavity is defined only by surgical clips, the radiation oncologist will construct a volume to represent the cavity. This may introduce some variability into the definition of the subsequent volumes of interest. In the large majority of cases, however, it is expected that the cavity will be easily visualized via CT, as the protocol mandates CT scan within 42 days of surgery, and recommends that it be performed within 14 days.

The PTV consists of the CTV plus an additional uniform 10 mm expansion to accommodate daily setup error and breathing motion. This volume will be used to generate the actual beam apertures (with a further margin added for beam penumbra which will depend on the accelerator used). This implies that this volume will be allowed to extend outside the patient and into the chest wall structures.

Since such a target volume is not appropriate for dose calculations (due both to including nontarget tissues and also occupying the build-up region, where the dose calculation becomes uncertain), an additional volume is defined: the PTV_EVAL. This volume starts with the PTV, but excludes any portion outside the patient, or lying within 5 mm of the skin surface, and re-excludes the pectoralis and ribs. It is the PTV_EVAL which is used for DVH analysis of the target, and the generation of constraints for coverage. (There are separate constraints for normal tissues, which are based on other regions of interest; see below.)

4.4.3 Beam Angles/Treatment Position

Typically three-, four-, or five-field non-coplanar beam arrangements using high-energy photons can be used (Baglan et al. 2003). No beams may be directed toward critical normal structures (heart, lung, contralateral breast). This implies that only quasitangential beams are allowed. Depending on the gantry- and table-angle limitations imposed by the geometry of the particular accelerator, this will make it difficult to meet the normal tissue dose constraints listed below for patients with small breasts or large cavities. Bolus should not be used.

4.4.4 Appropriateness for Treatment

There are a few more dosimetric constraints for this method than for the brachytherapy methods (see Table 4.3).

V90 is the coverage parameter, and has the same definition and allowable values described above for the brachytherapy methods. Of all the appropriateness parameters for 3D-CRT, it is the only one evaluated on the PTV_EVAL.

The uniformity criterion is the breast maximum dose. This can be demonstrated from the whole breast DVH, and is also commonly reported directly by the planning system.

4.4.5 Dose Prescription and Delivery

Dose prescription is 385 cGy per fraction, ten fractions, twice daily. The minimum time between fractions is 6 hours, and duration of treatment is 5–10 days. The dose in this case is prescribed to a reference point, usually the isocenter.

Ipsilateral breast constraints are defined at the 50% and 100% dose levels (V50 and V100). In addition to the V50 constraint defined for brachytherapy, no more than 35% of the breast reference volume is allowed to receive the prescription dose (385 cGy per fraction). Like the V50 constraint, the V100 constraint derives from a retrospective study of interstitial brachytherapy at William Beaumont Hospital (Baglan et al. 2003). In this study, the maximum percentage breast volume receiving the prescribed dose (40 Gy in eight fractions) was 38%.

Other constraints are as shown in Table 4.3. All of these should be relatively easy to meet. It is the constraints on the ipsilateral normal breast which will consume most of the planning effort.

Table 4.3 Evaluation parameters for 3D-CRT

Parameter	Allowed value	Evaluation of
V90[a]	≥90% of PTV_EVAL	DVH of PTV_EVAL
Ipsilateral breast maximum	≤120% of prescription dose (462 cGy/fraction)	Point dose
V50[a]	<60% of breast volume	DVH of ipsilateral breast
V100[a]	<35% of breast volume	DVH of ipsilateral breast
Contralateral breast maximum	<3% of prescription dose (12 cGy/fraction)	Point dose
V30[a]	<15% of lung volume	DVH of ipsilateral lung
V5[a]	<15% of lung volume	DVH of contralateral lung
V5[a] (right-sided lesions)	<5% of heart volume	DVH of heart
V5[a] (left-sided lesions)	<40% of heart volume	DVH of heart
Thyroid maximum	≤3% of prescription dose (12 cGy/fraction)	Point dose

[a] Vn is the volume of tissue treated to at least n% of the prescribed dose

4.4.6 Treatment Verification

Verification is via a written treatment verification record, to be submitted to the RPC at M.D. Anderson Hospital in Houston. In addition, for the first fraction, port films (or electronic images) of each treatment beam will be submitted, along with an orthogonal pair (AP and lateral). Subsequent portal films or images must be obtained on fraction numbers 2, 5, and 9.

4.5 Conclusions

Modern treatment planning software is required; this is generally available for external beam modalities, but more challenging for brachytherapy users. Additional software will often be required to electronically submit data for the protocol. The planning methods outlined for this protocol will certainly quickly become the benchmark for this type of treatment, so mastering it at this time is likely to be a good investment of time and effort.

References

1. Baglan KL, Sharpe MB, Jaffray D, Frazier RC, Fayad J, Kestin LL, Remouchamps V, Martinez AA, Wong J, Vicini FA (2003) Accelerated partial breast irradiation using 3D conformal radiation therapy (3D-CRT). Int J Radiat Oncol Biol Phys 55(2):302–311
2. Cheng CW, Mitra R, Li XA, Das IJ (2005) Dose perturbations due to contrast medium and air in MammoSite treatment: an experimental and Monte Carlo study. Med Phys 32(7):2279–2287

3. ICRU (1993) Prescribing, recording and reporting photon beam therapy (report no. 50). International Commission on Radiation Units and Measurements. Oxford University Press, Oxford

4. Pantelis E, Papagiannis P, Karaiskos P, Angelopoulos A, Anagnostopoulos G, Baltas D, Zamboglou N, Sakelliou L (2005) The effect of finite patient dimensions and tissue inhomogeneities on dosimetry planning of 192Ir HDR breast brachytherapy: a Monte Carlo dose verification study. Int J Radiat Oncol Biol Phys 61(5):1596–1602

5. Wazer DE, Lowther D, Boyle T, Ulin K, Neuschatz A, Ruthazer R, DiPetrillo TA (2001) Clinically evident fat necrosis in women treated with high-dose-rate brachytherapy alone for early-stage breast cancer. Int J Radiat Oncol Biol Phys 50(1):107–111

6. Wu A, Ulin K, Sternick ES (1988) A dose homogeneity index for evaluating 192Ir interstitial breast implants. Med Phys 15(1):104–107

The Radiobiology of Accelerated Partial Breast Irradiation

5

Simon N. Powell

Contents

5.1 Introduction

The combination of breast-conserving surgery and radiotherapy is a widely accepted treatment option for most women with clinical stage I or II invasive breast cancer or ductal carcinoma in situ. The optimal volume of breast-conserving irradiation is the subject of a current nationwide randomized trial: does the whole breast require radiotherapy, or is irradiating a limited volume of breast tissue surrounding the tumor bed adequate (McCormick 2005)? Accelerated partial breast irradiation (APBI) is a radiation technique that allows for shorter treatment schemes than with whole-breast irradiation (typically 1 week), and the expectation of reduced normal tissue toxicity by decreasing treatment volumes (i.e. cardiac damage and radiation pneumonitis). The currently available APBI treatment modalities include:

- Interstitial brachytherapy
  - Low dose-rate
  - High dose-rate
- Intracavitary therapy
  - Orthovoltage photons (Intrabeam, UK)
  - Intraoperative electrons (Milan)
  - Brachytherapy (MammoSite)
  - Ham applicator (MSKCC)
- External beam therapy
  - 3D conformal photons/mixed beam
  - Intensity-modulated radiation therapy
  - Protons

APBI as a treatment option will only succeed if normal tissue toxicity is reduced for the same local control benefit as demonstrated with whole-breast irradiation. Other potential benefits of APBI include patient convenience with the reduction in the length of the radiotherapy course, easier integration with chemotherapy, and potentially a reduction in the overall treatment cost (Suh et al. 2005). Furthermore, irradiation of the entire breast is viewed by most radiation oncologists as precluding subsequent breast radiotherapy (Freedman et al. 2005). Giving PBI initially may allow for a second chance at breast-conserving treatment in this setting.

Radiobiological aspects of APBI are in the process of optimization. The significant changes in treatment time raise uncertainties about the biologically equivalent dose (BED). The currently used doses were developed based on applications of dose equivalence models, such as the linear quadratic model, but whether these models truly apply to these novel treatment situations is not yet clear. Figure 5.1 shows an example of how BEDs can be calculated using the linear quadratic model. There are two main methods to represent biological equivalence: BED, which is a representation of dose equivalence using an infinite number of small fractions; and the dose in 2-Gy equivalents, which is an easier to understand concept with a currency that is well understood by radiation oncologists. At present, there is a wide spectrum of different dose-fractionation schedules used in APBI, and they are clearly not all biologically equivalent (Table 5.1). In this chapter a more detailed analysis of a number of these different approaches is presented.

Using Linear-Quadratic (LQ) model: Effect $= e^{(\alpha D + \beta D^2)}$

$$\frac{D1}{D2} = \frac{d2 + \alpha/\beta}{d1 + \alpha/\beta}$$

d1 = 2 Gy (or 0 for BED); d2 = dose per fraction using brachyRx
D2 = total dose with brachyRx; D1 = total dose equivalent

For example, with an HDR regimen: 32Gy/ 8#/ 4 Gy bid

For an α/β =10; and d2=4; $D1_{(2\,Gy)}$ = 37.3 Gy $\frac{D1}{32} = \frac{4+10}{2+10}$
                                     BED = 44.8 Gy

For an α/β =3; and d2=4; $D1_{(2\,Gy)}$ = 44.8 Gy $\frac{D1}{32} = \frac{4+3}{2+3}$
                                     BED = 74.7 Gy

Fig. 5.1 Calculation of biological equivalent dose

The biological consequences of dose inhomogeneity, with 10–20% variations in dose, have been analyzed. However, in APBI with implants, the dose inhomogeneity is significant, with 15–20% of the treatment volume receiving 150% of the dose (Das et al. 2004; Shah et al. 2004). The potential impact of these major inhomogeneities on tumor control and normal tissue complications is highlighted.

The use of radical radiation therapy schedules over a total treatment time of 1 week is also a treatment scheme with relatively little precedent. Early-stage head and neck cancers have been treated with about 60 Gy, using low dose-rate (LDR) brachytherapy over the course of 5–7 days, with effective local control of the primary site for tumors in the range of 1–2 cm (Nag et al. 2001; Shasha et al. 1998). The implication is that 60 Gy in 1 week is equivalent to at least 66–70 Gy over 6–7 weeks using fractionated external beam therapy. There are well-documented reasons why accelerated therapies may achieve some degree of dose discount in head and neck cancers, since the proliferation rates of the tumors are high as measured by their short potential doubling times. In breast cancers, postlumpectomy, the cell kinetics may be significantly different and

Table 5.1 Application of the linear quadratic model to clinically tested regimens – dose equivalence

Schedule		Acute	Late
Total dose (Gy)	Number of fractions	D1 for α/β = 10 (in 2 Gy fractions)	D1 for α/β = 3 (in 2 Gy fractions)
32	8	37.3	44.8
34	10	38.0	43.5
38.5	10	44.4	52.7
36.4	7	46.1	59.7
21	1	54.3	100.8
5	1	6.25	8
50	LDR	50	50
60	LDR	60	60

thus the potential advantage of the acceleration of therapy into 1 week of treatment is essentially unknown.

There are current trends in radiation oncology for a return to smaller and more focused treatment volumes, with the consequent use of accelerated and hypofractionated regimens. Recent evidence in prostate cancer suggests that an α/β ratio for these tumors may be as low as 1–2 Gy (Bentzen and Ritter 2005; Fowler 2005), suggesting that there would be radiobiological advantages for the use of hypofractionation. Although there are often similarities implied between prostate and breast cancer, in terms of hormonal dependent growth, wide variations in tumor growth rates and patterns of dissemination, it would be difficult to extend this similarity to the α/β ratio of breast cancer in the absence of data to support the conclusion. Since radiation therapy in the treatment of breast cancer is largely adjuvant postoperative, it is unlikely that the required data will ever be obtained.

Thus, although there are many uncertainties about the radiobiological effectiveness of APBI, the results of these therapies to date appear very satisfactory (Wallner et al. 2004). The effectiveness of targeting the area of the breast at risk may be improved by the use of APBI, perhaps allowing some degree of dose discount relative to whole-breast irradiation plus a tumor bed boost, where the techniques are associated with delivery inaccuracies. Although a tumor bed boost has been shown to improve local control in a large randomized trial (Bartelink et al. 2001), the accuracy of targeting the boost is still an open question, in spite of a quality assurance program for the EORTC study (Poortmans et al. 2004). The focus of this review is the radiobiological aspects of currently used approaches for APBI.

5.2 Advantages of Accelerated Therapy

The major perceived advantage of accelerated therapy, from the patient's perspective, is the convenience of completing treatment within 1 week. The selection of 1 week as the overall treatment time was based on the time patients could tolerate an implant within the breast, and the consequent inflammatory reaction to the foreign body. With the option of external beam radiotherapy for APBI, clearly the use of schemes over 2–3 weeks could be explored. At this stage, the published experience with external beam approaches is limited (Vicini et al. 2003, 2005), and the onus is to show equivalence to the implant experience.

The major reason to consider accelerated therapies from a radiobiological viewpoint is to prevent proliferation of the tumor during the course of therapy. The major evidence supporting an accelerated approach is from tumors of the head and neck and from cervix cancers (Awwad et al. 2002; Fyles et al. 1992), where delays in the overall treatment time have been shown to affect the outcome of treatment. However, the consequence of these analyses has been to consider the use of therapies with 3–5 weeks of treatment instead of 6–7 weeks. Whether there are advantages in accelerating all the way to 1 week of treatment is less clear. Even the impact of accelerated repopulation, an idea generated from analysis of local control of head and neck cancers (Maciejewski et al. 1996), would not support the use of schedules shorter than 3–4 weeks.

The major determinant of local control in breast-conserving therapy is the residual tumor burden, as predicted by the extent of surgical resection margin. The additional impact of the tumor growth rate on local control has not been demonstrated, although significant delays in the delivery of radiation therapy (beyond 12–16 weeks from surgery) has been shown to adversely affect outcome. However, converting this information into a potential advantage from highly accelerated therapy is difficult to model with any degree of certainty, since the actual number of residual clonogenic cells cannot be determined. Thus, the conclusion is that rapid acceleration of therapy is largely based on tolerance of an implant and patient convenience, rather than a clear radiobiological rationale.

The question could then be posed as to whether there are any disadvantages of accelerated therapy. Late normal tissue reactions have largely been thought to be independent of overall treatment time, so at first pass it could be surmised that there are no adverse effects of APBI. However, the evidence supporting relative independence of overall treatment time comes from Nominal Standard Dose (NSD) analyses, in which the majority of the data were derived from 3–6 week treatments. Using this model, the exponent relating the inverse of overall treatment time to late effects is 0.11, implying a relatively small impact. If we apply this figure to the change in overall treatment time from 6 weeks to 1 week, then the impact on late effects is $6^{0.11}$, which equals 1.218 or a 21.8% increase in effect. Thus, in spite of the uncertainty about the application of this model to these very short treatment times, the additional impact on effect is relatively small and more than offset by the reduction in dose used these protocols. As can be seen from the discussion below, there is significantly more impact from the use of hypofractionated treatment than from reduction in overall treatment time. The linear quadratic model, more frequently applied to the comparison of different fractionation schedules, does not take overall treatment time into account, and other limitations of this model include: the assumption of dose homogeneity; not considering volume as a variable; and limitations in the range of dose per fraction.

5.3 Volume of Breast Requiring Treatment in APBI

The pathological extent of tumor cells around the identifiable tumor within the breast has been studied by detailed analyses of mastectomy specimens, and simulating a lumpectomy (Holland et al. 1990). Although the simulation of the lumpectomy or wide excision may be somewhat idealized compared to real surgery, these analyses have revealed the patterns of disease around a main tumor mass as a useful concept in how breast cancers grow within the breast. The concept of an "extensive intraductal component" (EIC) was developed out of these analyses, and although the impact of EIC on local control can be neutralized by negative margins in the context of whole-breast irradiation, the concept is still useful in terms of describing a pattern of growth within the breast. In our studies of partial breast irradiation (Lawenda et al. 2003) we excluded EIC-positive tumors from eligibility, since we felt that the volume of breast requiring treatment with this tumor pattern was more extensive than the volumes conventionally covered using APBI. However, this criterion has not been used universally by the studies to date, and there are no published data that analyze the outcome in EIC-positive and EIC-negative tumors.

Therefore, using the data of Holland et al. (1990), we can suggest that the volume of breast to be included in the target volume for EIC-negative tumors should be 3 cm from the tumor edge, which in practical terms is 1.5–2 cm from the edge of an ideal wide excision. The aim of a wide excision is to remove the tumor with at least a 1 cm margin around the identifiable tumor. However, the major concern is that the 1 cm margin is rarely found evenly placed around the tumor, implying that the target volume should not be symmetrical around the resection cavity. In the absence of better evidence, the application of APBI by interstitial implant, MammoSite or external beam is based on a margin around the resection cavity. It would clearly be advantageous to map the location of the tumor on 3D reconstruction and then to map the residual breast tissue after resection, which is potentially feasible with current image fusion and deformable image registration procedures. The study of APBI needs data to analyze the extent of the margin and relate the finding to risk of recurrence. Only by continued analysis will we be able to determine the optimum margin requiring treatment after wide excision. The current guideline includes a range of 1–2 cm, but the extent of the radiation treatment volume has to be dependent on the volume of tissue resected in relation to the size of the tumor. In an analysis of the volume of resection and local control (Vicini et al. 1991), the JCRT found that local control rates were dependent on the final volume of resected breast tissue.

The induction of late tissue damage in the breast, such as fat necrosis, is dependent on whether the tissue is organized in parallel or series functional subunits (Withers 1986). This analysis has proved useful in a number of postradiation risk assessments, such as for the spinal cord and kidney, but whether it is broadly applicable to all tissue types is more questionable. A tissue that is organized in parallel in subunits, is much more tolerant of larger doses per fraction if only a small fraction of the total organ is irradiated. This situation could potentially apply to APBI, but there are insufficient data in relation to breast radiation treatments that could support or refute this idea. Further data acquisition from studying the doses delivered to target and non-target breast tissue is needed before conclusions can be drawn. The comparison of brachytherapy to external beam approaches will be useful since there will be a significant difference in the mean breast dose with the two techniques. The model predicts that each unit of volume carries its own probability of inducing fat necrosis, and that dose hot spots would be the major determinant of the probability of fat necrosis. However, external beam would significantly increase the mean breast dose, relative to brachytherapy, and this may manifest in a higher risk of fat necrosis. To date, this has not been observed using external beam APBI.

5.4 Dose Homogeneity

All brachytherapy used for APBI necessarily has significant dose inhomogeneity, whether an interstitial or intracavitary implant is used. This inhomogeneity of dose stems directly from the fact that small differences in distance from the sources used in brachytherapy make a big difference to the delivered dose. For an interstitial implant, the expected degree of inhomogeneity is that less than 25% of the volume receives greater than 150% of the prescribed dose. Indeed, for the RTOG trial of APBI by interstitial implant, the dose homogeneity index (DHI) was not allowed to be >25% for V150. This roughly translates into the idea that the 150% isodose lines stay separated around each catheter, and do not "coalesce". This guideline was based on idea that the larger the volume in any one hot-spot region the more likely the development of a complication such as fat necrosis. Although this is likely to be true, there are no analyses of the incidence of complications from APBI across the variety of published dose and fractionation schedules.

Dose inhomogeneity can also lead to the reported problem of "double-trouble", in which the biological effect of physical dose hot spots are amplified by the effect of the α/β ratio on large doses per fraction, not just at the prescribed dose, but at the 150% dose. In the example shown in Fig. 5.2, the impact of 6 Gy per fraction for the V150 (when the prescribed dose is 4 Gy) is shown to change the dose in 2 Gy equivalents to 86.6 Gy, with a BED of >100 Gy. Thus, even though the prescribed dose may only be 32–34 Gy, given in 3.2–4.0 Gy per fraction, the biological dose on normal tissues could be considered high in these hot-spot regions. It is in this context that there may be considerable differences between the different dose fractionation schedules that have been used for APBI, which will be discussed further below.

Even though there is a downside to dose inhomogeneity, there are positive contributions of the hot spots in terms of tumor control probability. If the tumor cells in each unit of volume of the treatment area are considered as independent entities, the ability to control the tumor cells in this volume unit will be proportional to dose. Therefore, in the regions receiving 150% of the dose, the probability of eradicating the tumor will be proportional to the dose applied. This effect can be demonstrated by the example shown in Fig. 5.3, in which we have estimated that the probability of controlling the tumor without radiation therapy is about 60%, and that 55 Gy in ten fractions (using a ten-fraction example) would give 100% control, then the ability of 34 Gy in ten fractions at the prescribed dose, with a DHI for V150 of 25%, would predict a 93% control rate for the implant, and a control rate of 86% if the prescribed dose were perfectly homogeneous. This example does not take account of the effect of any systemic therapy, such as hormonal therapy, which can clearly contribute to the local control probability. If the implant were to have any imperfections in the evenness of the implant, introducing incomplete coverage of the planning target volume (PTV), then there would be a significant negative impact on the tumor control probability.

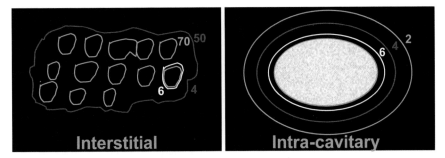

Fig. 5.2 Dose inhomogeneity: "double trouble". On the left an example is shown in which the volume covered by the 4 Gy prescribed dose is 8×7.5×3.5 cm, i.e. 210 ml. About 45 ml of this volume is seroma; therefore the volume of breast tissue being treated is 210−45=165 ml. The V150 (>6 Gy volume) is about 40 ml (V150 <25%). For the V150, the BED is calculated by the method shown in Fig. 5.1: 8×6 Gy, with an α/β ratio of 3, the dose in 2 Gy equivalents is 86.4 Gy. The ratio 86.4/48 is significantly higher than 44.8/32, emphasizing the role of double-trouble for large doses per fraction plus dose inhomogeneity. Using a low dose rate, the equivalent hot spot receiving 70 cGy per hour, the total dose becomes 63 Gy, and using an α/β ratio of 3, the LDR hot spots in 2 Gy equivalents is about 68 Gy. This highlights the potential radiobiological advantage of LDR therapy. For intracavitary implants, as shown on the right, the cavity receiving 4 Gy is 7×7×5 cm, i.e. a volume of 4/3×π×(3.5×3.5×2.5)=128.3 ml. The seroma cavity is 5×5×3 cm, i.e. 39.3 ml, leaving a treatment volume of 89 ml. The 6 Gy volume is 30 ml, observed in a rim around the cavity.

With intracavitary implants, using MammoSite, the dose inhomogeneity is somewhat different. The fraction of the PTV receiving 150% of the dose may be the same (about 25%), but all the V150 is adjacent to the balloon surface. This has been argued, by advocates of MammoSite, to be the reason why it is effective. However, the risk of residual tumor cells is not directly proportional to the distance from the edge of the resection, although there is undoubtedly a trend in that direction. More significant concerns in the use of MammoSite are that the V150 region is all contiguous; suggesting that treatment-induced fat necrosis may be more likely to happen. Even more practical concerns are the observations that the balloon catheter insertions frequently do not apply the surface of the balloon to the adjacent breast tissue, because of either air pockets or lack of adjacent breast tissue.

5.5 Dose Fractionation Schedules

The breakdown, in terms of their dose equivalence, of each of the published dose fractionation schedules for APBI is shown in Table 5.2. The two most commonly used schedules in terms of high dose-rate (HDR) implants are 34 Gy in ten fractions or 32 Gy in eight fractions. As can be seen in the table, these schedules have very similar BEDs. In terms of an antitumor dose, the equivalent dose in 2 Gy per fraction is about 38 Gy, which appears to be a relatively low dose. The dose was likely selected because of its equivalence to 45 Gy with an α/β ratio of three for late normal tissue complications, and therefore a likely safe dose. Given the importance of dose brought out by the EORTC boost trial (Bartelink et al. 2001) which indicated that 65–66 Gy is preferable to 50 Gy

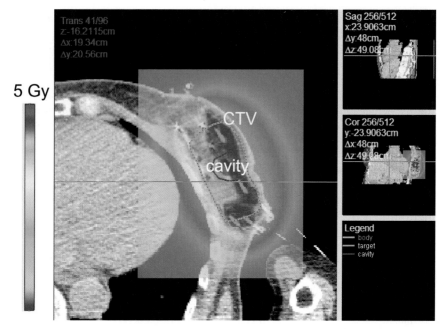

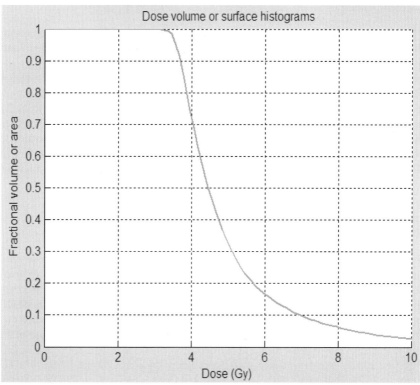

alone, why are these APBI schedules, which appear to deliver a somewhat low dose, effective? At present there is no clear-cut explanation for this apparent paradox, other than the APBI dose is delivered likely with greater precision than the traditional whole-breast and boost treatments.

The doses delivered in APBI with LDR implants are biologically somewhat higher. Studies have shown that doses in the range 45–50 Gy are well tolerated (Arthur et al. 2003; Vicini et al. 2002) and the prescribed doses are biologically higher than for HDR. Furthermore, there are fewer adverse effects of LDR against late reacting normal tissues, where a 0.5 Gy per hour dose rate appears to be equivalent to the same dose in 2 Gy per fraction. However, in spite of the theoretical advantages of LDR implants, this approach has fallen out of favor. Whereas remuneration may be part of the explanation, the other major explanation would appear to be that it is difficult to maintain the geometry of the implant over a continuous period of 5 days, and distortions of the implant would necessarily increase the DHI.

Outside of the commonly used regimens in the US, there is extensive experience in Italy using intraoperative radiotherapy, where a single fraction of electrons is delivered to a prescribed dose of 21 Gy (Veronesi et al. 2001). After quadrantectomy, the residual breast tissue at the surgical margin is partially mobilized to allow the placement of a chest wall shield. The total volume treated in this technique appears to be significantly smaller (about 50 ml) compared with 100+ ml with interstitial implants. Based on the fractionation schedule alone, the BED against late-reacting tissues appears to be very hot indeed. It will therefore be of considerable interest to see if this regimen is well tolerated with further follow-up. The reduction in treatment volume may be critical for its ability to be tolerated, but none of the current models satisfactorily takes volume into account. Conversely, the use of 5 Gy intraoperative radiotherapy using the IntraBeam device seems to be an extraordinarily low dose by any model calculations.

The use of seven fractions of 5.2 Gy has also been reported from Hungary (Polgar et al. 2004), and there is an ongoing randomized trial comparing this regimen with whole-breast irradiation. To date, there are no reported significant long-term complications of this regimen, despite its high BED. Again, it may be that the influence of dose and fractionation on outcome has to also take into account volume, before any real risk assessment can be determined. What is clear is that the more data we have reported, the better will be our insight into both tumor control probability and normal tissue complication probability using APBI.

◄ **Fig. 5.3** Dose inhomogeneity: contributes to tumor control probability. The calculation used assumes that 40% of patients have at least one subclinical microscopic focus; 55 Gy in ten fractions would cure all subclinical disease; and the probability of subclinical disease falls off exponentially with distance from surgical excision. The effect of hormonal therapy is excluded from this analysis. The estimated regional control rate is 93.9%. For perfect homogeneity by external beam, 34 Gy in ten fractions would give a control rate of 84.7%, and for 38.5 Gy in ten fractions the control rate would be 88%. In other words, the inhomogeneity contributes an additional 37.2% to local control efficacy

5.6 Accuracy of Treatment Delivery

In practical terms, the accuracy and reproducibility of treatment may be more important than the dose fractionation schedule. For interstitial implants, the accuracy is determined by how the implant is designed in relation to surgery. Most implants are now done after surgery as a separate procedure, but one advantage of intraoperative placement is direct communication with the surgeon about the location of the catheters. Information about which margin is potentially close can influence how the coverage of the close margin is managed. In the absence of this intraoperative cooperation, reconstructing where the margins are close or far cannot yet be done by postoperative imaging. The advantage of catheter placement postoperatively is that the healing process is enhanced and problems with postoperative seromas are less likely. Once the implant is placed, there is a limited amount of compensatory dose planning that can be achieved to adapt the implant to the PTV. HDR-based treatment planning has more flexibility to adapt to the PTV by altering the dwell times at different positions within the implant.

With the use of balloon intracavitary approaches, there is even less flexibility in treatment planning after the balloon catheter has been placed. The accuracy of treatment delivery is determined by the cavity created by the surgeon at the time of wide excision. For tumors in the central part of the breast, where there is adequate breast tissue all around the tumor, the balloon will apply satisfactorily to the at-risk margins. However, in thinner parts of the breast, when wide excision essentially removes the full thickness of breast tissue, the balloon will not treat the target volume on many aspects of its surface: the accuracy of treatment is determined by the location of the tumor in the breast and the cavity created by the surgeon.

With external beam approaches to APBI, a different concern arises. Given the usual limitations in defining the PTV in relation to the visualized seroma, for the first time there may be movement of the breast in relation to the external beam which could significantly impact the accuracy of treatment delivery. This results in a completely different technical challenge posed by external beam APBI. Can the breast PTV be accurately localized for each of the fractions, and does the breast move significantly within a fraction? We have investigated this by determining the accuracy of set-up using conventional skin markings and portal imaging, and then determining the isocenter localization in relation to internal fiducial markers (surgical clips placed at the time of wide excision). Our findings suggest that set-up errors are in the range of 2–8 mm with conventional isocenter placement techniques, which can have a significant impact on the dose–volume histogram for treatment delivered (not planned). With the use of a 3D camera to map the surface topology of the breast, the set-up error can be reduced to about 1 mm, which is the magnitude required for satisfactory delivery of therapy to the PTV. The fourth dimension of time shows that chest wall movement varies considerably between patients, and depends on the location of the tumor bed within the breast. Tumors which are more inferior and lateral tend to move more, secondary to diaphragmatic movement, whereas tumor in the superior and medial locations have very little movement in a relaxed breathing cycle. It is clear that monitoring movement is an important quality assurance that is needed to ensure treatment delivery that is not currently part of the strategy in external beam APBI.

The advent of image-guided radiation therapy with on-board imaging technologies will open up many new technical capabilities to improve the accuracy of treatment delivery. Cone beam CT images obtained prior to therapy on the treatment machine will likely significantly improve the accuracy of isocenter placement. However, how much it can improve upon what is achieved by surface topology mapping will need to be determined.

5.7 Summary

The process of optimizing the dose and fractionation schemes for APBI is still evolving. The use of 34 Gy in ten fractions by brachytherapy and 38.5 Gy in ten fractions by external beam, as utilized in the NSABP B-39 study, has been associated with excellent results. The period of follow-up for these clinical data can only be regarded as adequate for the interstitial implant data. Indeed, the longest follow-up is available for the LDR implants that were done early in the development of the procedure, where biological modeling would imply a higher tumor-controlling dose. The dose in 2 Gy equivalents for external beam APBI is 44.4 Gy, which is similar to the 45 Gy LDR experience, but without the extra component of hot spots to improve the tumor control probability. The use of external beam APBI can allow the exploration of dose fractionation schemes that deliver treatment over 2 or 3 weeks instead of 1 week.

Dose inhomogeneity is a major feature of all brachytherapy, and fully understanding the impact of these hot spots on the development of posttreatment changes in the breast needs more data. It is clear that more dose needs to be delivered when the dose is delivered homogeneously by external beam. Whether this will also result in fewer normal tissue complications, as predicted by the models, remains to be determined.

The final and perhaps most important point about the success of APBI is the ability to deliver the treatment accurately. A detailed discussion of BEDs is rendered irrelevant if the dose is not delivered accurately to the target volume. The use of external beam APBI, as allowed in NSABP B-39, does not have sufficient quality assurance for dose delivery, and it remains essential to continue to optimize delivery by this technique using the best of image-guided radiotherapy.

References

1. Arthur DW, Vicini FA, Kuske RR, Wazer DE, Nag S (2003) Accelerated partial breast irradiation: an updated report from the American Brachytherapy Society. Brachytherapy 2:124–130
2. Awwad HK, Lotayef M, Shouman T, Begg AC, Wilson G, Bentzen SM, Abd El-Moneim H, Eissa S (2002) Accelerated hyperfractionation (AHF) compared to conventional fractionation (CF) in the postoperative radiotherapy of locally advanced head and neck cancer: influence of proliferation. Br J Cancer 86:517–523
3. Bartelink H, Horiot JC, Poortmans P, Struikmans H, Van den Bogaert W, Barillot I, Fourquet A, Borger J, Jager J, Hoogenraad W, Collette L, Pierart M; European Organization for Research and Treatment of Cancer Radiotherapy and Breast Cancer Groups (2001) Recurrence rates after treatment of breast cancer with standard radiotherapy with or without additional radiation. N Engl J Med 345:1378–1387
4. Bentzen SM, Ritter MA (2005) The alpha/beta ratio for prostate cancer: what is it, really? Radiother Oncol 76:1–3

5. Das RK, Patel R, Shah H, Odau H, Kuske RR (2004) 3D CT-based high-dose-rate breast brachytherapy implants: treatment planning and quality assurance. Int J Radiat Oncol Biol Phys 59:1224–1228

6. Fowler JF (2005) The radiobiology of prostate cancer including new aspects of fractionated radiotherapy. Acta Oncol 44:265–276

7. Freedman GM, Anderson PR, Hanlon AL, Eisenberg DF, Nicolaou N (2005) Pattern of local recurrence after conservative surgery and whole-breast irradiation. Int J Radiat Oncol Biol Phys 61:1328–1336

8. Fyles A, Keane TJ, Barton M, Simm J (1992) The effect of treatment duration in the local control of cervix cancer. Radiother Oncol 25:273–279

9. Holland R, Connolly JL, Gelman R, Mravunac M, Hendriks JH, Verbeek AL, Schnitt SJ, Silver B, Boyages J, Harris JR (1990) The presence of an extensive intraductal component following a limited excision correlates with prominent residual disease in the remainder of the breast. J Clin Oncol 8:113–118

10. Lawenda BD, Taghian AG, Kachnic LA, Hamdi H, Smith BL, Gadd MA, Mauceri T, Powell SN (2003) Dose-volume analysis of radiotherapy for T1N0 invasive breast cancer treated by local excision and partial breast irradiation by low-dose-rate interstitial implant. Int J Radiat Oncol Biol Phys 56:671–680

11. Maciejewski B, Skladowski K, Pilecki B, Taylor JM, Withers RH, Miszczyk L, Zajusz A, Suwinski R (1996) Randomized clinical trial on accelerated 7 days per week fractionation in radiotherapy for head and neck cancer. Preliminary report on acute toxicity. Radiother Oncol 40:137–145

12. McCormick B (2005) Partial-breast radiation for early staged breast cancers: hypothesis, existing data, and a planned phase III trial. J Natl Compr Canc Netw 3:301–307

13. Nag S, Cano ER, Demanes DJ, Puthawala AA, Vikram B (2001) The American Brachytherapy Society recommendations for high-dose-rate brachytherapy for head-and-neck carcinoma. Int J Radiat Oncol Biol Phys 50:1190–1198

14. Polgar C, Major T, Fodor J, Nemeth G, Orosz Z, Sulyok Z, Udvarhelyi N, Somogyi A, Takacsi-Nagy Z, Lovey K, Agoston P, Kasler M (2004) High-dose-rate brachytherapy alone versus whole breast radiotherapy with or without tumor bed boost after breast-conserving surgery: seven-year results of a comparative study. Int J Radiat Oncol Biol Phys 60:1173–1181

15. Poortmans P, Bartelink H, Horiot JC, Struikmans H, Van den Bogaert W, Fourquet A, Jager J, Hoogenraad W, Rodrigus P, Warlam-Rodenhuis C, Collette L, Pierart M (2004) The influence of the boost technique on local control in breast conserving treatment in the EORTC 'boost versus no boost' randomised trial. Radiother Oncol 72:25–33

16. Shah NM, Tenenholz T, Arthur D, DiPetrillo T, Bornstein B, Cardarelli G, Zheng Z, Rivard MJ, Kaufman S, Wazer DE (2004) MammoSite and interstitial brachytherapy for accelerated partial breast irradiation: factors that affect toxicity and cosmesis. Cancer 101:727–734

17. Shasha D, Harrison LB, Chiu-Tsao ST (1998) The role of brachytherapy in head and neck cancer. Semin Radiat Oncol 8:270–281

18. Suh WW, Pierce LJ, Vicini FA, Hayman JA (2005) A cost comparison analysis of partial versus whole-breast irradiation after breast-conserving surgery for early-stage breast cancer. Int J Radiat Oncol Biol Phys 62:790–796

19. Veronesi U, Orecchia R, Luini A, Gatti G, Intra M, Zurrida S, Ivaldi G, Tosi G, Ciocca M, Tosoni A, De Lucia F (2001) A preliminary report of intraoperative radiotherapy (IORT) in limited-stage breast cancers that are conservatively treated. Eur J Cancer 37:2178–2183

20. Vicini FA, Eberlein TJ, Connolly JL, Recht A, Abner A, Schnitt SJ, Silen W, Harris JR (1991) The optimal extent of resection for patients with stages I or II breast cancer treated with conservative surgery and radiotherapy. Ann Surg 214:200–204; discussion 204–205

21. Vicini F, Baglan K, Kestin L, Chen P, Edmundson G, Martinez A (2002) The emerging role of brachytherapy in the management of patients with breast cancer. Semin Radiat Oncol 12:31–39

22. Vicini FA, Remouchamps V, Wallace M, Sharpe M, Fayad J, Tyburski L, Letts N, Kestin L, Edmundson G, Pettinga J, Goldstein NS, Wong J (2003) Ongoing clinical experience utilizing 3D conformal external beam radiotherapy to deliver partial-breast irradiation in patients with early-stage breast cancer treated with breast-conserving therapy. Int J Radiat Oncol Biol Phys 57:1247–1253

23. Vicini F, Winter K, Straube W, Wong J, Pass H, Rabinovitch R, Chafe S, Arthur D, Petersen I, McCormick B (2005) A phase I/II trial to evaluate three-dimensional conformal radiation therapy confined to the region of the lumpectomy cavity for stage I/II breast carcinoma: initial report of feasibility and reproducibility of Radiation Therapy Oncology Group (RTOG) Study 0319. Int J Radiat Oncol Biol Phys 63(5):1531–1537

24. Wallner P, Arthur D, Bartelink H, Connolly J, Edmundson G, Giuliano A, Goldstein N, Hevezi J, Julian T, Kuske R, Lichter A, McCormick B, Orecchia R, Pierce L, Powell S, Solin L, Vicini F, Whelan T, Wong J, Coleman CN (2004) Workshop on partial breast irradiation: state of the art and the science, Bethesda, MD, December 8–10, 2002. J Natl Cancer Inst 96:175–184

25. Withers HR (1986) Predicting late normal tissue responses. Int J Radiat Oncol Biol Phys 12:693–698

Surgical Considerations for Accelerated Partial Breast Irradiation

Henry M. Kuerer

Contents

6.1 Introduction

Much excitement and interest concerning accelerated partial breast irradiation (APBI) has been generated among the surgical community and patients. As a general rule, surgeons are always looking for new and improved techniques to offer their patients; however, the surgical community is also cautious about adopting novel local therapy approaches to disease. This type of caution, and sometimes even frank concern and skepticism, has most recently been expressed by the American College of Surgeons regarding novel laparo- and thoracoscopic procedures and, most notably, bariatric surgical procedures. As surgical oncologists, we want to control malignant disease with minimum morbidity and maximum survival and quality of life. Surgical oncologists are also committed to advancing the field of oncology, and like all academic physicians, they want to be able to counsel their patients regarding proposed treatments on the basis of data from adequate studies, preferably large randomized studies.

In the late 1980s and early 1990s, many clinicians were convinced that breast cancer treatments had reached their maximal potential. This, of course, was before we had sentinel lymph node biopsy, the taxanes, the wide use of breast ultrasonography, the aromatase inhibitors, and easily applied conformal radiation techniques. Many surgeons believe that APBI holds the promise of a shorter treatment course, greater patient convenience, utilization of fewer resources, and improved cost-effectiveness. Advocates of

APBI argue that these advantages may increase the use of radiation therapy as a standard component of breast-conserving therapy for breast carcinoma. APBI is now ripe for testing in large randomized trials. The surgical community is hopeful that it will turn out to be a true advance for some of our breast cancer patients.

There are some general as well as very specific surgical considerations associated with breast surgery and APBI. Some of these important considerations are highlighted in this chapter.

6.2 Volume of Breast Resection

Breast surgeons have different approaches to breast-conserving surgery. Many surgeons believe that margin width is like money—the more the better. In this approach, cosmesis takes the backseat. In fact, the field of collaborative "oncoplastic" multispecialty surgery was developed specifically to try to improve the cosmetic results associated with very large breast resections during conservative surgery (Anderson et al. 2005). On the other hand, many surgeons will cite the National Surgical Adjuvant Breast and Bowel Project long-term data showing acceptable local recurrence rates when a large margin width was not a prerequisite, or data from the Joint Center for Radiation Therapy showing that margin width may be irrelevant to local recurrence rates in patients receiving systemic therapy in addition to postoperative whole-breast radiation therapy (Park et al. 2000). Ideally, the surgical oncologist limits the extent of resection to ensuring negative margins, and therefore, both cosmetic and oncologic considerations become the primary aims in breast-conserving surgery (Chagpar et al. 2003).

Tumors are rarely situated at the center of the lumpectomy specimen, resulting in final margins that may be 3 or 4 cm on one side yet only a few millimeters on the opposite side. Therefore, the volume of resection is not always related to the margin width of the segmental resection. Some investigators have suggested that a more directed and limited resection can best be achieved by utilizing intraoperative ultrasonography (for tumors with mass lesions) or mammographically guided needle localization (for tumors with no mass lesions) to direct the surgery (Fornage et al. 2002; Rahusen et al. 2002). Singletary (2002) recently reviewed the effect of margin width on the rate of local recurrence in patients with invasive breast cancer and found that the size of the resection per se did not affect the rate of local recurrence in patients receiving whole-breast radiation therapy.

It is not clear at this point whether APBI will decrease, increase, or not affect the rate of local recurrence compared with conventional whole-breast radiation therapy in patients with close or even positive margins. There is some concern that surgeons may in fact do larger breast resections if they are planning on enrolling their patients in clinical trials evaluating APBI or treating them with APBI off protocol. That is, they may falsely assume that larger resections will prevent local recurrence in case the partial breast irradiation proves not to be as efficacious as whole-breast irradiation. For ductal carcinoma in situ (DCIS), there is compelling single-institution data that suggest that rates of local recurrence may be extremely low when margin widths are large in the absence of whole-breast irradiation (Silverstein et al. 1999). This, of course, is a controversial area, and the Radiation Therapy Oncology Group is testing this hypothesis in a randomized trial of whole-breast irradiation therapy versus observation for patients undergoing breast-conserving surgery for DCIS lesions of low or intermediate grade. At The University of

Texas M. D. Anderson Cancer Center, Pawlik et al. (2004) recently looked at the average volume of resected breast tissue in patients who had undergone breast-conserving surgery for DCIS or invasive cancers. The volume of resection was nearly identical for in situ disease and invasive breast cancer: about 65 cm^3 in each group.

When balloon-based intracavitary brachytherapy was introduced, there was an initial concern that surgeons would remove less breast tissue than might ordinarily have been considered necessary to create smaller cavities to accommodate the balloon sizes that were initially available (Pawlik et al. 2004). As different sizes and shapes of balloon catheters and new surgical techniques have been introduced, the volume of breast tissue removed by the surgeon is unlikely to be related to the use of intracavitary balloon catheter brachytherapy.

6.3 Brachytherapy

6.3.1 Interstitial Needle-Based Therapy

Although initial published reports on the use of brachytherapy as the sole type of radiation therapy after breast-conserving surgery are promising, standard catheter-based interstitial brachytherapy has a number of disadvantages (Jewell et al. 1987; King et al. 2000; Wazer et al. 2002). It is technically difficult, and only a limited number of clinicians in the United States are familiar with the technique. In addition, many patients and health-care providers find the placement of catheters and the appearance of the multiple puncture sites required for insertion of traditional brachytherapy catheters disturbing. For these reasons, the widespread use of traditional brachytherapy in patients with breast cancer has been limited. There has, however, recently been a large amount of interest in balloon-based intracavitary irradiation (see next section).

These disadvantages notwithstanding, there are a few surgical considerations related to interstitial based APBI delivery. Patients are more likely to develop a wound infection with an open-cavity needle placement compared with a closed-cavity interstitial needle placement. The open-cavity technique is performed either at the initial lumpectomy or at the time of re-excision for margin control. Benitez et al. (2004) reported an 8.5% infection rate with the open technique compared with a 2.5% infection rate with the closed technique.

6.3.2 Intracavitary Balloon-Based Brachytherapy

The MammoSite balloon intracavitary radiation delivery device (Proxima Therapeutics, Alpharetta, GA) allows for insertion of a high dose-rate radiation source at the center of an inflatable balloon. The device can be placed into the lumpectomy cavity at the time of surgery or after surgery when the definitive margin status is known. The MammoSite device is available in three versions—one designed to be inflated to a diameter of 4 to 5 cm with a maximum inflation volume of 70 cm^3, one designed to be inflated to 5 to 6 cm with a maximum inflation volume of 125 cm^3, and an ellipsoidal version measuring 4 by 6 cm with a maximum inflation volume of 65 cm^3. Because of its simplicity and acceptance by patients, balloon-based brachytherapy has been increasingly employed despite the lack of studies comparing its efficacy with that of standard postoperative external beam irradiation.

There are a few surgical considerations related to the use of the MammoSite device. To prevent skin injury, the device must be a minimum of 7 mm from the skin. It is interesting to note that this distance is not achievable in many cases without specific surgical planning and intervention. Some surgeons have advocated removing an elliptical area of skin over the tumor and then undermining the subcutaneous breast and fatty tissue and reapproximating it over the balloon catheter with one layer of interrupted sutures followed by a second subcuticular layer closure and by a third layer closure of the skin with a running suture. This technique may result in unsatisfactory cosmesis if the amount of skin removed results in pulling or repositioning the nipple–areola complex so that it is obviously different from the patient's healthy contralateral breast. At M. D. Anderson Cancer Center, we recommend removal of skin during lumpectomy only if the tumor is extremely close to or frankly involves the skin. However, to achieve sufficient skin spacing for MammoSite insertion, we routinely undermine the subcutaneous breast and fatty tissue and either reapproximate this tissue directly over the balloon catheter with one layer of interrupted sutures, if an open insertion technique is performed, or reapproximate the tissue if a postoperative catheter insertion is planned.

Deep closure of the breast and fatty tissues in an attempt to close the cavity where the seroma forms during breast-conserving surgery is considered to be poor surgical technique, as it often results in a very poor cosmetic result. However, we have not found that closing the superficial breast and fatty tissues above the catheter results in a poor cosmetic outcome when utilizing the MammoSite device. In fact, patients can return to the operating room for a rapid second procedure under local anesthesia if it is found that the skin spacing is inadequate for MammoSite treatment. If the breast was not closed appropriately in the first procedure, the breast tissue is undermined to allow for the breast and fatty tissue to be reapproximated with interrupted sutures to ensure adequate skin spacing. This second procedure can be very important for patients who are extremely committed to undergoing APBI with the balloon catheter device.

Many breast cancer multimodality treatment teams advocate the placement of metallic clips in the lumpectomy cavity to identify the region where the tumor was for treatment planning and follow-up. This is standard practice at M. D. Anderson. When using balloon-based catheters, however, metallic clips are not recommended because they may cause premature rupture of the catheter. To avoid this, we gently insert tiny microsurgical clips about 2 cm into the cavity wall so that the clips do not come into direct contact with the balloon.

Postlumpectomy insertion of the MammoSite device is preferred by many because final pathologic margin information is available at that time, and the patient does not have to wear the device in the immediate postoperative period. One simple method of postlumpectomy insertion devised by Stolier et al. (2005) is the so-called scar entry technique. In this technique, performed about 1 week after surgery, ultrasonography is performed just prior to MammoSite insertion, and the cavity is re-evaluated for appropriate size, shape, and cavity-to-skin distance. A 1.5-cm area of skin is anesthetized, and 10 cm^3 of local anesthetic is instilled into the lumpectomy cavity approximately 10 minutes prior to insertion of the device. The catheter is inserted through the corner of the incision or at the narrowest skin bridge, as identified by ultrasonography. The skin incision is opened about 1 cm with a hemostat, allowing the seroma to drain spontaneously. The catheter is then inserted through the opening and inflated with a saline-contrast solution. Every attempt is made to fill the balloon completely, without impinging on the balloon-to-skin distance or creating a problem with balloon symmetry. The volume of solution used to inflate the balloon is recorded. Ultrasonography is then used to check balloon conformance to the surrounding tissues, and the distance between the surface of the balloon and the skin is measured to confirm adequate skin spacing. The catheter is then completely deflated, and the skin on either side of the catheter is sutured to prevent the incision from opening further (Fig. 6.1). No sutures are used to secure the catheter, as the filled balloon prevents accidental dislodgment. The catheter is then reinflated to the previously recorded volume. Alternatively, Zannis et al. (2003) prefer to use the sharp metal trocar provided by the manufacturer of the MammoSite catheter to insert the catheter through a separate 1-cm incision just lateral to the lumpectomy scar under ultrasound guidance. Many clinicians also recommend low-dose oral antibiotics while the catheter is in place to minimize risk of infection.

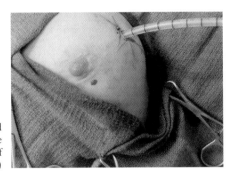

Fig. 6.1 The MammoSite device was inserted using the scar entry technique, and sutures were placed around the incision to prevent opening of the scar (from Stolier et al. 2005, with permission)

6.4 Intraoperative Radiation Therapy

Treatment with a single dose of radiation at the time of surgery is an extremely attractive alternative for patients undergoing lumpectomy for breast cancer. In fact, this "one-stop-shopping" approach to local control of breast cancer would be the preferred form of APBI for most clinicians and patients if intraoperative radiation therapy (IORT) proves to be efficacious with minimal short- and long-term complications. However, many questions remain among clinicians in the United States concerning assessing dosimetry and the long-term risk of fibrosis with IORT.

IORT can be delivered using mobile linear accelerators, which are easily positioned near the operating table and have a movable arm that can be appropriately positioned for irradiation. Mobile linear accelerators usually have a variable spectrum of electron energy (3 to 10 MeV) and can be used in any operating room without structural modifications. Cylindrical applicators with diameters of 4 to 10 cm and terminal angles between 0° and 45° are used to achieve electron-beam collimation (Kuerer et al. 2003). For radioprotection, mobile shields (2-cm-thick lead) are positioned around and beneath the operating table. The patient, therefore, does not need to be transferred from the operating table.

In general, IORT is easy to perform and only slightly prolongs the surgical procedure. Before IORT administration, the breast tissue must be separated from the subcutaneous tissue from 2.5 to 4.0 cm around the wound, with special care taken not to compromise the skin's blood supply. The breast tissue must also be separated from the pectoralis fascia so that lead shields can be put between the breast and the pectoralis major muscle to protect the chest wall, lungs, and heart. Although this wide mobilization of the breast tissue increases the total time of the operation slightly, some surgeons have argued that it facilitates postresection reconstruction, which can improve the cosmetic result of breast-conserving surgery (Intra et al. 2002).

The international TARGIT trial initiated in the United Kingdom is evaluating the use of definitive IORT with low-energy x-rays as the sole form of radiation therapy after segmental mastectomy. In this study, IORT is delivered using a minielectron beam-driven x-ray source called Intrabeam (Carl Zeiss SMT, Thornwood, New York). This device was approved by the Food and Drug Administration in the United States for radiation therapy in 1999. Low-energy x-rays (50 kV maximum) are emitted from the tip of a 10-cm-long, 3.2-mm-diameter probe that is enclosed in a spherical applicator (available in sizes ranging from 2.5 to 5.0 cm in diameter) that is inserted into the tumor bed (Fig. 6.2). IORT is delivered over 25 minutes. The prescribed doses at 1 cm and 0.2 cm, respectively, are 5 Gy and 20 Gy. Tungsten-impregnated rubber sheets are placed on the chest wall to protect the patient's heart and lungs and placed over the wound to stop any stray radiation. The skin dose is monitored with thermoluminescent detectors. It is extremely important to ensure that hemostasis is achieved prior to the intraoperative delivery of radiation, as the presence of blood could distort the cavity enough to change the dosimetry (Vaidya et al. 2005). The size of the sterile applicator used to deliver the intraoperative radiation is based on the size of the resection at the time of surgery. In the case of a very large resection, an advancement flap or other method of tissue mobilization may be necessary to bring the breast tissue into proper contact with the applicator.

Vaidya et al. (2005) have recently described several technical aspects of the IORT procedure: (1) different-sized applicators should be tried until one is found that fits snugly within the cavity; (2) a purse-string suture is needed to pass through the breast parenchyma and appose it to the applicator surface, without bringing the dermis too close to the applicator surface; (3) sometimes, one purse-string suture is required in the deep aspect of the cavity and another is needed more superficially; (4) nylon stitches can be used to slightly retract the skin away from the applicator (for skin further away from the edge that cannot be retracted without reducing the dose to target tissues, a piece of surgical gauze soaked in saline can be inserted deep to the skin to allow the dermis to be lifted off the applicator); and (5) the chest wall and skin can be further protected by radioopaque tungsten-filled polyurethane material, if necessary. These thin, rubber-like sheets are supplied as caps that fit on the applicator or that can be cut to size from a larger flat sheet on the operating table to fit the area of pectoralis muscle that is exposed and protect it from irradiation. These sheets provide effective protection (95% shielding) to intrathoracic structures.

The use of low-energy x-rays has advantages as well as potential disadvantages related to dose attenuation. Because the biologically effective dose of radiation delivered by this

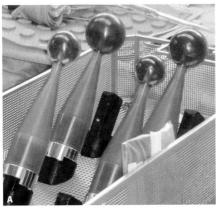
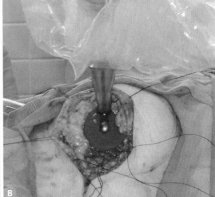
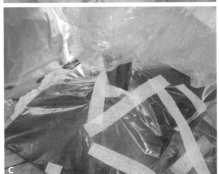

Fig. 6.2 Targeted intraoperative radiation therapy (TARGIT). **A** Various-sized sterile applicators for intraoperative delivery of radiation. **B** The applicator is in place and deep purse-string sutures have been placed to facilitate conformity of the applicator to the cavity wall. **C** Tungsten barrier in place just prior to treatment (photographs courtesy of Dr. Dennis R. Holmes, Kenneth Norris Comprehensive Cancer Center, Keck School of Medicine, University of Southern California)

source attenuates rapidly, specially designed operating rooms are not needed. However, the minielectron beam device has been criticized because the dose 1 cm from the margin is considered very low by many radiation oncologists and therefore may be ineffective in eradicating occult carcinoma cells.

6.5 External Beam Delivery of Conformal Radiation Therapy

Three-dimensional (3D) conformal radiation therapy combines digital diagnostic imaging and postimaging computer analysis to conform the radiation beam to the shape of the tumor. Treatment planning begins with computed tomography or magnetic resonance images that show the anatomy of the tumor and surrounding normal structures. These images are put into a treatment planning computer that produces an accurate 3D image of the tumor and surrounding organs so that multiple radiation beams can be aimed at the tumor from different directions, matching the contour of the treatment area. This delivers a prescribed dose across all three dimensions (height, width, and depth) of the tumor and allows the dose to be distributed across a wider range of surrounding normal tissue, minimizing the dose to any one area. The potential advantages of 3D conformal radiation therapy include improved dose homogeneity within the target volume, which may improve cosmetic results and reduce the risk of symptomatic fat necrosis.

In addition, whereas implant brachytherapy requires additional training and expertise, most radiation treatment facilities already have the technologic tools required to deliver 3D conformal radiation therapy. The Radiation Therapy Oncology Group recently completed a phase II multicenter trial evaluating 3D conformal partial breast irradiation, but the results have not yet been published.

Metallic clips are placed within the resection cavity at the time of surgery to facilitate 3D conformal radiation therapy planning. Otherwise, the surgical technique used for segmental breast resection is identical to that for patients treated with whole-breast irradiation.

6.6 APBI for Breast Preservation After Local Recurrence

At present, mastectomy is the standard of care for local recurrences in the breast in women who have undergone whole-breast irradiation. As APBI involves irradiating only a portion of the breast, in-breast local recurrences following APBI could potentially be treated with additional conservative surgery and radiation therapy. This approach might be most appropriate for women who have a larger amount of breast tissue and recurrences at sites other than the lumpectomy site. Theoretically, patients could receive either additional brachytherapy at the site of the recurrence or standard whole-breast irradiation. However, this concept would need to be tested in a carefully designed prospective study before it becomes widely adopted clinically. Whether or not APBI can be safely utilized following local breast recurrence and repeat segmental resection in patients previously treated with whole-breast irradiation is currently unknown and is the subject of a soon-to-be-opened clinical trial (Kuerer et al. 2004).

References

1. Anderson BO, Masetti R, Silverstein M (2005) Oncoplastic approaches to partial mastectomy: an overview of volume-displacement techniques. Lancet Oncol 6:145–157
2. Benitez P, Chen P, Vicini F, et al (2004) Surgical considerations in the treatment of early stage breast cancer with accelerated partial breast irradiation (APBI) in breast conserving therapy via interstitial brachytherapy. Am J Surg 188:355–364
3. Chagpar A, Yen T, Sahin A, et al (2003) Intraoperative margin assessment reduces reexcision rates in patients with ductal carcinoma in situ treated with breast-conserving surgery. Am J Surg 186:371–377
4. Fornage BD, Sneige N, Edeiken BS (2002) Interventional breast sonography. Eur J Radiol 42:17–31
5. Intra M, Gatti G, Luini A, et al (2002) Surgical technique of intraoperative radiotherapy in conservative treatment of limited-stage breast cancer. Arch Surg 137:737–740
6. Jewell WR, Krishnan L, Reddy EK, et al (1987) Intraoperative implantation radiation therapy plus lumpectomy for carcinoma of the breast. Arch Surg 122:687–690
7. King TA, Bolton JS, Kuske RR, et al (2000) Long-term results of wide-field brachytherapy as the sole method of radiation therapy after segmental mastectomy for T(is,1,2) breast cancer. Am J Surg 180:299–304

8. Kuerer HM, Chung M, Giovanna G, et al (2003) The case for accelerated partial-breast irradiation for breast cancer. Contemp Surg 59:508–516

9. Kuerer HM, Arthur DW, Haffty BG (2004) Repeat breast-conserving surgery for in-breast local breast carcinoma recurrence: the potential role of partial breast irradiation. Cancer 11:2269–2280

10. Park CC, Mitsumori MM, Nixon A, et al (2000) Outcome at 8 years after breast-conserving surgery and radiation therapy for invasive breast cancer: influence of margin status and systemic therapy on local recurrence. J Clin Oncol 8:1668–1675

11. Pawlik TM, Perry A, Strom EA, et al (2004) Potential applicability of balloon-catheter based accelerated partial breast irradiation after conservative surgery for breast carcinoma. Cancer 3:490–498

12. Rahusen FD, Bremers AJ, Fabry HF, et al (2002) Ultrasound-guided lumpectomy of nonpalpable breast cancer versus wire-guided resection: a randomized clinical trial. Ann Surg Oncol 9:994–998

13. Silverstein MJ, Lagios MD, Groshen S, et al (1999) The influence of margin width on local control of ductal carcinoma in situ of the breast. N Engl J Med 19:1455–1461

14. Singletary SE (2002) Surgical margins in patients with early-stage breast cancer treated with breast conservation therapy. Am J Surg 5:383–393

15. Stolier AJ, Furhman GM, Scoggins TG, et al (2005) Postlumpectomy insertion of the MammoSite brachytherapy device using the scar entry technique: initial experience and technical considerations. Breast J 3:199–203

16. Vaidya JS, Tobias JS, Baum M, et al (2005) TARGeted Intraoperative radiotherapy (TARGIT): an innovative approach to partial-breast irradiation. Semin Radiat Oncol 2:84–91

17. Wazer DE, Berle L, Graham R, et al (2002) Preliminary results of a phase I/II study of HDR brachytherapy alone for T1/T2 breast cancer. Int J Radiat Oncol Biol Phys 53:889–897

18. Zannis VJ, Walker LC, Barclay-White B, et al (2003) Postoperative ultrasound-guided percutaneous placement of a new breast brachytherapy balloon catheter. Am J Surg 4:383–385

The Virginia Commonwealth University (VCU) Technique of Interstitial Brachytherapy

7

Laurie W. Cuttino and
Douglas W. Arthur

Contents

7.1 History

The multicatheter interstitial technique was the brachytherapy technique used at the inception of accelerated partial breast irradiation (APBI) and is the technique that has been employed in all mature institutional experiences to date (Arthur and Vicini 2005; Arthur et al. 2003a; Cionini et al. 1993; King et al. 2000; Krishnan et al. 2001; Kuske et al. 2004; Lawenda et al. 2003; Polgar et al. 2002, 2004; Vicini et al. 2003a,b). The multicatheter technique is a universal technique that can be applied in any patient presentation provided the lumpectomy cavity is readily identifiable. Any lumpectomy cavity size, shape and location within the breast can be approached with a multicatheter technique.

The newer APBI techniques of MammoSite radiation treatment delivery system (RTS) and three-dimensional conformal radiotherapy (3D-CRT) are gaining in popularity, but are not technically universal and cannot be used in all patients as boundaries for the use of this device exist (Baglan et al. 2003; Keisch et al. 2003a,b; Vicini et al. 2003c). The MammoSite RTS requires a close working relationship between the surgeon and radiation oncologist to ensure that the lumpectomy cavity is created to provide the opportunity for proper balloon catheter placement allowing for balloon symmetry, inflation size and skin spacing (Arthur and Vicini 2004). In addition cavity location and small breast size may present as limitations. Unique challenges are faced in the use of the

3D-CRT technique as appropriate field design may not be possible due to cavity size and cavity location. Additionally the need and ability to counter breathing motion and daily set-up error have yet to be thoroughly understood.

The only obstacle to multicatheter brachytherapy is the ability to place the catheters in an appropriate distribution to ensure dosimetric target coverage, and this obstacle can be overcome with an appropriate approach to catheter placement. The essential component to any multicatheter technique is image guidance. Although this can be achieved with ultrasound, stereotactic mammography or computed tomography (CT), CT offers the advantage of being universally applicable and by improving the efficiency of the procedure. This chapter describes the CT image guidance technique used at the Virginia Commonwealth University (Cuttino et al. 2005).

Initially, multicatheter breast brachytherapy was employed as a boost following standard whole-breast radiotherapy and performed in the operating room using a free-hand insertion technique. Typically performed at the time of lumpectomy, the physician often implanted without final tumor histology, or nodal and margin status available complicating patient selection and target definition. Catheters were placed by direct visualization of the open lumpectomy cavity and/or with intraoperative fluoroscopic guidance after closure of the cavity. After completion of the procedure, catheter placement evaluation and dosimetric planning was performed with orthogonal films and two-dimensional treatment planning. Target delineation and dosimetric coverage of the target were difficult, relying heavily on experience and a degree of speculation. Improvements in technique were not possible until 3D brachytherapy planning software was commercially available and CT-based treatment planning became more widely accessible.

To demonstrate the importance of CT-based treatment planning, Vicini et al. reported on a series of eight patients who underwent multicatheter APBI using standard intraoperative cavity insertion techniques (Vicini et al. 1998). Although CT-based treatment planning was not available at this time, a postoperative CT scan was obtained in these eight patients for visual verification that the surgical clips (with an appropriate margin) were within the boundaries of the implant needles. These CT scans were later used for retrospective dosimetric analysis and determination of target coverage through 3D planning recreations of the treatment delivered. Despite meticulous catheter placement technique, without image guidance they found that a significant proportion of the target volume did not receive the prescribed dose. They reported that the median proportion of the target volume (the lumpectomy cavity plus a 1 cm margin) receiving the prescribed dose was only 68%. This clearly demonstrates the need for improved catheter placement techniques and verification of dosimetric target coverage prior to treatment initiation.

Image-guided catheter placement is possible using CT, ultrasound, or stereotactic mammography. At VCU, a CT-guided placement technique was developed to ensure target coverage and improve procedure efficiency (Cuttino et al. 2005). The procedure is performed entirely in the Radiation Oncology Department CT-simulation suite allowing complete procedure scheduling control and decreased time away from the department. This technique has proven feasible regardless of breast size, cavity shape, target location, overlying skin thickness or whether surgical clips are or are not present. As the quality of the implant construction is evaluated prior to procedure completion, an inexperienced brachytherapist can reliably obtain excellent target coverage in each case. In contrast to an experienced brachytherapist, those at the initial stages of a brachytherapy program may take additional time but will also be able to achieve excellent results. With additional experience, the time needed to complete the procedure quickly decreases. In outline form the procedure consists of a preprocedure evaluation, patient preparation, stainless steel trocar placement with intermittent CT guidance, flexible catheter exchange, final CT acquisition and CT-based 3D treatment planning.

7.2 Implantation Technique

7.2.1 Preprocedure Evaluation

To ensure an efficient and successful implant, the flow from consultation, that determines patient eligibility and technical feasibility, completely through the procedure and treatment delivery should be appropriate and well planned. At the time of initial consultation, each potential patient undergoes a CT scan in the Radiation Oncology Department to evaluate the lumpectomy cavity and determine patient eligibility and technical feasibility for APBI. This preimplant CT scan is evaluated with 3D planning software at which time the lumpectomy cavity is delineated. With both a 3D rendering of the cavity in respect to the ipsilateral breast as well as representative transverse slices, an initial design and approach for the multicatheter implantation can be determined that addresses catheter number, number of catheter planes and the optimal direction of placement. This information is printed and available at the time of the procedure and becomes a permanent part of the patient's medical record.

7.2.2 Patient Preparation

The VCU technique focuses around the use of the CT-simulator (Fig. 7.1). Although this technique could similarly be carried out on a diagnostic CT scanner, moving the procedure outside the department compromises the benefits of procedural control and efficiency to some degree. The procedure starts with proper patient positioning. With the patient supine the goal is to optimize access to the target site to facilitate catheter placement. This is best accomplished with the breast appropriately exposed. This is achieved typically with a wedge cushion placed under the ipsilateral shoulder and torso and the ipsilateral arm tucked low on the patients side. Once the patient is positioned then a test run through the CT scanner is needed to avoid future CT acquisition difficulties during the procedure.

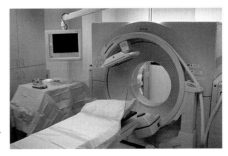

Fig. 7.1 CT simulator with optional fluoroscopy available

Proper patient comfort can be achieved with several varying methods and each patient may require a different level of anesthesia. As a result of our early experience with multicatheter breast implantation and the inability to predict a patient's anesthetic requirements, we have opted to incorporate the help of the mobile anesthesia team. This allows us to concentrate on completing the implant accurately and efficiently while the anesthesiologist monitors the patient and concentrates on patient comfort. Through a balance of conscious sedation and local anesthetic, patient comfort is effectively achieved. Once the patient is positioned and IV access established, the patient is prepped and draped in a sterile fashion. Although this is a minor procedure, infection of the breast in the face of APBI can be a difficult entity to manage and therefore it is recommended to pay considerable attention to sterile technique. It is our custom to closely model the sterile technique used in an ambulatory surgical setting and as a result have avoided any difficulties with breast infection to date.

7.2.3 Catheter Placement

Catheter orientation and direction of placement are individualized for each case to minimize the number of catheters needed to achieve target coverage as well as to optimize patient comfort. The positions of the catheter entrance and exit planes are determined using the 3D rendering and transverse CT images obtained at the time of consultation. These planes are drawn onto the skin with a sterile marking pen (Fig. 7.2). Once the size and location of the implant is delineated, then the local anesthetic can be administered. Several degrees of local anesthesia have been applied with success using 2% lidocaine or a mixture of equal parts 2% lidocaine and 0.5% bupivacaine. Sodium bicarbonate can be added to reduce the discomfort that accompanies injection. In all patients, local anesthetic is applied subcutaneously along the skin marks where the catheters will enter and exit (Fig. 7.3). The degree to which anesthetic is needed deep within the implant volume is dependent on the success of the conscious sedation and the patient's pain threshold. Caution must be exercised so as not to exceed recommended limits of lidocaine or, if using increased volumes of diluted lidocaine, to use excessive volumes that may temporarily distort the geometry of the target and complicate treatment planning or require the patient to return on a subsequent day for final CT acquisition and treatment planning. Typically, anesthetic is needed deep within the implant volume in addition to subcutaneous injection. This can be achieved by injecting a controlled volume around the periphery of the implant target, as surgeons do prior to lumpectomy, or with supplementary lidocaine injected through the open-ended trocar if, when placing, a sensitive area is identified.

Standard, commercially available stainless steel trocars with sharply beveled tips are used to establish the tract through the breast tissue prior to exchange with flexible afterloading catheters. For CT visualization and efficiency all trocars are placed in the breast and positions adjusted as necessary until the final positions have been verified and approved. Trocars can be cleaned, sterilized, and reused for additional procedures before requiring replacement, but the tips are quickly dulled and single use is recommended. The method of deep catheter placement varies from the method of superficial catheter placement and, following a few simple guidelines, helps to achieve placement goals. To accurately and safely place a deep catheter, the breast is firmly grasped (compressed) and

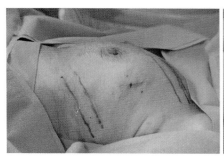 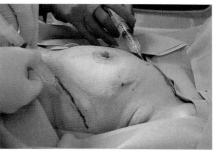

Fig. 7.2 Catheter exit and entrance planes are based on preimplant CT and delineated on the patient's skin for guidance

Fig. 7.3 Local anesthetic is placed subcutaneously to ensure painless skin entry and exit. Additional anesthetic is injected within the breast peripherally around the implant target

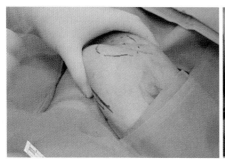 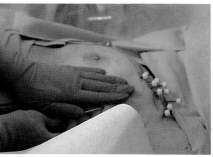

Fig. 7.4 Deep plane catheter placement. Compression with lift of breast improves control of trocar placement for accurate placement

Fig. 7.5 Superficial plane catheter placement. Utilizing a flat hand, the contour of the breast is controlled to allow the trocar to be placed at a consistence distance from the skin along its course

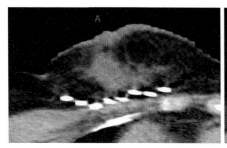 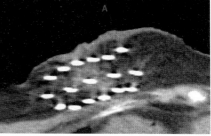

Fig. 7.6 CT scan for initial evaluation of trocar placement. Along the course of the deep plane trocars, the relationship of catheters to the chest wall and lumpectomy cavity is noted and adjustments in trocar location made as necessary

Fig. 7.7 CT scan for evaluation after implant construction for final assessment prior to flexible catheter exchange

lifted off the chest wall so that the trocar can be placed deep to the lumpectomy cavity while avoiding chest wall structures (Fig. 7.4). This technique will decrease the breast tissue distance that the trocar will traverse and provide the needed control over catheter depth and direction. In contrast, superficial catheters require placement so that the catheter to skin distance can be controlled along the course of the trocar. This is achieved by 'flattening' the skin surface so that the trocar can easily be placed and a consistent depth along its path is achieved with pressure from a flat hand after the superficial catheter enters past the skin (Fig. 7.5). A standardized approach to trocar placement and implant construction has been helpful and is based on the experience of the brachytherapist. It is recommended that those that are new to the technique first place two deep plane trocars and one superficial trocar as close to the level of the lumpectomy cavity as possible. After these three initial catheters are placed, a CT scan should be obtained for an initial evaluation of trocar orientation with respect to the lumpectomy cavity and target coverage goals. This is a focused CT, scanning over a minimal distance using 5 mm slices for rapid completion. The position of the trocars relative to the lumpectomy cavity is noted. If necessary, these positions can be adjusted. The remaining trocars are then placed to complete the deep and superficial planes pausing for CT evaluation for guidance as needed. With experience and preprocedure CT evaluation guidance, the need for periodic CT scans can be reduced to first obtaining a CT scan for evaluation of the completed deep plane (Fig. 7.6), adjusting if needed, and then after the implant has been completed (Fig. 7.7).

Trocars are placed according to standard principles of brachytherapy implant design (Zwicker and Schmidt-Ullrich 1995; Zwicker et al. 1999). Generally, trocars should be placed 1.0–1.5 cm apart, and the plane should extend 1.5–2.0 cm beyond the lumpectomy cavity. If the distance between the superficial and deep planes exceeds 3 cm, then a central plane is added. A typical implant will require between 14 and 20 trocars. Once all trocar positions have been reviewed on a CT scan and approved, the trocars are exchanged for flexible afterloading catheters. The catheters are secured in place with a locking collar (Fig. 7.8). Skin sutures are not required. Catheters are then trimmed with sterile scissors at a consistent length. Each catheter length is then carefully measured and recorded. Once all catheters are in their final position and cut to length, a final CT is performed. Thin metal wires are threaded into each catheter to facilitate tract visualization on the final CT scan. This scan encompasses the entire treated breast in 3 mm slices. Knowing all treatments will be delivered with the patient in the identical position in which the final CT scan was obtained, the position is noted for future reference. The final CT data set is then transferred to the brachytherapy planning software. An experienced radiation oncologist typically requires two to four CT scans and completes the entire procedure in less than 60–90 minutes.

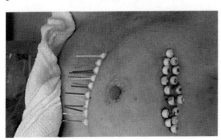

Fig. 7.8 External view of completed implant

Following the completion of the implant, the patient is observed in the department for approximately 1 hour. During that time period the implant site is cleaned and dressed and instructions for catheter care reviewed. Patients are discharged home with prescriptions for 10 days of an oral antibiotic and pain medication as needed. Pain medication is rarely needed and then rarely for longer than the first 1 or 2 days. Most discomfort is easily managed with nonsteroidal antiinflammatory medications.

7.3 Dosimetric Guidelines

Dosimetric guidelines have evolved over time. Using CT-based 3D brachytherapy treatment planning software, target volumes are delineated and dwell times determined to achieve dosimetric coverage goals (see Fig. 7.9). Once utilizing a planning treatment volume (PTV) defined as the lumpectomy cavity plus a 2.0 cm margin, our present standard is that the PTV is defined as the lumpectomy cavity expanded by 1.5 cm and bounded by the extent of breast tissue, the chest wall structures and to within 5 mm of the skin. Dosimetric guidelines that direct dwell positions and times are influenced by the goals

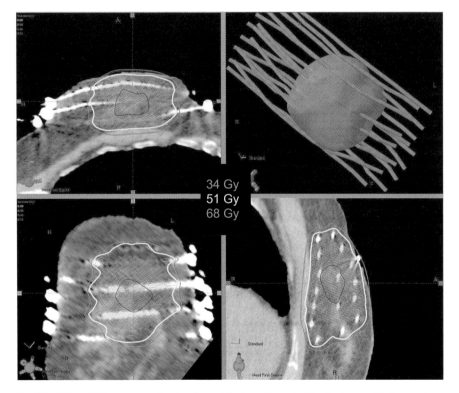

Fig. 7.9 CT-based 3D treatment planning for multicatheter interstitial brachytherapy. The lumpectomy cavity is outlined in red and the target shaded in orange (target defined as the lumpectomy cavity with 1.5 cm expansion)

of target coverage and dose homogeneity. Although 100% of the dose delivered to 100% of the target is the goal, this is difficult to achieve due to inherent error in lumpectomy cavity and PTV delineation. A realistic goal has rested on 90% of the target receiving 90% of the dose as acceptable and >95% of the target receiving >95% of the dose as desirable. The protocol requires that 90% of the PTV receives at least 90% of the prescription dose.

The character of dose distribution of a multicatheter implant has been associated with toxicity, illustrating the importance dose homogeneity (Arthur et al. 2003b; Wazer et al. 2002). For this reason, two absolute dose volume histogram (DVH) parameters have been established that are reproducibly achievable with proper catheter placement. These parameters include a DVH analysis evaluating how much tissue is receiving doses exceeding 100% of the prescription dose and a dose homogeneity index (DHI) defined as the ratio of the absolute volume of tissue receiving 150% of the prescribed dose to the volume receiving 100% (V150/V100) (Wu et al. 1988). The first parameter is based limiting the volume of breast tissue receiving 200% of the prescribed dose (V200) and limiting the volume of breast tissue receiving 150% of the prescribed dose (V150). With a prescribed dose of 34 Gy in ten fractions, this represents the volume of tissue receiving a fraction size of 6.8 Gy and 5.1 Gy, respectively. As these parameters are dependent on data utilizing a specific prescription dose, 34 Gy delivered in ten fractions, it is uncertain how to extrapolate this to alternative dose fractionation schemes. However, when using 34 Gy in ten fraction, it is recommended that the V200 does not exceed 20 cm^3, and that the V150 does not exceed 70 cm^3. However, with proper technique, these parameters are easily respected with the V200 rarely exceeding 15 cm^3 and the V150 rarely exceeding 50 cm^3. DHI is an associated entity that reflects the relative size of the areas receiving dose greater than the prescribed dose. To avoid toxicity the DHI should exceed 0.75.

Low dose-rate brachytherapy for breast cancer has been abandoned at VCU in favor of high dose-rate (HDR) brachytherapy which offers improved control of dosimetry, radiation safety and the ability to deliver treatment on an outpatient basis. Standard treatment at VCU now consists of treating with a commercially available HDR brachytherapy remote afterloader equipped with an Ir-192 HDR source and utilizing a treatment scheme comprised of 3.4 Gy fractions, twice-daily over 5 days, for a total prescription dose of 34 Gy.

7.4 Results

Although target coverage and dose homogeneity can be improved through CT-based treatment planning software and dose optimization, there is a limited degree of dose improvement that can be achieved with 3D treatment planning. The manipulation of dwell position and times cannot compensate for poor implant geometry, thus stressing the importance of image-guided catheter placement and immediate postoperative CT imaging.

To evaluate the feasibility and dosimetric reliability of the VCU CT-guided method of catheter insertion a dosimetric comparison of APBI cases completed before and after the initiation of the CT-guided method was performed (Cuttino et al. 2005). In this evaluation, 29 patients were identified as having the necessary data available for complete comparison. All patients presented with early-stage invasive breast cancer and were treated with HDR partial breast brachytherapy following lumpectomy and had CT scans of the brachytherapy implant available for analysis. All 29 patients were treated to 34 Gy delivered in ten twice-daily fractions over 5 days. The daily interfraction interval was 6 hours. Treatment was performed using an HDR afterloading device with a 5–10 Ci Ir-192 source. Catheter placement was completed by one of two approaches.

During the period 1995–2000, 15 patients had catheters placed in the operating room with traditional methods based on clinical evaluation and aided by orthogonal fluoroscopic films. Dosimetric planning was two-dimensional and derived from orthogonal films of the implant obtained the day following catheter placement. Homogeneity and target coverage were evaluated in the coronal and cross-sectional views at the center of the implant as well as representative cross-sectional views above and below the center of the implant. The dosimetric goal was to deliver 100% of the prescription dose to the lumpectomy cavity, as delineated by the six surgical clips, plus a 2 cm margin in all directions, restricted by the anatomical extent of breast tissue. During the period 2000–2002, 14 patients had catheters placed with CT-guidance in our department and dosimetry planned with 3D planning software (Brachyvision Planning System, Varian, Palo Alto, California) based on the final CT scan obtained at the completion of the procedure. The lumpectomy cavity was first contoured and this volume expanded by 1 cm and designated as PTV 1 cm (PTV1cm). Similarly, PTV 2 cm (PTV2cm) was delineated by expanding the contour of the lumpectomy cavity by 2 cm. These volume expansions were bounded by the extent of breast tissue. Three dosimetric goals were established to evaluate overall implant quality as represented by target coverage and dose homogeneity. Target coverage was determined to be acceptable if 100% of the prescribed dose was delivered to >95% of PTV1cm, >90% of the dose is delivered to >90% of PTV2cm. Dose homogeneity was deemed acceptable if the DHI was >0.75. DHI is in this study was defined as (V150–V100)/V100, where V100 is the absolute volume of tissue receiving 100% of the prescribed dose, and V150 is the volume receiving 150% of the dose.

To facilitate comparison between the two catheter placement techniques it was necessary to retrospectively reconstruct the implants from the traditional catheter placement cohort within the 3D treatment planning software. The post-placement CT scans from this cohort were entered into the 3D planning system and the volumes for the lumpectomy cavity, PTV1cm and PTV2cm, were delineated. DVHs analyzing dose delivered to normal breast tissue volumes were generated for the purpose of comparing the quality of implants constructed with the traditional catheter placement technique and the CT-guided catheter placement technique. The percent of the PTV1cm volume covered with 100% of the dose, the percent of the PTV2cm volume covered with 90% of the dose, and the DHI were generated for each case and compared.

In this comparison, the CT-guided technique proved superior in achieving an optimized brachytherapy implant by the parameters used in this study. When the CT-guided technique was used, the percentage of implant cases that satisfied all three dosimetric goals increased from 42% to 93%. Mean dose coverage, defined as the percentage of PTV2cm receiving 90% of the prescribed dose, increased from 89% to 95% ($P=0.007$) and the mean DHI increased from 0.77 to 0.82 with the new technique ($P<0.005$). There was a correlation between the improved dosimetry achieved and the cosmetic outcome and risk of fat necrosis in this small group of patients, but the findings need confirmation in a larger group of patients for the dosimetric improvements to definitively translate into clinical outcome.

7.5 Conclusion

Multicatheter interstitial brachytherapy was the original technique used to deliver APBI and is the technique on which the concept of APBI was initiated. Although newer techniques, MammoSite RTS and 3D-conformal radiation therapy, have now been established with the promise of simplifying APBI, these techniques have not yet been shown to be as universal as the multicatheter approach. Out of all the APBI techniques reported, the multicatheter technique continues to be the most adaptable and universally applicable approach and can be applied regardless of breast size or lumpectomy cavity size, shape or location. If a treatment center desires the ability to offer APBI to any patient who is eligible, then the ability to appropriately construct a multicatheter implant continues to be necessary—even if this option is held in reserve until the newer forms of APBI have proven unable to meet dosimetric goals of target coverage.

The VCU method of CT-guided catheter insertion ensures that optimal implant geometry is confirmed at the completion of the procedure, therefore avoiding the need for additional time in the department and minimizing the time to treatment initiation. Through a direct dosimetric comparison, the VCU method of CT-guided catheter insertion has been shown to improve target coverage and dose homogeneity as compared to non-image guided techniques (Cuttino et al. 2005). With the assurance of optimal catheter placement, subsequent catheter manipulation is avoided and the need for relying on creative dwell time manipulation due to sub-optimal catheter placement is minimized. The CT-guided catheter placement technique is a reliable method of implant construction resulting in reproducible target coverage and dose homogeneity that promises to translate into improved disease control and reduced toxicity.

References

1. Arthur DW, Vicini FA (2004) MammoSite RTS: the reporting of initial experiences and how to interpret. Ann Surg Oncol 11:723–724
2. Arthur DW, Vicini FA (2005) Accelerated partial breast irradiation as a part of breast conservation therapy. J Clin Oncol 23:1726–1735
3. Arthur DW, Koo D, Zwicker RD, et al (2003a) Partial breast brachytherapy after lumpectomy: low-dose-rate and high-dose-rate experience. Int J Radiat Oncol Biol Phys 56:681–689
4. Arthur D, Wazer D, Koo D, et al (2003b) The importance of dose-volume histogram evaluation in partial breast brachytherapy: a study of dosimetric parameters. Int J Radiat Oncol Biol Phys 57:S361–S362
5. Baglan KL, Sharpe MB, Jaffray D, et al (2003) Accelerated partial breast irradiation using 3D conformal radiation therapy (3D-CRT). Int J Radiat Oncol Biol Phys 55:302–311
6. Cionini L, Pacini P, Marzano S (1993) Exclusive brachytherapy after conservative surgery in cancer of the breast. Lyon Chir 89:128
7. Cuttino LW, Todor D, Arthur DW (2005) CT-guided multi-catheter insertion technique for partial breast brachytherapy: reliable target coverage and dose homogeneity. Brachytherapy 4:10–17
8. Keisch M, Vicini F, Kuske RR, et al (2003a) Initial clinical experience with the MammoSite breast brachytherapy applicator in women with early-stage breast cancer treated with breast-conserving therapy. Int J Radiat Oncol Biol Phys 55:289–293

9. Keisch M, Vicini F, Kuske RR (2003b) Two-year outcome with the MammoSite breast brachytherapy applicator: factors associated with optimal cosmetic results when performing partial breast irradiation. Int J Radiat Oncol Biol Phys 60 [Suppl 1]:s315

10. King TA, Bolton JS, Kuske RR, et al (2000) Long-term results of wide-field brachytherapy as the sole method of radiation therapy after segmental mastectomy for T(is,1,2) breast cancer. Am J Surg 180:299–304

11. Krishnan L, Jewell WR, Tawfik OW, et al (2001) Breast conservation therapy with tumor bed irradiation alone in a selected group of patients with stage I breast cancer. Breast J 7:91–96

12. Kuske RR, Winter K, Arthur D, et al (2004) A phase II trial of brachytherapy alone following lumpectomy for stage I or II breast cancer: Initial outcomes of RTOG 95-17. Proceedings of the American Society of Clinical Oncology, 40th Annual Meeting 23:18

13. Lawenda BD, Taghian AG, Kachnic LA, et al (2003) Dose-volume analysis of radiotherapy for T1N0 invasive breast cancer treated by local excision and partial breast irradiation by low-dose-rate interstitial implant. Int J Radiat Oncol Biol Phys 56:671–680

14. Polgar C, Sulyok Z, Fodor J, et al (2002) Sole brachytherapy of the tumor bed after conservative surgery for T1 breast cancer: five-year results of a phase I-II study and initial findings of a randomized phase III trial. J Surg Oncol 80:121–128; discussion 129

15. Polgar C, Major T, Fodor J, et al (2004) High-dose-rate brachytherapy alone versus whole breast radiotherapy with or without tumor bed boost after breast-conserving surgery: seven-year results of a comparative study. Int J Radiat Oncol Biol Phys 60:1173–1181

16. Vicini FA, Jaffray DA, Horwitz EM, et al (1998) Implementation of 3D-virtual brachytherapy in the management of breast cancer: a description of a new method of interstitial brachytherapy. Int J Radiat Oncol Biol Phys 40:629–635

17. Vicini FA, Kestin L, Chen P, et al (2003a) Limited-field radiation therapy in the management of early-stage breast cancer. J Natl Cancer Inst 95:1205–1210

18. Vicini F, Arthur D, Polgar C, et al (2003b) Defining the efficacy of accelerated partial breast irradiation: the importance of proper patient selection, optimal quality assurance, and common sense. Int J Radiat Oncol Biol Phys 57:1210–1213

19. Vicini FA, Remouchamps V, Wallace M, et al (2003c) Ongoing clinical experience utilizing 3D conformal external beam radiotherapy to deliver partial-breast irradiation in patients with early-stage breast cancer treated with breast-conserving therapy. Int J Radiat Oncol Biol Phys 57:1247–1253

20. Wazer D, Berle L, Graham R, et al (2002) Preliminary results of a phase I/II study of HDR brachytherapy alone for T1/T2 breast cancer. Int J Radiat Oncol Biol Phys 53:889–897

21. Wu A, Ulin K, Sternick E (1988) A dose homogeneity index for evaluating (192Ir interstitial breast implants. Med Phys 15:104–107

22. Zwicker RD, Schmidt-Ullrich R (1995) Dose uniformity in a planar interstitial implant system. Int J Radiat Oncol Biol Phys 31:149–155

23. Zwicker RD, Arthur DW, Kavanagh BD, et al (1999) Optimization of planar high-dose-rate implants. Int J Radiat Oncol Biol Phys 44:1171–1177

The William Beaumont Hospital Technique of Interstitial Brachytherapy

Peter Y. Chen and Greg Edmundson

8

Contents

8.1 History

Multiple randomized trials have proven the equivalency of breast conservation therapy (BCT) compared to mastectomy with published results of some of the trials with 20-year follow-up (Arriagada et al. 1996; Blichert-Toft et al. 1992; Fisher et al. 2002; Jacobson et al. 1995; Van Dongen et al. 2000; Veronesi et al. 2002). However, only 10–60% of women who are candidates for BCT actually receive such treatment (Morrow et al. 2001; Nattinger et al. 2000). Such under-utilization of BCT can be attributed to many factors which are related in part to the time, toxicity and inconvenience of delivering 6 to 7 weeks of daily external beam radiation therapy (EBRT) to the whole breast following partial mastectomy.

In an effort to offer the breast conservation option to more women and to improve the quality of life of breast cancer patients treated with BCT, we began, in March 1993, a pilot study to treat selected early-stage breast cancer patients with accelerated partial breast irradiation (APBI) using an interstitial low dose-rate (LDR) brachytherapy implant with iodine-125 sources as the sole radiation therapy (RT) modality (Vicini et al. 1997, 1999). In June 1995, we began a parallel trial of outpatient high dose-rate (HDR) brachytherapy as the sole source of RT (Baglan et al. 2001). Both the LDR and HDR treatment regimens have the same eligibility criteria of age >40 years, infiltrating ductal carcinoma ≤3 cm in maximum dimension, negative surgical margins ≥2 mm and surgically staged axilla with not more than three positive nodes [this last criterion was changed in 1997 to negative nodes based upon the documented survival benefit of regional along with local RT plus chemotherapy in node-positive women after mastectomy compared to chemotherapy alone from the Danish and British Columbia trials (Overgaard et al. 1997, 1999; Ragaz et al. 1997)].

All patients underwent a partial mastectomy to achieve negative surgical margins of at least 2 mm; if this was not obtained at the initial operative procedure, re-excision of the biopsy cavity was undertaken.

8.2 Physics

The dosimetric goal of brachytherapy implantation, whether LDR or HDR, was to cover the partial mastectomy excisional cavity with a 1- to 2-cm margin of normal breast tissue. This was done with the interstitial implant placed via either an open or a closed cavity technique, the former at the time of initial surgical excision or at re-excision and the latter in a delayed setting after all pathological findings were confirmed with a brachytherapy implant done under a separate anesthesia using CT and ultrasonic guidance.

8.2.1 LDR Dosimetry

The LDR implants were template-guided to enable interstitial placement of one, two or three planes and loaded with iodine-125 seeds. Dosimetric planning consisted of placement of inert sources into each afterloading catheter to assist in 3D geometric localization. Anterior-posterior and lateral radiographs were taken at the time of simulation for computerized reconstruction. The Nucletron planning system (Nucletron, Veenendaal, The Netherlands) was used for isodose calculations. With the use of iodine-125 seeds, dose homogeneity of the implant volume was optimized by adjusting the spacing of seeds in the individual catheters (Clarke et al. 1989). A dose of 50 Gy delivered at 0.52 Gy/h was prescribed as a minimum dose within the prescription volume; a dose constraint of having no contiguous area (i.e. confluent around multiple catheters) of 150% of the prescribed dose in the central plane isodose distribution was instituted for every LDR patient (Vicini et al. 1997).

No iodine-125 sources were placed in the proximal or distal ends of the afterloading catheters, beyond the treatment volume. Seeds were placed a minimum of 5 to 7 mm from the skin surface in order to prevent excessive dose to the skin.

8.2.2 HDR Dosimetry

As all HDR brachytherapy implants were template-based with afterloading needles which were not replaced by flexible catheters, implantation geometry was rigid with consistently straight paths within the volume of interest allowing for better uniformity. A post-implant CT scan was obtained to verify adequate coverage of the target volume.

At the time of simulation, orthogonal plain films were taken to allow for 3D reconstruction of the needle implant. The target volume was the partial mastectomy excisional cavity plus a 1- to 2-cm margin of normal breast tissue. The Nucletron planning system generated the treatment plan and isodose distribution. With a standard step size of 5 mm, the HDR Iridium-192 source dwell times were optimized to deliver a uniform dose throughout the target volume. Avoidance of excessive skin dose was achieved by restricting the closest dwell position to skin to a distance of 5 mm. The target volume received a minimum dose of either 32 Gy in eight fractions of 4 Gy delivered twice daily over 4 consecutive days or 34 Gy in ten fractions of 3.4 Gy twice daily over 5 days. The minimal interfraction time interval was 6 hours.

8.3 Implantation Technique

Since April 1995, all such interstitial brachytherapy implants for breast APBI have been done via the HDR technique. Those implants done via the LDR technique followed a similar placement technique except for replacement of the interstitial needles by afterloading catheters, which were loaded with I-125 sources, after 3-D treatment planning.

The procedure of needle placement is either performed with an open cavity at the time of partial mastectomy/axillary nodal procedure or as a closed cavity with a preplanning CT scan done prior to the time of interstitial needle placement. Whether open or closed cavity, the goal is to implant a volume 1 to 2 cm beyond the excised cavity. Although such margins are achievable in width, length, cephalad and caudad directions, these margins may not be attained in the deep and superficial planes (this is due to the anatomical limits of the chest wall and overlying skin).

The desired minimum distance from the superficial plane of needles to the skin is 5 mm; if the implanted superficial row is less than this distance, that plane of needles may not be required. The underlying chest wall limits the deep plane; indeed, if the excised cavity is down to the pectoralis fascia, the deep plane of needles may need to be inserted just deep to the musculature. If in the judgment of both the surgeon and radiation oncologist the deep plane of needles may not adequately cover the deep extent of the target volume, the interstitial procedure may need to be aborted.

All implants with the interstitial needle technique at Beaumont are template-based (Fig. 8.1). The templates have 13 needle apertures in the two-plane system, i.e. 7 deep and 6 superficial with an interplane distance of 1.4 cm and a spacing of 1.5 cm between needles. The three-plane template consists of 7 deep, 6 intermediate and 5 superficial needle apertures arranged in the same distance configuration as the two-plane system. For generous anatomical breasts, Beaumont has a specially machined template with interplane and needle distances of 2 cm configured in three planes with 18 apertures.

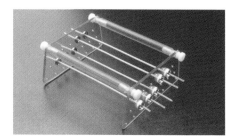

Fig. 8.1 Brachytherapy template

8.3.1 Open Cavity Technique

After the axillary procedure and the partial mastectomy are completed, the reference radiation oncologist enters the operating room. The radiation oncology service ascertains that surgical clips are placed to delineate all borders of the excisional cavity. These are placed to delineate the cephalad, caudad, medial, lateral, as well as anterior and posterior margins. With a surgical marking pen, the margins of the excised cavity are projected onto the skin and outlined.

Based on the location and depth of the partial mastectomy site, a rigid two- or three-plane breast brachytherapy template is selected; connecting bars of variable length, i.e. 12, 14, 16, 18 or 20 cm, are chosen. Once fastened together, the template with connecting bars is orientated along the excisional site to ensure adequate coverage in terms of width, length and depth. Due to the just-completed axillary procedure, the template is angled away from the apex of the axilla to avoid undue pressure on or trauma to the axillary incisional wound. The deep row of needles is inserted with the central needle placed first to allow for proper alignment of the template in relation to the excised cavity (Fig. 8.2).

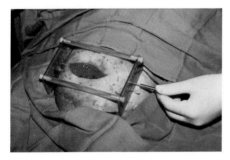

Fig. 8.2 Central needles placed first

Once the template is confirmed to be anchored by the central needle for adequate coverage of the cavity in all directions, the remainder of the deep plane needles are placed. Upon completion of the deep row of needles, the surgeon may desire to close the cavity before the intermediate and superficial plane of needles are inserted. If this is the case, a single central intermediate as well as superficial plane needle are placed to ensure that the entire depth of the cavity is appropriately covered. Indeed, if breast tissue superficially is noted to be beyond the extent of what the template would cover, slight manual compression of the overlying breast may then allow for adequate coverage of the more superficial tissue.

If cavity closure is to be done upon completion of the interstitial procedure, the intermediate and superficial plane needles are inserted under direct visualization to ensure adequate cavity coverage. As each needle is inserted, a yellow H clamp is placed on the sharp needle end to secure it in place. The open needle end is closed off with a sterilization cap (Fig. 8.3).

Prior to closure of the wound cavity, the surgeon is requested to confirm the appropriateness of the interstitial HDR needle placement; if any needles need repositioning, this can be accomplished prior to closure of the cavity. DuoDerm pads are applied to relieve any pressure points caused by the template; bacitracin is applied at each of the en-

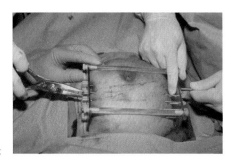

Fig. 8.3 Open cavity technique: securing implant

trance/exit skin sites of the interstitial needles. Two ABD pads are used to dress the site of interstitial implantation. A specialized Velcro type brassiere is given to the patient for use during the duration of the interstitial application. A course of antimicrobial therapy is maintained for the duration of the brachytherapy treatments and for 7 to 10 days afterwards.

A dosimetric simulation as well as post-implant CT scan is obtained within 24 to 48 hours. The surgical specimens are sent to pathology and a minimum turn-around time of 48 hours is needed to adequately process the submitted specimens. If not all the pathological criteria are met for treatment via interstitial brachytherapy alone, the interstitial brachytherapy is converted to boost irradiation to be then followed by a course of whole-breast external beam RT (EBRT).

8.3.2 Closed Cavity Technique

Any potential candidate for a closed cavity interstitial implantation must have had cavity-delineating clips placed at the time of the partial mastectomy/ipsilateral axillary procedure. The patient returns 7 to 10 days after the lumpectomy for a preplanning CT scan with fiducial markers placed on the breast of interest (Fig. 8.4). Radioopaque angiographic catheters are placed and taped longitudinally on the involved breast. A central catheter is placed along the nipple followed by a series of such markers spaced 2 cm apart to cover the full extent of the breast, both medially and laterally (Fig. 8.4).

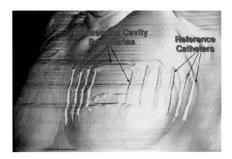

Fig. 8.4 Closed cavity technique

A free-breathing CT scan is obtained for purposes of delineating the clinical target volume as well as for preplanning with a virtual template. Upon completion of the CT scan, the excisional cavity is outlined on all the CT slices. Once input of this information is completed, a virtual simulation is undertaken. Through the efforts of dosimetry, a virtual template with virtual needles of appropriate length is used to computer-simulate the forthcoming implantation (Fig. 8.5) (Vicini et al. 1998). On skin surface anatomically rendered 3D reconstructed images, the orientation of the virtual template as well as entrance and exit points of the virtual needles are well-defined in relation to the previously placed radioopaque fiducial markers. Various parameters needed to perform the implantation are obtained, such as the angulation of the template, length of the needles required, and depth needed to adequately cover the deep margin of the excisional/partial mastectomy cavity (Fig. 8.6).

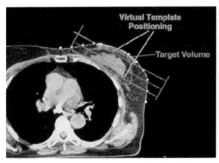 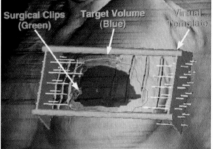

Fig. 8.5 Closed cavity technique   **Fig. 8.6** Closed cavity technique

Paper printouts are made of the virtual treatment plan(s) including the anatomical data of entrance/exit sites of the needles, template angulation and required depth of the implant—all of these are taken to the operating room on the day of closed cavity placement. Under general anesthesia, the implantation is undertaken with the guidance of the virtual treatment plan along with real-time intraoperative ultrasound (DeBiose et al. 1997). Based upon the parameters of the virtual plan, the appropriate template, whether two or three planes, and needles of proper length are selected. Longitudinal stippled marks are placed on the skin of the breast of interest to correspond to the prior fiducial opaque markers used in preplanning. An intraoperative ultrasound unit is then employed to delineate the margins of the excisional cavity, and this is outlined on the skin with a surgical marker pen.

From the technical details off the virtual plan, the template is orientated across the involved breast via the longitudinal marks on the breast skin corresponding to the virtual fiducial markers. Via ultrasound guidance, each needle of the deep plane is inserted under constant ultrasound viewing to ensure adequate depth of placement and that the needles are implanted no deeper than the chest wall (ideally, ultrasound can be used to monitor the entire placement of each deep-plane needle in relation to the underlying chest wall and lung; on rare occasions, we have requested a radiologist to be in the OR for assistance) (Fig. 8.7). The remainder of the deep-plane needles are placed, again under the guidance of ultrasound.

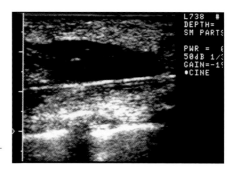

Fig. 8.7 Intraoperative ultrasound image of needle placement

One intermediate as well as superficial plane needle are inserted under constant ultrasound viewing to ensure that the depth of the cavity is adequately covered by the three planes; if the superficial tissues are not appropriately implanted, manual compression of the breast may be required to achieve adequate needle placement. The remainder of the intermediate and superficial plane needles are implanted. As in the open cavity procedure, once each needle is inserted, a yellow H clamp is placed on the sharp needle end and a sterilization cap is placed on the open needle end. Just prior to terminating the procedure, one more view of the completed interstitial implant is done with the ultrasound unit.

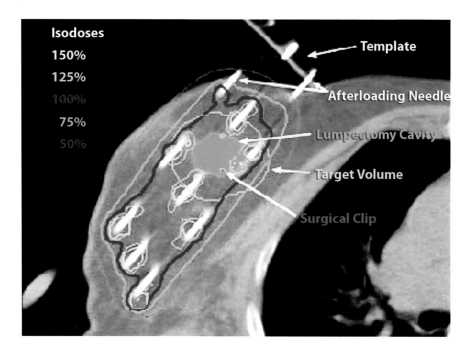

Fig. 8.8 Dosimetric treatment planning

As in the open technique, DuoDerm is applied to relieve any pressure points caused by the template. Bacitracin is applied at each of the entrance/exit sites of the HDR needles. The template/implant is dressed with two ABD pads. The patient will remain on antibiotics for the duration of the implantation and an additional 7 to 10 days after implantation. As with the open technique, a postimplantation CT scan is obtained at 24 to 48 hours to ensure adequate coverage of the clinical/planning target volume (Fig. 8.8). Final dosimetric calculations with optimization may be performed on the CT-acquired dataset. The patient is instructed not to shower, place undue pressure on the implant, or sit in the front seat of the car for fear of airbag deployment with the interstitial needles within the breast when she travels in for the twice-daily treatments.

The dose prescription for the HDR breast protocol is either eight fractions of 400 cGy per fraction for a total of 3200 cGy prescribed to the clinical target volume given on a twice-daily schedule with a minimal interfraction time interval of 6 hours, or ten fractions of 340 cGy twice-daily for a total dose of 3400 cGy. Prior to each fraction, needle positions are re-verified in reference to the skin; this is done by both caliper measurements of the template-to-skin distances of each needle or via a Mylar overlay which delineates the entrance point of each needle through the skin.

8.4 Clinical Results

Between 1993 and 2001, 199 patients were treated at William Beaumont Hospital with interstitial brachytherapy alone (120 with LDR and 79 with HDR). With a median follow-up of 6.4 years, the 5-year local acturial recurrence rate was 1.2% with an elsewhere breast failure rate of 0.6% (Chen et al. 2006). To compare potential outcome differences based upon the volume of breast irradiated, the patients treated with interstitial brachytherapy alone were matched with 199 patients treated with whole-breast RT. The match criteria included tumor size, lymph node status, patient age, margins of excision, estro-

Table 8.1 Toxicities with resolution or stabilization over time

Toxicity	Interval								
	≤6 months (n=165)			2 years (n=128)			≥5 years (n=79)		
	Grade			Grade			Grade		
	I	II	III	I	II	III	I	II	III
Breast pain (%)	27	0	0	13	1	0	8	1	0
Breast edema (%)	50	1	0	12	0	0	6	1	0
Erythema (%)	35	1	0	11	0	0	11	0	0
Hyperpigmentation (%)	67	2	0	39	2	0	37	0	0
Fibrosis (%)	22	1	0	48	2	1	46	5	1
Hypopigmentation (%)	18	0	0	34	0	0	38	0	0

gen receptor status and use of tamoxifen. The rate of local recurrence was not significantly different between the two groups: those receiving whole-breast RT demonstrated a 1% recurrence rate and those receiving partial breast irradiation a similar 1% risk of local recurrence (P=0.65). Furthermore, no statistically significant differences were seen in the 5-year actuarial cause-specific survival (97% versus 97%, P=0.34) and overall survival (93% versus 87%, P=0.23) between those receiving whole-breast RT and those receiving accelerated partial breast irradiation alone (Vicini et al. 2003a).

In terms of toxicities and cosmetic outcome, the toxicity parameters examined in our cohort of patients included breast edema, erythema, fibrosis, hyperpigmentation, hypopigmentation, breast pain, breast infection, telangiectasia, and fat necrosis. Toxicities were graded using the Radiation Therapy Oncology Group (RTOG)/Eastern Cooperative Oncology Group (ECOG) late radiation morbidity scoring scheme (Cox et al. 1995) for skin, subcutaneous tissues, pain, radiation dermatitis, and dermatology/skin from the Common Toxicity Criteria (CTC) version 2.0 (Trotti et al. 2000). As per the guidelines of CTC version 2, toxicities were graded using the acute/chronic radiation morbidity scale: grade 0 = no observable radiation effects, grade I = mild radiation effects, grade II = moderate radiation effects, and grade III = severe radiation effects. Cosmetic evaluation was based on standards as set out by the Harvard criteria (Rose et al. 1989). An excellent score was given when the treated breast looked essentially the same as the contralateral untreated breast. A good score was assigned for minimal but identifiable radiation effects on the treated breast. Scoring a fair result meant significant radiation effects readily observable. A poor score was used for severe sequelae of normal tissue.

Breast toxicities including pain, edema, erythema, and hyperpigmentation were nearly all mild and diminished over time (Table 8.1). Breast pain diminished from 27% at 6 months to 8% at 5 years. Breast edema decreased from 50% at 6 months to 12% at 2 years and 6% at 5 years. Similarly, erythema demonstrated the following pattern: 35% at 6 months to 11% at 2 years with stabilization thereafter. Hyperpigmentation followed a similar downward trend in frequency: 67% at 6 months to 37% at 5 years. All of these were statistically analyzed using Pearson's chi squared test and were found not to be chance occurrences (Chen et al. 2006)

Breast sequelae which increased until the 2-year mark and then stabilized included breast fibrosis (22%, 48% and 46% at 6 months, 2 years and 5 years, respectively) and hypopigmentation (18%, 34% and 38% at 6 months, 2 years and 5 years). Of note, any slight degree of periscar induration was scored as mild fibrosis regardless of whether or not post surgical changes may have contributed. Nearly all the pigmentary changes, whether hyper- or hypopigmentation were mild and pinpoint rather than diffuse, and corresponded to the sites where the LDR catheters or HDR needles had been placed. Likewise, the chi squared analysis verified these trends. The time-course trend of hypopigmentation followed that of fibrosis with an increase in frequency out to 2 years with a subsequent plateau occurring with further passage of time.

The frequency of fat necrosis and telangiectasia increased with time; the time course of fat necrosis was 9% at 2 years and 11% at 5 years. The median time to occurrence of fat necrosis was 5.5 years (range of 0.25 to 8.2 years; Table 8.2). Telangiectasias, nearly all of which were grade I, were evenly distributed between the LDR and HDR treatment modalities at 5 years being 34% for both LDR and HDR (P=0.983).

Good to excellent cosmetic outcomes were noted in 95% to 99% of patients depending on the time of assessment (Table 8.3). At 6 months the percentage of good scores

Table 8.2 Toxicities with increased incidence over time

Toxicity	Interval								
	≤6 months (*n*=165)			2 years (*n*=128)			≥5 years (*n*=79)		
	Grade			Grade			Grade		
	I	II	III	I	II	III	I	II	III
Telangiec-tasia (%)	5	0	0	21	2	0	34	1	0
Fat necrosis (% of all patients)[a]		1			9			11	

[a] Fat necrosis is not graded. Median time to occurrence: 5.5 years (0.25–8.2 years).

was 85%. However, between 6 months and 2 years, the percentage of excellent scores increased from 10% to 29%. Comparison of cosmetic results at 2 and 5 years demonstrated stabilization of scores with the percentage of excellent scores increasing out to 5 years. The percentage of good to excellent cosmetic outcome scores never fell below 95%.

Table 8.3 Cosmetic outcome over time with APBI

≤6 months (*n*=165)[a]			2 years (*n*=129)[a]			≥5 years (*n*=134)[a]		
Excellent	Good	Fair	Excellent	Good	Fair	Excellent	Good	Fair
10%	85%	1%	29%	68%	2%	33%	66%	1%
	95%			97%			99%	

[a] Four percent and 1% of cosmetic outcomes were unreported for ≤ 6 months and 2 years, respectively.

No statistically significant difference was noted in the incidence/severity of any toxicity or cosmetic outcome with the following parameters: tamoxifen, type of brachytherapy (LDR versus HDR), and tumor size (T1 versus T2) (Pearson's chi squared analysis). However, the incidence of breast erythema at 2 and 5 years and the incidence of delayed infections were higher for those patients receiving chemotherapy (*P*=0.015, 0.016, and 0.003, respectively). Cosmetic assessment at 6 months was better in those patients not receiving chemotherapy than in those who received chemotherapy (100% versus 94%, *P*=0.005) (Chen et al. 2006).

8.5 Future Directions

Patients undergoing HDR interstitial brachytherapy for APBI have been treated using a fixed rigid template system with interstitial needles in place. Beaumont is now in the transition phase of replacing the rigid needle system with afterloading flexible catheters. Although the advantage of the template-based needle system is that a library of dosimetric plans can be quickly calculated for each patient, the flexible catheter system should allow for more individualization of the implanted volume. The goal of such a multicatheter system would be optimal dosimetric coverage of the target volume while sparing normal surrounding tissues which need not be in the high-dose volume.

Additionally, the brachytherapy interstitial implantation technique is operator-dependent; skill is required for such implant placement which can be a technically demanding clinical challenge. Thus, less complex systems of obtaining the same dosimetric dose coverage include 3D conformal external beam radiotherapy (3D-CRT) delivered in 5 days or within 10 days (Baglan et al. 2003; Vicini et al. 2003b; Formenti et al. 2002, 2004). Such conformal technology has been investigated by the RTOG in a phase I/II trial (RTOG 0319) on partial breast irradiation using 3D-CRT, which completed accrual in late April 2004. Another means of brachytherapy which is technically less demanding than the multicatheter/needle technique is the MammoSite RTS applicator. Approved by the US Food and Drug Administration (FDA) in May 2002, this allows dosimetric coverage of the target volume of interest via a balloon catheter system which can be placed either in an open or closed cavity setting (Kreisch, et al, 2003).

Although the MammoSite RTS applicator as well as 3D-CRT are now available, the experience at Beaumont Hospital would suggest that not all patients would qualify for either of these two newer techniques. Depending on the cavity location, cavity configuration, cavity to skin distance and the relationship of the cavity to the chest wall, there will remain patients who will benefit from the more customized/individualized dosimetry afforded by multicatheter/multineedle type interstitial implantations. Thus, although the operator-independence of the newer techniques including MammoSite and 3D-CRT treatments is quite appealing, we at Beaumont still believe there remains a role for the multicatheter system based on an individualized case-by-case assessment.

Currently, our policy is that any patient who is eligible for partial breast irradiation is entered into the randomized phase III clinical trial sponsored jointly by the National Surgical Adjuvant Breast Project and RTOG [NSABP B-39/RTOG 0413 trial: "A randomized phase III study of conventional whole breast irradiation (WBI) versus partial breast irradiation (PBI) for women with stage 0, I or II breast cancer"] to provide definitive class I evidence as to the efficacy of APBI compared with that of whole-breast irradiation. Enrollment was initiated in March 2005.

References

1. Arriagada R, Le MG, Rochard F, et al (1996) Conservative treatment versus mastectomy in early breast cancer: patterns of failure with 15 years of follow-up data. Institut Custave-Roussy Breast Cancer Group. J Clin Oncol 14:1558–1564

2. Baglan K, Martinez A, Frazier R, et al (2001) The use of high-dose rate brachytherapy alone after lumpectomy in patients with early-stage breast cancer treated with breast-conserving therapy. Int J Radiat Oncol Biol Phys 50:1003–1011

3. Baglan K, Sharpe M, Jaffray D, et al (2003) Accelerated partial breast irradiation using 3D conformal radiation therapy (3D-CRT). Int J Radiat Oncol Biol Phys 55:392–406

4. Blichert-Toft M, Rose C, Andersen JA, et al (1992) Danish randomized trial comparing breast conservation therapy with mastectomy: six years of life-table analysis. Danish Breast Cancer Cooperative Group. J Natl Cancer Inst Monogr 11:19–25

5. Chen P, Vicini F, Benitez P, et al (2006) Long-term cosmetic results and toxicity after accelerated partial breast irradiation (APBI): a method of radiation delivery via interstitial brachytherapy in treatment of early-stage breast cancer. Cancer 106:991–999

6. Clarke DH, Edmundson G, Martinez A, et al (1989) The clinical advantages of I-125 seeds as a substitute for Ir-192 seeds in temporary plastic tube implants. Int J Radiat Oncol Biol Phys 17:859–863

7. Cox J, Stetz J, Pajak T (1995) Toxicity criteria of the Radiation Oncology (RTOG) and the European Organization for Research and Treatment of Cancer (EORTC). Int J Radiat Oncol Biol Phys 31:1341–1346

8. DeBiose D, Horwitz E, Martinez A, et al (1997) The use of ultrasonography in the localization of the lumpectomy cavity for interstitial brachytherapy of the breast. Int J Radiat Oncol Biol Phys 38:755–759

9. Fisher B, Andersen S, Bryant J, et al (2002) Twenty-year follow-up of a randomized trial comparing total mastectomy, lumpectomy and lumpectomy plus irradiation for the treatment of invasive breast cancer. N Engl J Med 347:1233–1241

10. Formenti S, Rosenstein B, Skinner K, et al (2002) T1 stage breast cancer: adjuvant hypofractionated conformal radiation therapy to tumor bed in selected postmenopausal breast cancer patients – pilot feasibility study. Radiology 222:171–178

11. Formenti S, Truong M, Goldberg J, et al (2004) Prone accelerated partial breast irradiation after breast-conserving surgery: preliminary clinical results and dose-volume histogram analysis. Int J Radiat Oncol Biol Phys 60:493–504

12. Jacobson JA, Danforth ND, Cowan KH, et al (1995) Ten-year results of a comparison of conservation with mastectomy in the treatment of stage I and II breast cancer. N Engl J Med 332:907–911

13. Keisch M, Vicini F, Kuske RR, et al (2003) Initial clinical experience with the MammoSite breast brachytherapy applicator in women with early-stage breast cancer treated with breast-conserving therapy. Int J Radiat Oncol Biol Phys 55:289–293

14. Morrow M, White J, Moughan J, et al (2001) Factors predicting the use of breast conserving therapy in stage I and II breast carcinoma. J Clin Oncol 19:2254–2262

15. Nattinger AB, Hoffmann RG, Kneusel RT, et al (2000) Relation between appropriateness of primary therapy for early-stage breast carcinoma and increased use of breast conserving surgery. Lancet 356:1148–1153

16. Overgaard M, Hansen PS, Overgaard J, et al (1997) Postoperative radiotherapy in high-risk premenopausal women with breast cancer who receive adjuvant chemotherapy. Danish Breast Cancer Cooperative Group 82b Trial. N Engl J Med 337:949–955

17. Overgaard M, Jensen MB, Overgaard J, et al (1999) Postoperative radiotherapy in high-risk postmenopausal breast-cancer patients given adjuvant tamoxifen: Danish Breast Cancer Cooperative Group DBCG 82c randomised trial. Lancet 353:1641–1648

18. Ragaz J, Jackson SM, Le N, et al (1997) Adjuvant radiotherapy and chemotherapy in node-positive premenopausal women with breast cancer. N Engl J Med 337:956–962

19. Rose M, Olivotto I, Cady B, et al (1989) Conservative surgery and radiation therapy for early stage breast cancer: long-term cosmetic results. Breast Cancer 124:153–157

20. Trotti A, Byhardt R, Stetz J, et al (2000) Common toxicity criteria: version 2.0. An improved reference for grading the acute effects of cancer treatments: impact on radiotherapy. Int J Radiat Oncol Biol Phys 47:13–14

21. Van Dongen JA, Voogd AC, Fentiman IS, et al (2000) Long-term results of a randomized trial comparing breast conserving therapy with mastectomy: European Organization for Research and Treatment of Cancer 10801 trial. J Natl Cancer Inst 92:1143–1150

22. Veronesi U, Cascinelli N, Mariani L, et al (2002) Twenty-year follow-up of a randomized study comparing breast conserving surgery with radical mastectomy for early breast cancer. N Engl J Med 347:1227–1232

23. Vicini F, Chen P, Fraile M, et al (1997) Low-dose rate brachytherapy as the sole radiation modality in the management of patients with early-stage breast cancer treated with breast-conserving therapy: preliminary results of a pilot trial. Int J Radiat Oncol Biol Phys 38:301–310

24. Vicini F, Jaffray D, Horwitz E, et al (1998) Implementation of 3D-virtual brachytherapy in the management of breast cancer: a description of a new method of interstitial brachytherapy. Int J Radiat Oncol Biol Phys 40:629–635

25. Vicini F, Kini V, Chen P, et al (1999) Irradiation of the tumor bed alone after lumpectomy in selected patients with early-stage breast cancer treated with breast conserving therapy. J Surg Oncol 70:33–40

26. Vicini F, Kestin L, Chen P, et al (2003a) Limited-field radiation therapy in the management of early stage breast cancer. J Natl Cancer Inst 95:1205–1210

27. Vicini F, Remouchamps V, Wallace M, et al (2003b) Ongoing clinical experience utilizing 3D conformal external beam radiotherapy to deliver partial breast irradiation in patients with early stage breast cancer treated with breast-conserving therapy. Int J Radiat Oncol Biol Phys 57:1247–1253

Brachytherapy Techniques: the University of Wisconsin/Arizona Approach

9

Robert R. Kuske

Contents

9.1 Introduction: a 14-year Historical Perspective on the Evolution of APBI

"If only you listen to your patients, new ideas will emerge" (Aron 1984). In October 1991, a woman from Venezuela with a stage T2N0M0 ductal carcinoma of the right supra-areolar breast presented before the multidisciplinary Conference and Clinic at the Ochsner Clinic in New Orleans. Aware that there were alternatives to mastectomy, and that there were no linear accelerators in her home country at the time within 8 hours of her home, she insisted that her physician consultants come up with an alternative to the standard 6.5 weeks of external beam breast irradiation. The surgical oncologist at the Clinic, John Bolton, suggested that we consider offering her wide-volume brachytherapy, similar to how we had been treating soft-tissue sarcomas. He noted that the published local control rates with single-plane implants covering the surgical bed with generous margins were excellent, allowing limb preservation (Brennan et al. 1987). Our soft-tissue sarcoma brachytherapy results in New Orleans mirrored those published in this series. The low dose-rate (LDR) brachytherapy was designed to deliver a radiation dose capable of sterilizing microscopic extensions of sarcoma beyond the surgical margin, which was microscopically clear. An inherently hotter central dose inside the peripheral envelope offers a built-in boost dose to the surface area at greatest risk for tumor cells after surgical excision. An added benefit particularly attractive to this patient was that, since the treatment is delivered with LDR iridium seeds within plastic catheters embedded directly within the tissues that harbored the malignancy, a tumoricidal dose could be given much more quickly, in 3 to 5 days instead of the conventional 6 to 7 weeks of external beam whole-breast irradiation.

Since the margins were unevaluated in Venezuela, Dr. Bolton took her back to surgery for a reexcision in New Orleans, and an axillary dissection for staging was also planned. In the operating room, with the wound open and exposed, multiple brachytherapy catheters were inserted, with 1.5 cm between each catheter within a plane, and approximately 2.5 cm between the two planes, superficial and deep. The goal was to bracket the lumpectomy cavity between two planes of catheters, and extend them peripherally 2 cm beyond the surgical edge in all directions, except superficial and deep where the skin and pectoralis major fascia provide anatomic limits to coverage.

The prescription dose was 45 Gy in 3 days with LDR seeds. The seeds were loaded 1 cm deep to the skin surface on both the proximal and deep sides of the implant. This is in contrast to modern three-dimensional treatment planning, where the seed positions in the z-plane are placed from each edge of the target volume. The seed strength was 1 mCi per seed, and the dose was delivered in 3 days on an inpatient basis with shielding and radiation precautions. On day 4, the patient was on a plane back to Venezuela, her family, and her business. Photos of her breast immediately after catheter removal and at the time of her 10-year follow-up are shown in Figs. 9.1 and 9.2, respectively.

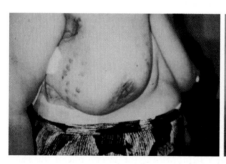
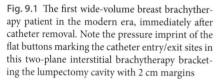
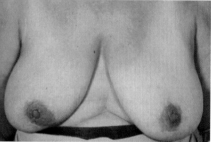

Fig. 9.1 The first wide-volume breast brachytherapy patient in the modern era, immediately after catheter removal. Note the pressure imprint of the flat buttons marking the catheter entry/exit sites in this two-plane interstitial brachytherapy bracketing the lumpectomy cavity with 2 cm margins

Fig. 9.2 The same patient as in Fig. 9.1, 10 years after APBI

The breast team at the Ochsner Clinic was encouraged by the results in this patient, the first patient treated with wide-volume breast brachytherapy alone in the modern era. Her breast maintained its softness over time, in contrast to the woody induration seen with brachytherapy as a boost. The cosmetic outcome was favorable.

We submitted a phase II trial to the institutional review board (IRB). Initially, 50 patients were to be treated by interstitial brachytherapy, followed by a 2-year hiatus to evaluate acute and subacute toxicity and cosmesis. The study was then extended to 163 patients after a favorable review of the initial data. We treated women with LDR brachytherapy in alternating blocks of ten patients each to avoid selection bias. The HDR dose (32 Gy in eight fractions over 4 days, or 34 Gy in ten fractions over 5 days) was independently calculated by prominent biologists/physicists to be equivalent to the LDR regimen for tumor control probability and late tissue effects. The published results for the first 50 patients presented a matched pair analysis comparing select brachytherapy patients to whole-breast irradiation patients selected by the same criteria (Table 9.1) and the same physicians, with similar stage, age and follow-up intervals (King et al. 2000). Tumor control, toxicity, and cosmesis were similar between the matched pairs. There was no significant difference between LDR and HDR results, so the subsequent study extension was primarily HDR.

Table 9.1 APBI selection criteria for the original Ochsner Clinic trial and the subsequent Radiation Therapy Oncology Group phase II trial

Criterion	Ochsner	RTOG
Tumor size (cm)	≤4	≤3
Ductal carcinoma in situ	Included	Excluded
Positive nodes	0–3	0–3
Extracapsular nodal extension	Allowed	Prohibited
Inked surgical margins	Negative	Negative
Extensive intra-ductal component	No restrictions	Prohibited
Lobular carcinoma in situ or lobular histology	Allowed	Prohibited
Collagen vascular disease	Allowed	Prohibited

After IRB review, the trial was extended to 163 patients, including 19 ductal carcinoma in situ, 116 invasive ductal, 7 invasive ductal with extensive intraductal component (EIC), 11 lobular, 6 tubular, and 4 mucinous histologies; 24 were node-positive. Overall, 71% of the patients were treated with HDR brachytherapy. Five patients (3%) had breast, 4 nodal (2.5%), and 7 distant ((4.3%) recurrence at a median follow-up of 65 months (Kuske et al. 2004a).

The New Orleans excellent outcomes were mirrored by those from the William Beaumont Hospital (Baglan et al. 2001), providing impetus towards Radiation Therapy Oncology Group (RTOG) Trial 95-17. RTOG 95-17 is the first cooperative group phase II trial of partial breast irradiation (PBI). This trial accrued 100 patients (99 eligible) from ten institutions. At 4 years, the ipsilateral breast recurrence rate was 3%, the same as the contralateral new primary cancer rate (Kuske et al. 2004b).

Research in APBI is blossoming, with at least five international randomized trials ongoing. Investigation in APBI has followed an ideal path, from a single patient giving us the concept, to single institution trials at two hospitals, to a national phase II cooperative group trial, to multiple international phase III trials. Soon, we will have direct comparisons between conventional 6-week whole-breast irradiation and 5-day PBI.

9.2 A New Hypothesis and a Potential Paradigm Shift

There has been a 109-year tradition of treating the entire breast in all breast cancers, no matter what stage or how early they were detected. Sir William Halstead proposed the original hypothesis, that the entire organ needed to be treated and all possible extensions of the malignancy, including nodal regions.

In the early 1980s, the Halstead hypothesis was challenged, but only to the extent that the entire breast could be treated by a comprehensive radiation beam rather than the scalpel.

Attempts at partial breast surgery, not followed by whole-breast irradiation, were failures, with local recurrence rates in the range of 30–40% (Morrow and Harris 2000).

A principle of radiation oncology is: When treating large volumes or entire organs, a lower dose per fraction improves tolerance by decreasing the late effects (e.g. fibrosis, microvessel damage, telangiectasis, necrosis) of irradiation. In consideration of the goal of optimizing cosmetic outcome in the treatment of early-stage breast cancer with breast-preserving approaches, the original pioneers of breast conservation therapy chose to treat the ipsilateral breast with daily doses of irradiation in the range 180–200 cGy per fraction. The whole breast was treated to 4500–5000 cGy, followed usually by a boost to the excision site plus a margin to 6000–6600 cGy over 6–7 weeks.

We hypothesized in 1991 that:
1. In select breast cancers, true biologically significant multicentricity is rare, and more recent improvements in breast imaging (e.g. breast MRI) and pathology (e.g. margin assessment) may further reduce the risk of disconnected multiquadrant disease.
2. Virtually extending the surgical margins by eliminating interconnected breast cancer extensions beyond the surgical edge with focused dose-intense radiation might lower the true local recurrence rate.
3. Since the radiation source is immediately in the vicinity of the tissue at risk, brachytherapy can be given in a shorter time period, accelerating the treatment time, potentially making breast conservation radiotherapy more accessible to eligible women.
4. As a result of the physics of brachytherapy, the dose falls off rapidly away from the source dwell positions, decreasing normal tissue exposure to radiation, potentially preventing sequelae to the heart, lung, chest wall, skin, lymphatic, and uninvolved breast irradiation.
5. The shorter overall treatment duration allows all the local therapy for breast cancer to be given upfront, with systemic therapy to follow without delay, potentially maximizing local and systemic control of the malignancy.
6. PBI may allow more options for salvage therapy in the event of local relapse.

APBI represents a potential paradigm shift. The existing paradigm assumes that the entire breast needs to be treated by either surgery or limited surgery followed by whole-breast irradiation. APBI introduces the concept that in appropriately selected breast cancers, only the affected portion of the breast needs to be treated. Since the treatment volume is limited, the treatment can be dramatically shortened from 6 weeks to 4–5 days.

9.3 The Target Volume

Based upon the pathological and clinical literature available to us at the time we stated the new hypothesis, we decided to embark upon initial clinical trials treating 2 cm beyond the surgical edge, unless the skin or pectoralis fascia intervened. Later, after the advent of the balloon intracavitary catheter, considerable discussion and thoughtful analysis ensued about whether 1 cm might be sufficient in carefully selected patients. An analysis by Vicini et al. (2002) led to a hypothesis that a 1-cm margin may be sufficient in carefully selected patients.

Currently, the choice of appropriate margin of irradiation is purely conjectural. It is clear that 0 cm, or no radiation at all, results in unacceptably high local breast recurrence rates in the range of 30–40% even with negative surgical margins. The local recurrence rates with treating an additional 2 cm are 3% at 7 years in the author's prospective clinical trials and 3% at 4 years in the RTOG 95-17 multiinstitutional prospective cooperative group phase II trial. Preliminary short-term local recurrence rates with the balloon intracavitary catheter are acceptable, and we will see if the 7- and 10-year outcomes match interstitial results.

For the phase III trial, considerable thought and discussion went into choosing the ultimate criterion of treating 1.5 cm out for interstitial brachytherapy, 1.0 cm out for balloon intracavitary brachytherapy, and 2.5 cm out for the 3D conformal option on this study. We rationalized that if the balloon compresses the breast tissue on average by 0.5 cm, then the breast tissue treated may be 1.5 cm beyond the surgical edge, which would match that achieved with interstitial brachytherapy. With 3D conformal PBI, we had to take breathing motion and set-up uncertainty into account, resulting in the more generous treatment margin around the lumpectomy cavity with this technique.

The research in the field of PBI is currently very active, so it is anticipated that delineation of the appropriate radiation margin around the excision cavity will be clearer. Perhaps the margin will vary from patient to patient in the future, depending on tumor and patient characteristics. As seen in specimen radiographs, the tumor is frequently eccentrically located within a specimen, with a generous margin on one side and a close margin on another. It is conceivable that the radiation margin in the future may vary geometrically, based upon accurate and reliable pathological determination of surgical margin width in three dimensions.

9.4 Irradiating the Target Volume

Once the decision is made as to the amount of tissue surrounding the lumpectomy edge that needs to be irradiated, there are many different means to deliver the radiation dose.

Interstitial Brachytherapy

This is actually the oldest radiation delivery method, used shortly after Madame Curie discovered radium. Geoffrey Keynes applied interstitial brachytherapy to a wide variety of breast cancers in the 1920s, long before the first linear accelerators or even cobalt-60 units were brought into clinical use (Keynes 1937). The first modern-day PBI technique was developed at the Ochsner Clinic, and the initial studies there provide the longest follow-up and evidence-based medicine for APBI (King et al. 2000; Kuske et al. 2004a). Balloon intracavitary and especially 3D conformal or intensity-modulated radiation therapy PBI techniques have less-mature data supporting their use. Interstitial brachytherapy can cover any shape or size of lumpectomy cavity, and the radiation margin is freely controllable. Interstitial brachytherapy provides the ultimate conformal radiation delivery, with the least dose to surrounding normal tissues.

Balloon Intracavitary Brachytherapy (MammoSite)

This is the simplest method of APBI, with one catheter centered inside a spherical or elliptical balloon, and usually one dwell position or a limited number of linear dwell positions. Insertion and physics calculations are much easier than with interstitial brachytherapy. Because of the limitations of a single dwell position (or linear array), the dose can be prescribed only 1 cm beyond the surface of the balloon, and symmetrically around the central catheter. Even with tissue compression, the dose does not reach out as far as with interstitial brachytherapy, and narrow skin separations (<7 mm), irregular shaped cavities, or air/fluid loculations pose significant difficulties with this technique. For carefully selected patients and cavities, however, the simplest solution may be the best solution.

Three-Dimensional Conformal External Beam PBI

This is the newest technique, with the least data to support it (Vicini et al. 2003). It is designed for radiation oncologists who are uncomfortable with and unable to perform brachytherapy. Breathing motion and set-up uncertainty pose technical challenges. There is not the dose inhomogeneity inherent in brachytherapy, with a hotter central dose, so the prescribed dose must be greater with this technique (385 cGy per fraction). Exit dose to other parts of the body is possible. In our experience, skin reactions can be quite symptomatic with this technique. It is, however, a popular APBI method because radiation oncologists and their physicists are comfortable with their linear accelerators. This technique requires a substantial investment in physics and dosimetry time in order to meet all the dose constraints and normal tissue limits.

Electron Beam

The only published study with PBI using electron beam is a negative study with high local recurrence rates, especially for lobular carcinomas (Ribeiro et al. 1990). Covering a defined target volume with quality assurance and documentation is a significant challenge. An Italian trial and various institutions in the US are experimenting with single-dose intraoperative electrons. The radiobiology of a single large fraction may be suboptimal, but the convenience is undeniable.

Soft X-Rays (Intrabeam)

This technique treats approximately 2 mm of breast tissue surrounding the cavity to a very low dose.

9.5 Brachytherapy Techniques

9.5.1 Open Freehand Interstitial Catheter Insertion

Open freehand technique depends upon the skill of the brachytherapist to insert catheters or needles in an array that both covers the target volume, and provides a spacing that will insure a homogeneous dose distribution. It was the original method of breast brachytherapy, used by Geoffrey Keynes in England in the 1920s as the original breast conservation therapy (Keynes 1937), Samuel Hellman from the Joint Center for Radiotherapy in the late 1970s and early 1980s as a boost, and myself in the early 1990s as the first modern day APBI technique.

At the time of a lumpectomy or reexcision, the radiation oncologist goes to the operating room with the surgeon. With the skin incision open, the extent of the surgical excision can be determined by probing the cavity with an index finger. A sterile magic marker delineates the edges of the cavity onto the skin surface. A single, double, or rarely triple plane implant is then designed by marking the planned needle entry and exit sites on the skin (Figs. 9.3 and 9.4).

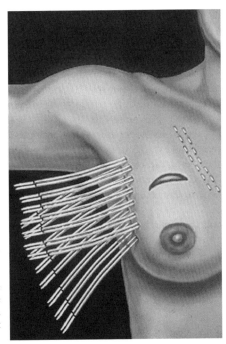

Fig. 9.3 Two-plane interstitial implant as performed on the RTOG 95-17 phase II trial. With the wound open, the edges of the lumpectomy cavity are marked on the skin. Deep and superficial planes are placed posterior and anterior to the cavity, extending 2 cm beyond the cavity in all dimensions. In the study, the end dwell positions of the radioactive source(s) were planned 1 cm from the skin surface on both sides, in contrast to modern 3D planning where the positions span the target volume only

A single-plane implant is indicated if the thickness of the tissue to be covered is 1.5 cm or less. This typically is the case for very medial lesions near the parasternal breast tissue or in very small breasts or in augmented breasts (Fig. 9.5). It is appropriate to design a single-plane implant for one side of the target volume, and broaden it out in a "Y" pattern where the breast becomes thicker, such as under the nipple. A double plane is

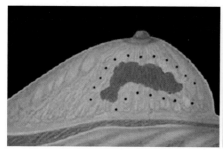 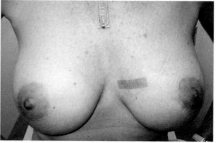

Fig. 9.4 Sagital cross-sectional view of a two-plane implant with the cavity in *purple* and the catheters represented by *black dots*

Fig. 9.5 Prebrachytherapy photograph of a parasternal medial tumor excision site in an augmented breast. Ultrasound-guided catheter insertion is preferred, and the thin breast tissue can usually be covered by either a single plane or Y-shaped single plane branching out to a second plane laterally towards the nipple

necessary if the tissue thickness is greater than 1.5 cm but less than 3 cm. A third plane is added when the target tissue exceeds or equals 3 cm.

The spacing between needles within a plane varies with the size of the implant. Smaller volumes require closer spacing and larger volumes can be cover with wider spacing. For example, when using a single-plane implant, the needle spacing typically is 1.0–1.2 cm. For double-plane implants, the spacing is 1.5 cm. In high-risk areas such as directly under the lumpectomy scar, smoother dose distributions under the skin can be obtained by adding extra catheters in between the original marks at a superficial depth. By adding these extra catheters, called the "gauntlet under the skin," the dose under the skin can be feathered by varying the dwell times without overdosing the skin surface and running the late risk of telangiectasia.

General principles of freehand technique include:
1. When in doubt about coverage, add an extra catheter in the OR, because you can always pull it or not use it if the dose distribution is acceptable without it, but it is harder (but not impossible!) to add it later after the patient has awoken.
2. Catheter entry and exit locations should be selected at least 1 cm away from the target volume, or a source dwell will need to be in the skin, guaranteeing a telangiectatic spot.
3. Ideally, the needles are perfectly straight and parallel to each other.
4. At the ends of the implant, placing an extra catheter in between the two planes will prevent bowing in of the isodose curves.
5. Crossing needles in a perpendicular orientation near the catheter entry and exit sites can be helpful in contouring the dose at these ends of the target volume, so that you do not have to past-load dwell positions in each catheter to prevent a scalloping in of the dose at the ends of a line source (Fig. 9.6).

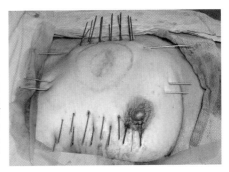

Fig. 9.6 An ultrasound-guided implant illustrating: (1) triangulation between the superficial and deep planes, where the superficial needles are in between pairs of deep needles, and (2) the use of crossing needles at right angles and between the two planes, at the periphery of the target volume, benefiting dosimetry in the z-plane of the implant and avoiding medial sources too close to the skin

Clearly, freehand techniques require skill and experience from the brachytherapist. For this reason, this technique is less commonly used than the other image-guided techniques discussed in this chapter. This technique is still frequently used with augmentation mammoplasty where seeing the silicone surface as you guide each needle across the target volume is helpful in avoiding augmentation implant puncture and subsequent rupture. For the target volume not visible within the cavity at the right and left sides, however, it is much safer to have intraoperative ultrasound in order to avoid puncture.

9.5.2 Ultrasound-Guided Supine Catheter Insertion

Ultrasound can be very helpful in guiding needle insertion in a closed lumpectomy cavity. In the presence of a seroma, the surgical excision cavity is readily seen by ultrasound. Using real-time ultrasound, it is feasible to guide each brachytherapy needle millimeter by millimeter across the breast at a chosen depth (Figs. 9.7 and 9.8). The deep plane is inserted either along the surface of the pectoralis major muscle or 5 mm deep to the lumpectomy cavity. The superficial plane is inserted at a depth of 0.75 to 1.0 cm from the skin surface (Fig. 9.9). A middle plane is added when the separation between the two planes, easily measured by the ultrasound device, exceeds 3 cm, or at the ends of the implant to prevent bowing in of the isodose curves as described above.

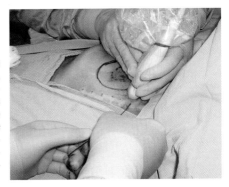

Fig. 9.7 Ultrasound-guided needle insertion. The lumpectomy cavity is marked by the *dotted oval*, and the target 2 cm beyond by the *solid oval*. Catheter deep and superficial entry sites are marked as dots on the skin. The needle is bent for the deep plane to facilitate its exiting on the other side. The ultrasound transducer, inside a plastic sleeve containing gel, guides each needle millimeter by millimeter across the pectoralis fascia, avoiding pneumothorax and aiding precise localization

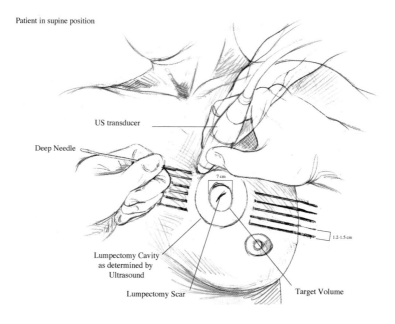

Patient in supine position

US transducer

Deep Needle

7 cm

1.2-1.5 cm

Lumpectomy Cavity
as determined by
Ultrasound

Lumpectomy Scar

Target Volume

Fig. 9.8 Ultrasound-guided needle insertion, illustrating freehand technique and catheter separation

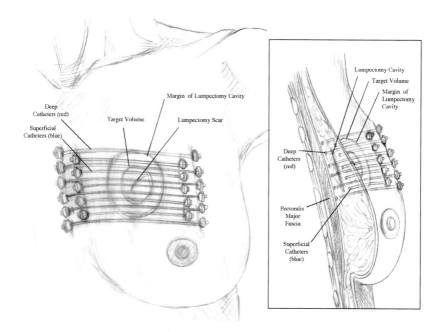

Margin of Lumpectomy Cavity

Deep
Catheters (red)

Target Volume

Lumpectomy Scar

Superficial
Catheters (blue)

Lumpectomy Cavity

Target Volume

Margin of
Lumpectomy
Cavity

Deep
Catheters
(red)

Pectoralis
Major
Fascia

Superficial
Catheters
(blue)

Fig. 9.9 Typical catheter distribution with supine ultrasound guidance. Note the medial location

Needles should be chosen that are easily seen by the ultrasound transducer. The challenge is to make each needle go straight and parallel to the others while looking at the ultrasound monitor for proper depth. Some brachytherapists will have a diagnostic radiologist present to hold the transducer and monitor depth and target volume coverage, while others will use their dominant hand for needle insertion and the other hand to hold the transducer.

This technique is also skill-dependent, since it is still a freehand technique without a template to ensure a geometrical array of catheters across the target volume. It can be done under local anesthesia with analgesia, or under conscious sedation. Unless you are performing the implant at the time of axillary surgery or a excision/reexcision, general anesthesia is not required.

Ultrasound catheter insertion in the supine position usually requires fewer catheters than the template-guided insertions below, because the breast flattens out in the supine position and there is no compression to elongate the lumpectomy cavity and subsequent target volume. This fact makes hook-up to the HDR iridium-192 remote afterloading machine simpler (Fig. 9.10).

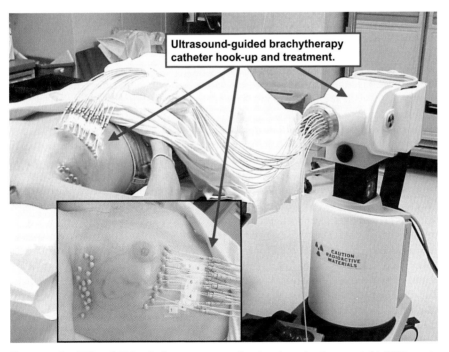

Ultrasound-guided brachytherapy catheter hook-up and treatment.

Fig. 9.10 After CT-based 3D brachytherapy treatment planning, the patient is connected to HDR remote afterloader for treatment

9.5.3 Image-Guided Prone Catheter Insertion with a Special Breast Template

In 1996, the lead breast imager at the Ochsner Clinic, Dr. Gunnar Cederbom, asked me if I had ever considered brachytherapy in the prone position on a stereotactic core needle breast biopsy table. He pointed out the major advantages of such an approach:

1. In the prone position the breast hangs by gravity, pulling the breast tissue away from the pectoralis major muscle, ribs, and pleura.
2. The built-in mammography equipment under the table could be used to image the breast, facilitating image-guided breast brachytherapy.
3. Prior to the procedure, under ultrasound guidance, a small amount (about 3–5 ml) of nonionic contrast such as Omnipaque along with 2 ml air can be injected directly into the lumpectomy cavity, highlighting the seroma as well as all its crevices and outpouchings.
4. Attaching a template to the breast and taking a mammographic image directly down the holes should allow reliable, reproducible coverage of the target volume.
5. Any margin around the lumpectomy cavity can be chosen (e.g. 1, 1.5, 2.0, 2.5 cm, etc.) and theoretically one could have broader coverage on one side of the cavity, where the margin is perhaps tighter, and a smaller margin on the other side where the surgical margin is generous.
6. The procedure can be performed totally under local anesthesia with analgesia.
7. The resultant catheter distribution is a volume implant, rather than one or two planes, allowing much more flexibility for dosimetry and coverage of odd cavity shapes.
8. Assuming the template is attached in the same way, a radiation oncologist in a different state, or even a resident in training, would perform exactly the same implant as a very experienced brachytherapist would do.

A typical procedure would go as follows. The patient or a nurse applies topical lidocaine cream (EMLA) to the involved breast 1 to 2 hours before the start time. One hour before start time, the patient takes 5/325 mg Percocet and 5 mg Valium. The patient is taken to the ultrasound suite, where the seroma is identified. An ultrasound-compatible needle is inserted at least 2 cm away from the seroma, to avoid leakage of contrast agent later, after a small amount of local anesthetic has been injected to raise a skin wheal and along the planned path of the needle. The needle is positioned in the middle of the seroma, and approximately 80% of the seroma fluid is aspirated into a syringe. This decreases the target volume. Then 3 ml nonionic contrast agent and 2 ml air are injected directly into the cavity. The needle is withdrawn. The patient is taken to the stereotactic core biopsy suite in the Radiology Department, the surgeon's office, or your department, wherever the device is located. The table and underlying mammography equipment are draped in sterile fashion. The patient's breast is prepped with povidone-iodine or a similar solution. The patient is asked to lower her breast through the hole in the table, so that the nipple is centered and the breast hangs by gravity underneath the table (Fig. 9.11). The radiation oncologist or surgeon then palpates the seroma and faces the lumpectomy scar (Fig. 9.12). The template is positioned on the breast so that the surgical scar is between the two plates and visible to the physician (Fig. 9.13). The surgical scar should not be up against one of the plates because the catheters need to be parallel to the skin under the lumpectomy scar, not perpendicular, for dosimetry reasons. For smaller breasts, tincture of benzoin or an equivalent may be applied to the skin before the template is attached to prevent slippage. Usually, the upper edge of the template is placed tightly up against the chest wall so adequate deep coverage is provided. A mammographic image is taken with the line of the X-rays aligned along the holes in the template (Fig. 9.14). Since the mammography unit below the table is rotatable, the correct angle can be chosen so that front and back holes of coordinate C12, for example, are superimposed on the image (Fig. 9.15). The breast/template image obtained is remarkable, because the seroma is clearly seen with air/contrast and the template coordinates covering the target volume are easily identified (Figs. 9.16 and 9.17). Half-strength buffered local anesthetic is injected just under the skin surface to raise a skin wheal, and more dilute tumescent local anesthetic with epinephrine is injected directly down the planned holes of insertion for a relatively painless and bloodless procedure (Fig. 9.18). Since moderate compression is applied by the template, the cavity is somewhat spread out and elongated, causing the use of many more catheters than is usually seen with the old-style one- or two-plane implants. An average of 20 catheters are inserted with this procedure. After the needles

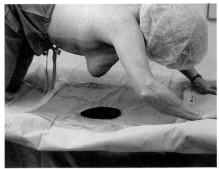

Fig. 9.11 Patient lowering herself onto the sterilely-draped stereotactic core biopsy table with her prepped breast hanging by gravity

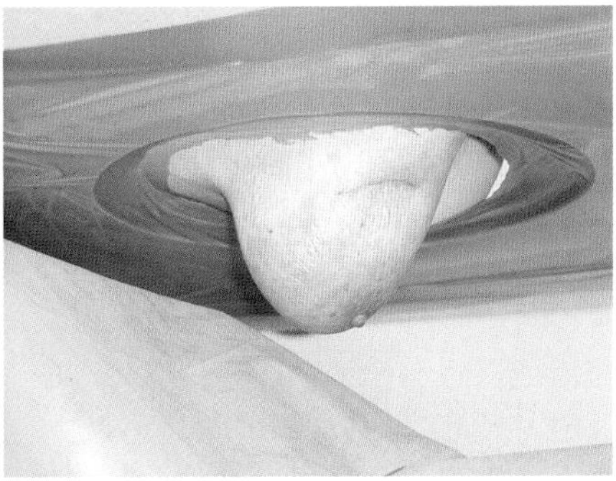

Fig. 9.12 Underneath the table, the breast separates from the chest wall, lungs, and pleura. The physician faces the lumpectomy scar in preparation for attaching the template

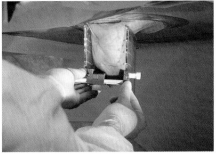

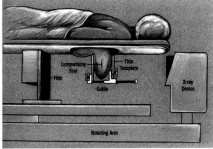

Fig. 9.13 The template is attached with the scar facing outward and the base of the template usually up against the ribs

Fig. 9.14 Overview of prone patient positioning and the underlying rotatable mammography equipment with drapes removed for clarity

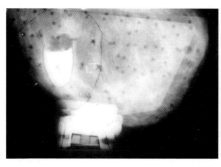

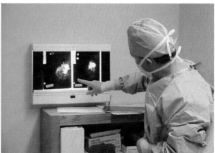

Fig. 9.15 Mammographic image with the front and back template holes approximately aligned. Note the air-contrast level in the lumpectomy cavity. The target volume is delineated, and some of the proposed coordinates are marked by an X

Fig. 9.16 The radiation oncologist or surgeon reviews the films, noting the relation between the contrast and the lumpectomy scar marked by a wire, and plans the implant

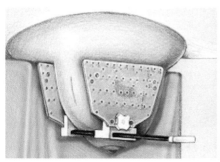

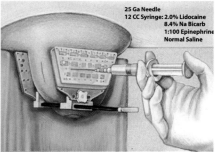

Fig. 9.17 Illustration with the contrast-enhanced lumpectomy cavity in magenta, and the target volume in gray, facilitating image-guided brachytherapy

Fig. 9.18 Tumescent local anesthesia is injected directly down the path of all planned needles before any needles are placed, making sure that a skin wheal is raised on both sides

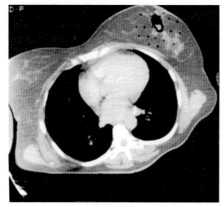

Fig. 9.19 A breast CT is obtained the day after the procedure for 3D treatment planning. Note how the deep plane can be positioned across the pectoralis fascia with this prone technique. The even distribution of catheters around the cavity promotes excellent dosimetry with a high dose homogeneity index

are in place, the template is disassembled and removed from the breast. Plastic Comfort catheters are then inserted inside each needle and pulled until the needle is out and a distal hemispherical button touches the skin at the entry position. A button is placed at the other end of each catheter and attached to the catheter, securing it in place, and the catheter is trimmed to the button. Bacitracin ointment is applied at each entry/exit site, and a Surgibra is used to hold ABD pads in place over the implant so no tape is necessary. A treatment-planning CT scan is obtained of the involved breast on the next day, after any swelling has subsided (Fig. 9.19). The contrast-enhanced lumpectomy cavity is contoured on each CT slice, and this volume is expanded the desired amount (usually 1.5–2 cm) on the computer as the planning target volume (PTV). Within each catheter, dwell times are selected at 0.5-cm intervals so that the PTV is covered by the prescription isodose line, with an acceptable (>0.75) dose homogeneity index. Treatment systems have dose optimization algorithms that facilitate PTV coverage, but it is important to make sure that none of the 150% isodose curves connect between one catheter and an adjacent one.

Since the catheter insertion with this technique is done in the prone position, and the CT-planning and HDR treatments are done in the supine position, there will be some change in the geometry of the catheters as the patient changes position. This is acceptable, because the treatment is done in the same position as the CT-planning. A practical advantage of treating the patient in the supine position is that the deep row of catheters usually drapes across the pectoralis major muscle and chest wall, insuring excellent deep coverage (Fig. 9.19) that is usually the most problematic issue with freehand techniques. Also, pneumothorax occurs in a small percentage of freehand procedures, either from the thin local anesthetic needle or the brachytherapy needle itself, but in the prone position with a parallel plate template system, pneumothorax should never be seen as a complication.

Figure 9.20 demonstrates the typical cosmetic outcome 6 months after brachytherapy with this technique. Note the absence of radiation skin changes, and pock marks that will continue to become fainter and more subtle over time. This is a soft breast.

9.5.4 CT-Guided Supine Catheter Insertion with a Special Breast Template

Not every radiation oncologist or surgeon has easy access to a stereotactic core biopsy table in order to perform prone brachytherapy catheter insertion. The procedure can

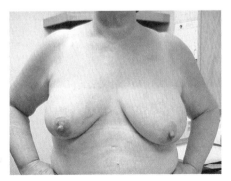

Fig. 9.20 The appearance of the breast 6 months after template interstitial breast brachytherapy

be performed on the radiation oncologist's own treatment-planning CT scanner in the supine position.

Contrast is injected directly into the lumpectomy cavity as described above under ultrasound guidance. The CT table and the patient's breast are draped and prepped in a similar fashion to that described above. The patient is positioned supine on the CT table, with the arm up or down (Fig. 9.21). Tincture of benzoin is applied to the breast to make it sticky and facilitate latching the template onto the skin. The radiation oncologist locates the lumpectomy scar and palpates the seroma. While an assistant pulls up on the breast, separating it from the chest wall, the same breast brachytherapy template is attached to the breast with the upper edge as close to the chest wall as possible.

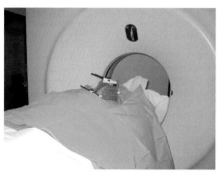 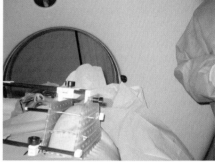

Fig. 9.21 Supine CT-guided breast brachytherapy with the special template (feet to left, head inside the CT aperture). After a prep and sterile draping, the left breast has been pulled up and away from the chest wall as the template is attached

Fig. 9.22 CT-compatible wires are placed in specific template holes to orient the template. One is directly over the lumpectomy scar

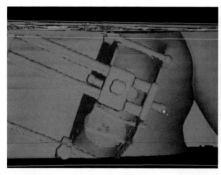 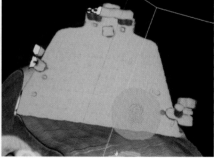

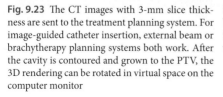

Fig. 9.23 The CT images with 3-mm slice thickness are sent to the treatment planning system. For image-guided catheter insertion, external beam or brachytherapy planning systems both work. After the cavity is contoured and grown to the PTV, the 3D rendering can be rotated in virtual space on the computer monitor

Fig. 9.24 Using the three skin wires, circled here in blue, and the entry/exit holes, it is simple to rotate the image until a "needle's eye view" is visualized with the cavity and PTV evident

CT-compatible catheters or needles can be placed within specific template holes on the skin surface or through breast tissue to also anchor the template and prevent slippage (Fig. 9.22). These marker needles help orient the template and label coordinates on the subsequent images. A CT of the breast is obtained. The images are electronically transferred to the treatment-planning computer. The contrast-enhanced lumpectomy cavity is contoured on each CT slice, and the PTV is grown to the desired margin. A color wire frame illustrates the lumpectomy cavity when the treatment planning computer is put in 3D mode (Figs. 9.23 and 9.24). This visualization works with external beam planning systems such as Pinnacle or brachytherapy planning systems such as Plato. The patient can be rotated in virtual space until the holes in the template are aligned with the marker

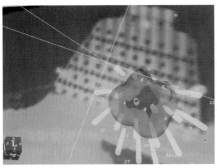
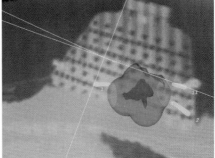

Fig. 9.26 This technique for catheter insertion allows real-time image guidance to check coverage of the PTV. Changes to catheter distribution can be planned and checked as you go along. In this case, the PTV extended deep to the "A" row of the template, so an additional three catheters were inserted underneath the template while an assistant lifted the template further off the chest wall. Depth for coverage and avoidance of the pleura can be measured off the CT image, and all the previous needles provide spatial orientation to help keep the free-hand insertion parallel and straight

Fig. 9.25 For smaller breasts, three pre-CT brachytherapy needles can be inserted through the template and breast tissue after local anesthesia, providing fiduciary markers as well as anchors preventing template slippage

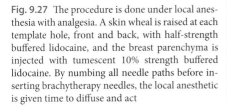

Fig. 9.27 The procedure is done under local anesthesia with analgesia. A skin wheal is raised at each template hole, front and back, with half-strength buffered lidocaine, and the breast parenchyma is injected with tumescent 10% strength buffered lidocaine. By numbing all needle paths before inserting brachytherapy needles, the local anesthetic is given time to diffuse and act

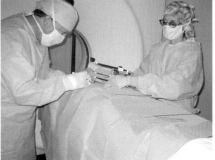

needles helping this process (Fig. 9.25). The coordinates of holes to be implanted are then determined by where the PTV overlaps with the holes in the template in the aligned position (Fig. 9.26). A rule of thumb for any template catheter insertion method is to add a catheter beyond the PTV if the closest hole is inside the PTV. If the template hole is at the edge of the PTV, no additional catheter is necessary.

This technique provides real-time documentation of coverage of the target volume, and allows immediate adjustments or additional catheters. Deep coverage is not as reliable as with the prone technique, but by having an assistant grasp the template, pulling it off the chest wall, an additional row of deep needles can be added using CT guidance (Fig. 9.27). By staying parallel to the previous needles and checking the desired additional depth on the CT scan, pneumothorax can be avoided. If in doubt, a few CT images can be taken after the needles are part-way through the breast.

All needles are inserted with the same analgesia and tumescent local anesthetic procedure described above. At the end, it is advisable to add a few closely spaced superficial catheters flanking the lumpectomy scar, the "gauntlet," ensuring good coverage under the skin without the prescription isodose line going beyond the surface (Fig. 9.28). At the end of the procedure, the catheters do not protrude beyond the skin surface (Fig. 9.29), and connection to the HDR remote afterloader is easily accomplished (Fig. 9.30).

9.5.5 Balloon Intracavitary Catheter Insertion

The MammoSite balloon can be inserted at the time of surgery or later as a separate procedure. In the first couple of years after the catheter became available, most of our MammoSite catheters were inserted at the time of surgery for the patient convenience of having everything done at once. Now, closed wound catheter insertion is preferred because the pathology report is available confirming that the patient is indeed a candidate for APBI or the balloon. We can also perform a preimplant ultrasound or CT to check the skin flap thickness and shape of the cavity, maximizing our success rate with balloon insertion. There are fewer aborted procedures, down from approximately 20% with intraoperative insertion to 10% with a closed wound. Finally, the sutured lumpectomy wound has fully healed and hemostasis has occurred, which further ensures the success of the balloon and in our opinion provides a better cosmetic outcome.

We insert the MammoSite either with the scar-entry technique (SET) or the lateral trocar tunneling technique. In the SET a #11 blade is used to reopen the lumpectomy scar approximately 0.75 cm under local anesthesia. The seroma is rarely more that 1–2 cm deep to the lumpectomy scar, making entry into the seroma easy. After the blade nick, a hemostat or Kelly clam is inserted under ultrasound guidance into the wound and gently opened, and this process repeated until a gush of seroma fluid emanates out of the hole. All the seroma is expressed with the hemostat in place. Immediately upon removal of the hemostat, it is replaced with the deflated MammoSite catheter, checking its position using the ultrasound. The balloon is inflated while the ultrasound image is observed. After the balloon is inflated, Steristrips are placed across the rest of the lumpectomy scar so that the wound does not propagate causing a dehiscence.

There are advantages and disadvantages of SET. SET is an easier technique that avoids the large sharp threatening trocar. Since the ends of a line source are relatively colder, the anisotropy of the isodose curves helps pull the dose away from the skin, which is usually

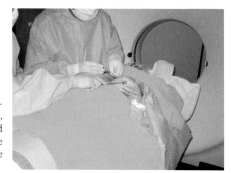

Fig. 9.28 After the template is removed, the physician and physicist survey the needle distribution, looking for potential gaps that could create cold spots. Usually, additional superficial needles are inserted freehand so that there is a smooth isodose curve under the skin near the lumpectomy scar

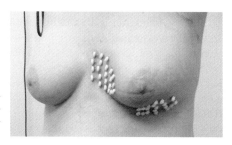

Fig. 9.29 With a catheter-within-a-catheter system, there is no catheter protruding past the buttons, making bandaging easier and enhancing patient comfort between treatments

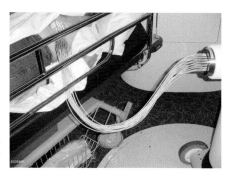

Fig. 9.30 Treatment delivery with a HDR iridium-192 source using a remote afterloading machine. Treatment times are typically 5–10 minutes for a source strength of 4–10 Ci

the biggest problem with MammoSite, and the chest wall. An additional cosmetically detrimental scar on the breast is avoided. On the other hand, some surgeons sometimes object on basic surgical principles to reopening and entering through the same wound. The catheter enters normal to the skin, which can produce bandaging and patient comfort issues. In a worst case scenario, usually happening if the insertion is performed too early for wound healing, the lumpectomy scar can propagate after the MammoSite is put in, causing a wound dehiscence.

The lateral trocar tunneling method is simpler if done at the time of lumpectomy or reexcision, but intraoperative insertions are plagued with the issues noted above. This procedure can be performed with a closed wound using ultrasound guidance. Since breast tissue tends to collapse after a lateral dissection, the large trocar is necessary to provide a path for the catheter into the lumpectomy cavity. This trocar results in a larger scar on the breast, typically 2 cm or larger.

With either technique, good tissue conformance to the balloon surface must be checked. Separations of the breast tissue requiring treatment from the prescription iso-dose curve by air gaps or seroma/hematoma fluid collections are to be avoided.

9.6 Judgment: Selecting the Optimal Technique for a Particular Patient

The major decision trees are:
1. When to offer external beam PBI techniques or breast brachytherapy.
2. If you have decided that breast brachytherapy is preferable, do you select balloon intracavitary or interstitial breast brachytherapy techniques?

For issues and concerns highlighted in the summary section of this chapter, most of the author's patients will receive brachytherapy over external beam PBI. Note that these are theoretical concerns, and more data will be required before one can apply these selection criteria uniformly. The phase III trial does not ask participants to choose patients in the same way that the author selects patients in his clinic; otherwise selection bias would preclude meaningful data analysis to see if these issues withstand the test of randomized scrutiny.

In the author's clinic, those patients who are offered external beam PBI are usually women with large breasts or subareolar primaries, and favorable tumor factors such as older age, generous surgical margins >0.5 cm, and smaller tumors lacking EIC or lymphovascular invasion (LVI).

Similarly, patients who are offered balloon intracavitary brachytherapy have more favorable tumors in breasts that have a thick skin–cavity separation as determined by pretreatment ultrasound. The prescription point for the balloon catheter is only 1 cm beyond the balloon surface, in contrast to the prescription point for interstitial brachytherapy at 2 cm or whatever distance the radiation oncologist and physics team choose. Despite one paper in the literature (Edmundson et al. 2002) implying that breast tissue is compressible, and the balloon can treat as much as 1.6 cm of breast tissue beyond the surgical margin, there are data from the University of Wisconsin indicating that interstitial consistently treats more breast tissue than the balloon catheter (Patel et al. 2005). Furthermore, the compressibility of breast tissue varies between premenopausal dense breasts and postmenopausal fatty breasts.

Because of the physics of balloon intracavitary brachytherapy, prescribing beyond 1 cm results in extraordinary high doses in the breast tissue touching the balloon, so this is strictly forbidden. Interstitial brachytherapy is only limited by the number of catheters inserted, and is determined by geographic coverage. By its nature, interstitial brachytherapy can cover any size or shape cavity, so it is much more dose-controllable than the balloon catheter. As a result, most patients who cannot be treated by the balloon, because it does not fit the cavity or has too narrow a skin separation, can have the balloon pulled, and be treated with interstitial breast brachytherapy.

To decide between balloon intracavitary and interstitial breast brachytherapy, ultrasound is performed in the radiation oncology clinic or radiology after excision with negative margins. In our experience, if the thinnest skin separation at this time is less than 1.0 cm, it is rare that the balloon will fit with a minimum of 7 mm skin separation, given tissue compression after the balloon is expanded. Potential exceptions would be: (1) a good separation in every place except one focal location, and SET is performed to insert the balloon catheter through that thin spot, and (2) a breast surgeon who is willing to go back in and resect an ellipse of skin over the thin section to widen the skin flap, realizing that this maneuver could adversely affect the cosmetic outcome.

An attempt will be made to insert a balloon catheter, and breast CT evaluation the next day will indicate whether it will work or not. If the skin and pleura separations are at least 10 mm the treatment is a go, if the separations are 7–10 mm one is in the gray zone, and if the separations are less than 7 mm abandoning the balloon procedure and proceeding to interstitial or 3D conformal techniques is recommended.

In all cases, a thorough discussion with the breast surgeon, preferably in a multidisciplinary breast oncology clinic/conference, is important. As a team, you must decide if you will offer the balloon or 3D external techniques to young women (e.g. <45 years of age), or EIC- or LVI-positive patients, or to those with surgical margins less than 2–5 mm. You may decide, as we have, to offer interstitial brachytherapy to such higher risk patients and balloon or 3D techniques to the favorable patients with acceptable skin separations or 3D locations.

The clinical judgment and decision-making offered above represents the experience and theoretical concerns of the author and his breast oncology team. Ongoing clinical trials should shed light in the future on appropriate selection criteria for each technique and indeed breast PBI in general.

9.7 Summary

Five techniques of covering the target volume with brachytherapy are reviewed in this chapter. Each has its advantages and disadvantages, and a *strong recommendation* is for the radiation oncology/surgical team to have many, if not all, techniques of delivering PBI in their armamentarium. If a patient who is otherwise a candidate for PBI is unable to receive it by one technique, it is far preferable to be able to take care of her by another technique than to resort back to 6 weeks of whole-breast external beam radiotherapy. For the ongoing phase III clinical trials, it is critically important to keep the patient on the appropriate arm of the study even if technical issues make one PBI technique problematic.

There are theoretical reasons why brachytherapy may result in better outcomes than external beam PBI techniques, such as 3D conformal or intensity-modulated radiotherapy. First, brachytherapy is prescribed to the periphery of the target volume, with all tissue inside this envelope receiving a significantly higher dose of radiation. We call this the inherent "boost" provided by the dose inhomogeneity that is part and parcel of brachytherapy. Indeed, the radiation dose immediately adjacent to a source dwell position within a catheter can be very high. The central higher radiation dose with brachytherapy can improve local control, but also result in possible fat necrosis, fibrosis, telangiectasia, or other late effects of irradiation. Second, the rapid fall off of dose away from the catheter(s) should reduce the exposure of normal tissue to radiation. External beam PBI techniques can traverse significant amounts of normal tissue to get to the target, such as the thyroid gland, opposite breast, lung, heart, chest wall, uninvolved breast tissue, skin, or other organs that simply get in the way of the beam. Low doses of irradiation may be even more carcinogenic than therapeutic doses; so long term effects must be watched for the next 10 to 25 years on these organs. Third, the typically homogeneous dose distribution with external beam PBI has inspired the experts in the field to recommend higher prescribed doses than with brachytherapy, 385 cGy per fraction in contrast to 340 cGy per fraction, for example. The net effect is a higher total prescribed dose, a higher dose per fraction, and more normal tissue exposure to radiation with external beam PBI techniques. There is little or no long-term data with PBI at these doses per fraction and a formal radiobiological review of the potential effect on late tissue effects and tumor control probability has not been published. Only the clinical trials will shed ultimate light on the impact these theoretical concerns will have on outcomes.

One issue that has not been resolved involves our current practice of uniformly treating a certain margin (1–2 cm) around the lumpectomy cavity, regardless of where the tumor is centered or where the pathologic margin is closest. When viewing specimen radiographs, it is rare that the lesion is centered within the fat, like a sunny-side-up egg. Instead the visible lesion tends to be more commonly eccentrically located near one aspect of the specimen, with a large area of uninvolved fat or normal breast tissue at one end and the tumor approximating the edge on the other end. Ideally, one would want to generously treat the breast tissue adjacent to the close margin and minimize treatment to the breast tissue on the side that has generous surgical margins. Practically, however, contouring PBI in this manner has technical challenges, and it is easier to simply treat all margins to a given distance.

The future of breast brachytherapy is promising, with many techniques for accomplishing target volume coverage, and more innovations to come as industry interest in this expanding technology blossoms. Meticulous attention to detail in selecting patients and covering the target volume is key to future success. Learning the above techniques is essential to serving your patients and participating in the ongoing clinical trials. Avenues for learning these techniques include studying this textbook, visiting the clinics of experienced breast brachytherapists, formal schools offered by societies and equipment manufacturers, and of course building your own clinical experience.

References

1. Aron BS (1984) Teaching of radiation oncology residents. University of Cincinnati College of Medicine, Cincinnati, Ohio
2. Baglan KL, Martinez AA, Frazier RC, et al (2001) The use of high-dose brachytherapy alone after lumpectomy in patients with early-stage breast cancer treated with breast-conserving therapy. Int J Radiat Oncol Biol Phys 50:1003–1011
3. Brennan MF, Hilaris B, Shiu MH, et al (1987) Local recurrence in adult soft tissue sarcoma: a randomized trial of brachytherapy. Arch Surg 122:1289–1293

4. Edmundson GK, Vicini FA, Chen PY, et al (2002) Dosimetric characteristics of the MammoSite RTS: a new breast brachytherapy applicator. Int J Radiat Oncol Biol Phys 52:1132–1139

5. Keynes G (1937) Conservative treatment of cancer of the breast. BMJ 2:643

6. King TA, Bolton JS, Kuske RR, et al (2000) Long-term results of wide-field brachytherapy as the sole method of radiation therapy after segmental mastectomy for T(is,1,2) breast cancer. Am J Surg 180:299–304

7. Kuske RR, Boyer C, Bolton JS, et al (2004a) Long-term results of the Ochsner Clinic prospective phase II breast brachytherapy trial. San Antonio Breast Meeting

8. Kuske RR, Winter K, Arthur D, et al (2004b) A phase II trial of brachytherapy alone following lumpectomy for stage I or II breast cancer: initial outcomes of RTOG 95-17. American Society of Clinical Oncology

9. Morrow M, Harris JR (2000) Local management of invasive breast cancer. In: Harris JR, Lippman ME, Morrow M, Osborne CK (eds) Diseases of the breast, 2nd edn. Lippincott Williams and Wilkins, p 528, Table 6

10. Patel R, et al (2005) Presented at the 3rd Annual School of Breast Brachytherapy, Las Vegas, Nevada, March

11. Ribeiro GG, Dunn G, Swindell R, et al (1990) Conservation of the breast using two different radiotherapy techniques: interim report of a clinical trial. Clin Oncol (R Coll Radiol) 2:27–34

12. Vicini FA, Baglan K, Kestin L, et al (2002) The emerging role of brachytherapy in the management of patients with breast cancer. Semin Radiat Oncol 12:31–39

13. Vicini FA, Remouchanps V, Wallace M, et al (2003) Ongoing clinical experience utilizing 3D conformal external beam radiotherapy to deliver partial-breast irradiation in patients with early-stage breast cancer treated with breast-conserving therapy. Int J Radiat Oncol Biol Phys 57:1247–1253

The MammoSite Technique for Accelerated Partial Breast Irradiation

10

Martin E. Keisch and Frank A. Vicini

Contents

10.1 Introduction

The MammoSite RTS (Cytyc Surgical Products) is an inflatable balloon breast brachytherapy applicator. The introduction of the MammoSite RTS has overcome some of the perceived technical barriers of the multicatheter approach, such as the steep learning curve, and challenging quality assurance (Arthur 2003). The device fills the surgical cavity giving a dose of radiation that is highest on the surface and falls off rapidly covering the immediately surrounding 1 cm of breast tissue (Edmundson et al. 2002). Since the FDA approval of the MammoSite, the device has become the most frequently employed method of partial breast irradiation (PBI) with over 3000 physicians in more than 700 centers trained in its use. More than 12,000 patients are estimated to have been treated using the device.

    The original device is a dual lumen spherical balloon catheter inflatable to 4–5 cm with a central lumen for the high dose-rate (HDR) iridium-192 (Ir^{192}) source. The catheter is a silicone balloon and shaft approximately 6 mm in diameter and 15 cm in length (see Fig. 10.1). The shaft contains a small inflation channel and a larger central "treatment" channel for passage of the HDR source. A needleless injection port is attached to the inflation channel, and a Luer fitting is attached to the treatment channel. An adapter is provided separately, to connect with any brand of commercially available HDR remote afterloading device. Additional sizes and shapes are available and are addressed below. The applicator is placed into the lumpectomy cavity, inflated to fill the cavity, and used to treat the lumpectomy margin.

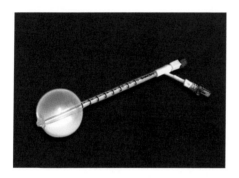

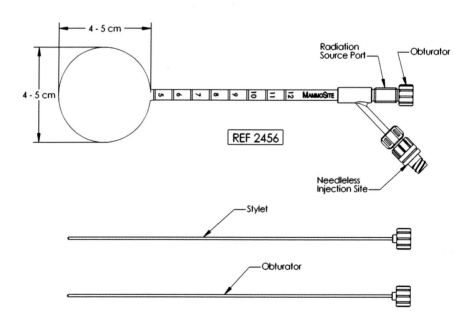

Fig. 10.1 MammoSite Dual Lumen Breast Brachytherapy Catheter (with permission of Cytyc Surgical Products)

10.2 History of the Applicator

The MammoSite was developed as a sister product to an inflatable balloon brain brachytherapy applicator, the GliaSite (Dempsey et al. 1998). After modifying the liquid iodine-125 design for HDR and developing the concept into a functional device, animal testing was performed both to determine functionality and to begin understanding the tissue effects of radiation delivered via this novel approach (Spurlock et al. 2000). After completing animal studies, a human phase I/II trial was performed (Keisch et al. 2003).

10.2.3 MammoSite and the FDA Trial

Between May 2000 and October of 2001, 70 patients were enrolled in a multi-institution prospective phase I/II trial approved by the investigational review board (IRB) designed to test the MammoSite device's safety and performance in preparation for attempted FDA approval either as the sole modality of irradiation (PBI) or as a boost dose after whole-breast irradiation (Keisch et al. 2004). However, all patients entered on the trial were enrolled in the PBI arm at the treating physician's choice.

Eligibility requirements included: age ≥45 years, tumor ≤2 cm, invasive ductal histology, negative nodal status, negative marginal status (National Surgical Adjuvant Breast and Bowel Project definition), applicator placement within 10 weeks of final lumpectomy procedure, and a cavity post-lumpectomy with one dimension of at least 3.0 cm. Ineligibility criteria included: an extensive intraductal component, pure intraductal cancers, lobular histology, or collagen vascular disease. Additionally, patients were deemed ineligible for technical issues including inadequate balloon–skin distance, excessive cavity size, or poor balloon–cavity conformance. Patients could be enrolled prior to final lumpectomy to allow device placement in an open fashion during that procedure; other patients were enrolled post-lumpectomy and implanted using a closed technique (typically under ultrasound guidance).

Final determination of suitability for HDR brachytherapy treatment was made after device placement using computed tomography (CT) imaging in all patients to measure the applicator–skin distance (minimum requirement 5 mm). Conformance was assessed by CT imaging after device placement, and was deemed acceptable if the balloon was in contact with the lumpectomy margin uniformly, without air or fluid-filled gaps. CT and fluoroscopic simulation were used for treatment planning, both to determine the single dwell position in the center of the balloon and for daily confirmation of balloon diameter. Acceptable diameters ranged from 4 to 5 cm, corresponding to a fill volume of 35–70 ml. In all cases, 34 Gy was delivered at a point 1 cm from the surface of the balloon in fractions of 3.4 Gy twice daily over 5–7 elapsed days with various commercially available remote afterloaders. Interfraction separation was a minimum of 6 hours.

A total of 70 patients were enrolled, 54 patients were implanted, and 43 patients were ultimately eligible for and received brachytherapy as the sole radiation modality after lumpectomy. Figure 10.2 shows the distribution of patients from enrollment through treatment and the reasons for not being implanted or treated. In most patients not treated, failure to treat was due to either technical or pathologic features. Patients implanted after lumpectomy were more likely to be treated than those implanted at the time of lumpectomy due to knowledge regarding final pathology. The patients tolerated therapy well. The most commonly reported radiation effects were limited to mild or moderate erythema without desquamation. In addition, other less common but significant events included moist desquamation in three patients, two infections including an abscess requiring drainage, and three seromas requiring drainage due to patient discomfort. No definite serious device-related events were reported. In four patients, serious adverse events were noted that were potentially related to the device; these were the previously mentioned abscess and seromas. The trial led to United States FDA approval of the device in May 2002 (Keisch et al. 2003).

10.3 Physics of the MammoSite

10.3.1 General

The 4–5 cm spherical device is the best characterized in the literature. It was originally used with a single dwell position in the center of the balloon. The FDA trial used a prescription point 1 cm from the balloon surface at the equator. The depth dose profile is such that the 4 cm diameter volume (35 ml) has a balloon surface dose of 225% when prescribed to 1 cm. Due to the inverse square law the balloon surface dose is lower with increasing fill volumes. Additionally, the total volume receiving the prescription dose increases with increasing fill volumes and balloon diameter. Figure 10.3 shows the PDD curves around the spherical balloon normalized to the prescription point for inflation diameters of 4, 5, and 6 cm.

Data exist comparing the dosimetry of the MammoSite to that of traditional interstitial catheter-based implants (Edmundson et al. 2002). This study confirmed that coverage of the target (D90) is generally equal to or superior to catheter implants. The dose homogeneity with the MammoSite seen across all balloon fill volumes appears to be acceptable when compared to criteria understood to be important in avoiding soft-tissue complications. Dose homogeneity as measured by the dose homogeneity index (DHI) is not as uniform as with a modern CT-planned multicatheter implant. The volume receiving over 200% of the prescription is negligible, and the volume receiving 150% falls below the volume found by Wazer et al. (2001) to correlate with a higher incidence of fat necrosis. Dosimetric studies by Edmundson et al. (2002) and Dickler et al. (2004) both demonstrate that the effective treatment depth is often higher than 1 cm due to stretching of the breast tissue forming the cavity wall. The depth can be over 1.5 cm quite frequently, depending on the lumpectomy cavity size and the balloon inflation volume. The actual volume of the tissue receiving the prescription dose is comparable to that of a catheter-based implant (Edmundson et al. 2002).

10.3.2 Single Dwell vs. Multiple Dwell

As noted above the device was designed for a single dwell position in the center of the balloon. When treated and prescribed in this fashion, the dose nearly matches the shape of the balloon in all directions. After the FDA trial, patients were treated with multi-

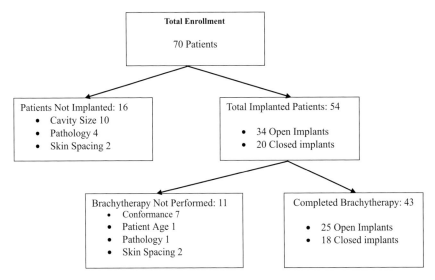

Fig. 10.2 FDA Trial patients (Keisch et al. 2003)

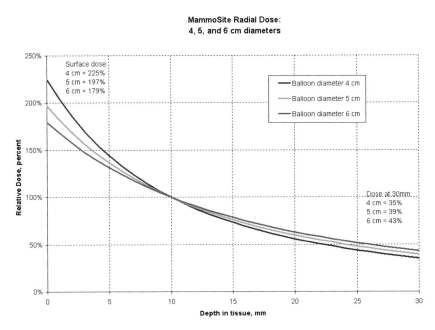

Fig. 10.3 Radial dose distribution around various diameter spherical balloon applicators (courtesy of G. Edmundson)

ple dwell positions, optimized by a variety of methods (Astrahan et al. 2004; Dickler et al. 2005). Physicians were motivated to optimize using multiple dwell positions to improve coverage of the planning target volume (PTV), to decrease skin dose, and to attempt to recover implants with less than perfect balloon geometry. Although studies have shown that optimizing multiple dwell positions can improve coverage and other dosimetric challenges, it is generally at some cost, whether over- or under-dosing some breast tissue (Fig. 10.4). The issue has been explored in depth by the group from Tufts-Brown (Cardarelli et al. 2005), who demonstrated the ability of a plan with multiple dwell positions to improve both homogeneity and coverage in the setting of less than perfect anatomy. An example would be in a patient with a cavity in proximity to the chest wall, or skin. Another setting potentially benefiting from an optimized plan would be a patient with an air- or fluid-filled cavity. In the authors' experience a combination of preplanning the angle of approach during device placement, and optimizing multiple dwell positions with either the elliptical or spherical balloon offers the most flexibility in anatomically challenging situations. However, with an ideal implant geometry and anatomy a single dwell position is best.

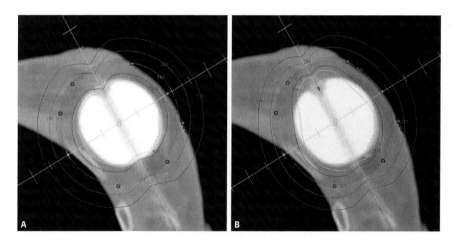

Fig. 10.4 Single dwell position (**A**), and Optimized multiple dwell positions (**B**) demonstrating sparing of skin and deep tissues at the expense of increased inhomogeneity within the PTV (Astrahan et al. 2004)

10.3.3 Elliptical MammoSite

The elliptical balloon measures 4×6 cm and requires multiple dwell positions for appropriate dosimetry. It was designed to improve the filling of the sometimes irregularly shaped lumpectomy cavity. The standard weighting of five dwell positions loaded 50:66:100:66:50 matches the 200% isodose to the balloon surface. Depending on the angle of balloon entry the weightings can be optimized to potentially spare superficial or deep structures such as the skin or chest wall, while still providing good coverage of the PTV. Unlike the spherical balloons, there is a limited fill range of 60–65 ml inflation requiring care in determining its appropriateness as an applicator. Additionally, the elliptical balloon must be oriented nearly along the long axis of the cavity, making the surgical approach more limited. Nevertheless, the device can be useful in some clinical situations.

10.3.4 Contrast Effect

The recommended mixture for filling the balloon is an approximately 5–10% mixture of contrast agent and saline to allow visualization of the balloon on plain radiographs, without significant artifact on CT imaging. It has been reported that excessive concentrations of contrast agent can lead to significant underdosing due to absorption by the contrast solution (Cardarelli et al. 2005). Clinically, this problem should not arise as excessive concentrations of contrast agent would degrade the CT image to a degree such that determination of appropriateness for treatment would be difficult.

10.4 Implantation Techniques

There are three general placement methods: the lateral techniques (either open or closed), and the scar entry technique or SET. The guidelines are summarized below.

For balloon placement at the time of removal of the breast tumor (open lateral technique), the device should be inserted lateral to the lumpectomy cavity opening using a small skin incision and a trocar-created pathway while the wound is still open. The trocar is then removed and the deflated balloon is inserted through the pathway. The MammoSite balloon is then inflated with a mixture of contrast agent and saline (approximately 5–10%) to approximate the balloon surface to the inside of the lumpectomy cavity. The cavity and balloon are inspected visually for good conformance and the lumpectomy opening is closed using standard technique with the exception of an additional deep layer closer in the breast tissue to ensure adequate skin spacing (Fig. 10.5). No suturing of the external portion of the MammoSite to the skin surface is recommended.

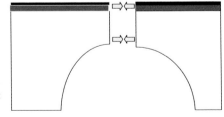

Fig. 10.5 Schematic drawing showing both sub-cuticular closure and deep closure within breast tissue employed to improve skin spacing.

For implants after the tumor has already been removed, the balloon can be placed using one of two techniques. An 8-mm trocar is guided into the center of the cavity using ultrasound imaging (with proper local anesthesia). The trocar is then replaced with the deflated MammoSite. The seroma is allowed to drain. The MammoSite is expanded using the 5–10% contrast agent/saline mixture. No external suture is required to hold the balloon in place. The external portion of the MammoSite is then dressed. Alternatively, the device can also be implanted after lumpectomy surgery through the surgical scar. The procedure is referred to as the SET method. It is accomplished under local anesthesia by opening the surgical scar and carefully dissecting down to the lumpectomy cavity. Once the lumpectomy cavity is penetrated, the seroma fluid in the cavity is drained. The MammoSite is then inserted through this opening. The MammoSite is inflated with fluid to fill the cavity. Stitches on either side of MammoSite along the surgical scar are placed to prevent propagation of the wound opening.

For closed placement, the cavity should still be closed at the time of lumpectomy with a superficial and deep closure to improve the likelihood of a successful placement. A typical placement takes less than 15 minutes whether performed at time of lumpectomy or as a closed procedure. The patient is then imaged with CT to determine appropriateness for treatment.

The device is simple and with simplicity comes a degree of limitation. An appropriate cavity is necessary. The configuration of the cavity is determined by direct inspection or by use of a disposable sizing device at the time of lumpectomy, or by CT or ultrasound prior to a delayed placement. The cavity must have an appropriate size, configuration, and depth to assure a favorable dosimetry. Surgeons are trained to close the cavity subcutaneously to improve results by improving the depth to the balloon surface, thus reducing skin dose. Balloon orientation can also improve dosimetry by taking advantage of the source anisotropy, if placed directly through the point of minimal skin thickness (Edmundson et al. 2002). Placement in this fashion can reduce the skin dose significantly if the entry angle and placement site are carefully chosen (Fig. 10.6).

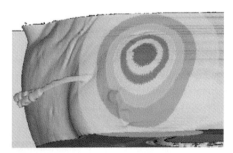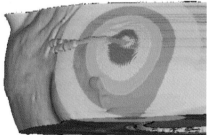

Fig. 10.6 Demonstration of the relative reduction in skin dose due to placement approach to take advantage of the anisotropy of the source (Edmundson et al. 2002)

10.5 Other Considerations

The balloon occasionally ruptures as a result of balloon abrasion by needles, surgical clips, or perhaps friction with fibrous tissue. Some early experiences have had significant rupture rates, while others have had low rates (Harper et al. 2005; Keisch et al. 2003; Kirk et al. 2004). When rupture occurs the balloon must be replaced, reimaged and replanned, and treatment continues. A second-generation spherical balloon has been FDA-cleared and appears more resistant to rupture. Since the release the original device, the manufacturer has developed and released to additional devices, a 5- to 6-cm variable volume sphere and a 4×6-cm elliptical balloon with a single volume. The new devices are also FDA-approved. The larger balloon allows larger cavities to be filled completely improving conformance after larger lumpectomies (Richards et al. 2004). The elliptical balloon provides additional flexibility for irregularly shaped or unusually located lumpectomy cavities. The elliptical balloon requires multiple dwell positions for routine treatment, adding a slightly higher level of complexity to the treatment planning, but at the same time additional flexibility in dosimetric coverage by allowing variable treatment depths along the long axis of the ellipse.

10.6 Appropriateness for Treatment

Final determination of suitability for HDR brachytherapy treatment is made after the device is placed using CT imaging in all patients to measure the applicator–skin distance, and to assess conformance and balloon symmetry. Skin spacing is an approximate surrogate for skin dose. With a distance of 5 mm from the balloon surface to the skin, the dose ranges from a maximum of 145% for a 4-cm sphere to 130% for a 6-cm sphere, not accounting for any dose reduction due to potential effect of anisotropy, or increases due to optimization of multiple dwell positions. Conformance is a descriptor of the degree to which the balloon is in direct contact with the lumpectomy margin, and as such relates to the degree of uniform coverage of the PTV. The recommended minimally accepted conformance is that which results in a D90 of 90%.

Two methods exist for determination of acceptable conformance. First, the air- or fluid-filled spaces around the balloon can be contoured and measured. The resulting volume must be less than 10% of the volume of the PTV as determined by expanding the balloon by 1 cm and subtracting the balloon volume (Fig. 10.9). The second method is performed by contouring a 1-cm rim of tissue in all directions around the balloon (Fig. 10.7), planning the dose to a prescription point 1 cm from the balloon surface at the equator, and directly measuring the D90 from a dose–volume histogram. The latter method is more accurate and allows assessment of the ability of volume optimization calculations to improve coverage. Asymmetry of the balloon can be subtle and inconsequential, such as in the case of local deformation due to the surrounding tissue impinging on the applicator (Fig. 10.8), or it can be due to central lumen deviation from tissue and cavity entry effects leading to significant variation in dose from one side of the balloon to the other (Fig. 10.9). Central lumen deviation of 2 mm or less results in variability in dose of 15% or less, and is deemed clinically acceptable.

10.7 Clinical Results

The FDA study patients continue to be followed for local control, toxicity, and cosmetic endpoints. Of the initial 43 patients, 40 are enrolled in the long-term follow-up trial. Information from a 48-month follow-up was presented in October 2005 (Keisch and

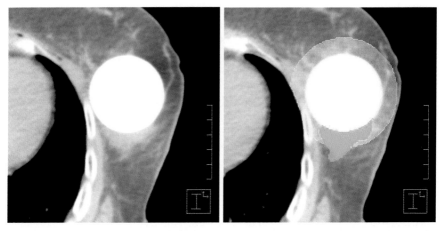

Fig. 10.7 CT scan for determination of suitability for treatment due to a small seroma. In this case the seroma measured less than 10% of the PTV and the implant was acceptable for treatment

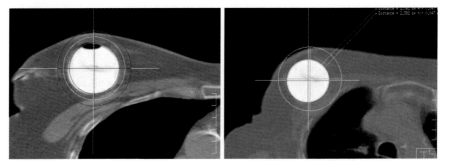

Fig. 10.8 Minimal asymmetry of little dosimetric consequence

Fig. 10.9 Central lumen deviation of 3mm in a 42 mm diameter balloon.

Vicini 2003) and to date tolerance and cosmesis remains excellent. No local failures have occurred. Of the 40 patients, 33 (82.5%) were reported to have a good/excellent cosmetic result. A correlation exists between rated cosmetic outcome and skin spacing, a surrogate measure of skin dose. At the last update, skin spacing was associated with an improved cosmetic result at cut-offs of 7 and 8 mm in separate 2×2 analyses (P=0.13 and P=0.04, respectively). There was a significant correlation between skin spacing and cosmesis as a continuous variable (Wilcoxon Rank Sum test, P=0.03). Among all 41 patients, the cosmetic results were excellent/good in 85% of those with a skin spacing ≥7 mm and in 57% of those with a skin spacing 5–6 mm. The cosmetic results were excellent/good in 89% of patients with a skin spacing ≥8 mm and in 58% of those with a spacing of 5–7 mm. Although some concern has been expressed over the relatively high incidence of telangiectasias (40% at 48 months), it should be noted that these occurred over an area typically limited to an area of 3×3 cm or smaller. Of the 40 patients, 16 (40%) had local telangiectasias and 14 had localized fibrosis (35%). Fibrosis was not associated with any variable examined. Telangiectasias occurred more frequently in patients who had a skin spacing of 5–7 mm (67%) than in those with a spacing of ≥7 mm (29%, $P=0.03$). The median skin spacing of patients with and without telangiectasias was 0.75 cm and 1.15 cm, respectively ($P=0.00009$). Local breast tissue retraction was noted in five patients in whom the median skin spacing was 0.72 mm compared with 1.15 mm in those not developing retraction ($P=0.04$). Local breast tissue retraction occurred in 25% of patients with a skin spacing of 5–7 mm and in 7% of those with a spacing of >7 mm ($P=0.15$). Three patients (7.5%) experienced fat necrosis, but this was not symptomatic and did not require treatment (radiographic findings only). No patient has developed adverse sequelae requiring surgical correction or chronic analgesics. Patient satisfaction was rated excellent or good 100% of the time.

Since FDA approval, additional MammoSite clinical research has continued. Several single-institution series are ongoing, and a large multi-institution registry trial has accrued approximately 1500 patients and is maturing (Keisch et al. 2005; Vicini et al. 2005). A combined study of results in 11 single-institution trials and the FDA trial is underway (Keisch et al. 2003). To date, all the studies support the initial FDA trial results.

The manufacturer initiated a registry trial in 2002 after FDA approval for the device was obtained. The American Society of Breast Surgeons has assumed full responsibility for the trial including all accrual registration, data collection, analysis, and quality assurance. The trial closed to accrual in August 2004. All currently available information from this dataset supports the acceptability of the treatment with regard to tolerance and cosmesis (Keisch et al. 2005). The preliminary data on 1419 patients with a median follow-up of 5 months shows a similar relationship between skin spacing and cosmetic outcome as seen in the FDA trial. Additionally, infection can have an impact on cosmesis. The infection rate was 8% overall with 5% felt to be device-related. Over time, more patients were implanted in the closed setting leading to a lower explantation rate due to adverse pathology. No statistically significant difference in infection rates was noted for open versus closed placement techniques (Keisch et al. 2005; Vicini et al. 2005).

In September 2004, 12 institutions representing a combined experience of 577 patients with a median follow-up of over 17 months and a minimum follow-up of 6 months met at an independent meeting sponsored by Virginia Commonwealth University (VCU) to review the combined experience. The data continue to support the safety and utility of the device. Infection rates and other adverse events were well within acceptable limits. The infection rate was approximately 7%. The local recurrence rate was 0.9%. It is anticipated that the results of this collaborative meeting will be published in the near future (Arthur D, personal communication). The institutions included several that had already published their initial experiences (Kirk et al. 2004; Richards et al. 2004).

Toxicity is an important end-point and traditionally is broken down into acute and chronic and/or delayed toxicity. Several acute side effects are common with the MammoSite RTS including erythema and subsequent hyperpigmentation of the skin overlying the implant, seroma formation, and breast tenderness (Keisch et al. 2003). Less frequently seen are the side effects of moist desquamation, delayed healing and infection. Chronic or delayed toxicities include fat necrosis, skin atrophy, telangiectasias, and fibrosis (Keisch and Vicini 2003). From the data available, the incidences of the common and self-limited side effects of erythema, hyperpigmentation and breast tenderness are similar to those found with interstitial multicatheter-based brachytherapy (Keisch 2005). These symptoms effect small volumes of tissue and resolve quickly. Seroma formation is common (10–30%) when assessed by imaging such as ultrasound, but symptomatic seromas are relatively rare (Chen et al.; Harper et al. 2005; Kirk et al. 2004). Of interest is the incidence of persistent seromas in patients not undergoing MammoSite balloon-based brachytherapy, which is as high as 30% at 6 months after lumpectomy (Dowlatshahi et al. 2004). Management of seromas should be conservative. Although they can be aspirated, caution is advised due to the potential increased risk of infection.

When dealing with an indwelling catheter, proper measures to avoid infection are an important consideration. Published infection rates vary from 5% to 16% (Harper et al. 2005; Keisch et al. 2003, 2005; Kirk et al. 2004; Zannis et al. 2003). The VCU meeting pooled data showing an infection rate of 7 % of the 577 patients treated by experienced physicians. It should be noted that some of these patients are included in multiple datasets including the FDA trial, the MUSC study, the St. Vincent's study and the ASBS registry trial. The strength of the VCU data lies in the experience level of the treating physicians. All in attendance felt that infection rates are directly related to the level of catheter site care, which should include strict dressing changes and keeping the site dry. The use of prophylactic antibiotics was controversial but may be helpful. Very few complications requiring surgical intervention have been documented, however, it should be noted that some alarming case reports exist including flap necrosis and persistent infections requiring drainage. The most common intervention is aspiration of seromas, whether for symptoms or for diagnostic evaluation. The incidence is not clear, but from the authors experience is approximately 5–10 % in the community, though far less at high volume centers. Fat necrosis is an important delayed toxicity that can cause tender induration in a limited local area at the site of brachytherapy and cause patient alarm (Wazer et al. 2001). Both asymptomatic and symptomatic fat necrosis occurs, with many more asymptomatic events noted. Overall, fat necrosis is rare with symptomatic events recorded in less than 5 % of cases (Keisch et al. 2003, 2005; Vicini et al. 2005), comparing favorably to multi-catheter brachytherapy (Keisch 2005; Wazer et al. 2001). Regardless, it appears to be a most commonly a temporary, self-limited toxicity that may occur and resolve one to two years after treatment. Rarely fat necrosis may cause significant symptoms, requiring intervention. Surgical removal of the necrotic tissue typically allows the symptoms to resolve. Overlying skin changes can occur and may have a lasting impact on cosmesis as noted above. The changes include both telangiectasias and atrophy, which are located focally at the brachytherapy site. When evaluating the patients with the longest follow-up, the FDA trial patients, with follow-up out to over four years, these skin changes appear stabilize after two years.

10.8 Conclusions

The MammoSite RTS devices are a relatively new, but commonly employed method of partial breast irradiation. The device has reported experiences with follow up as long as 40 months (Keisch et al. 2003), and patient numbers as high as 1500 (Vicini et al. 2005). It is the most readily available form of partial breast irradiation at the current time. The technique requires close interaction between the surgeon and the radiation oncologist for optimum use. Compared to multicatheter based brachytherapy the device placement, dosimetry, and physics is relatively simple, and at the same time somewhat less flexible. The resultant dose distribution is less homogenous, but more conformal than both external beam, and multicatheter based approaches. The MammoSite is currently one of three forms of partial breast irradiation employed on the National Cancer Institute sponsored phase III trial randomizing between whole and partial breast irradiation.

References

1. Arthur D (2003) Accelerated partial breast irradiation: a change in treatment paradigm for early stage breast cancer. J Surg Oncol 84(4):185–191

2. Astrahan MA, Jozsef G, Streeter OE (2004) Optimization of MammoSite therapy. Int J Radiat Oncol Biol Phys 58(1):220–232

3. Cardarelli GA, Rivard MJ, Tsai J (2006) Multiple dwell positions for the MammoSite HDR ^{192}Ir brachytherapy applicator. Brachytherapy (in press)

4. Chen P, Vicini F, Kestin L, et al (2006) Long-term cosmetic results and toxicity with accelerated partial breast irradiation (APBI) utilizing interstitial brachytherapy. Cancer 106:991–999

5. Dempsey JF, Williams JA, Stubbs JB, et al (1998) Dosimetric properties of a novel brachytherapy balloon applicator for the treatment of malignant brain-tumor resection-cavity margins. Int J Radiat Oncol Biol Phys 42(2):421–429

6. Dickler A, Kirk M, Choo J, et al (2004) Treatment volume and dose optimization of the MammoSite breast brachytherapy applicator. Int J Radiat Oncol Biol Phys 59(2):469–474

7. Dickler A, Kirk M, Chu J, Nguyen C (2005) The MammoSite breast brachytherapy applicator: a review of technique and outcomes. Brachytherapy 4(2):130–136

8. Dowlatshahi K, Snider HC, Gittleman MA, et al (2004) Early experience with balloon brachytherapy for breast cancer. Arch Surg 139:603–608

9. Edmundson GK, Vicini FA, Chen PY, et al (2002) Dosimetric characteristics of the MammoSite RTS, a new breast brachytherapy applicator. Int J Radiat Oncol Biol Phys 52(4):1132–1139

10. Harper JL, Jenrette JM, Vanek KN, et al (2005) Acute complications of MammoSite brachytherapy: a single institution's initial clinical experience. Int J Radiat Oncol Biol Phys 61(1):169–174

11. Keisch M (2005) MammoSite. Expert Rev Med Devices 2(4):387–394

12. Keisch M, Vicini F (2003) In response to Drs. Kuerer, Pawlik, and Strom (editorial). Int J Radiat Oncol Biol Phys 57(3):900–902

13. Keisch M, Vicini F, Kuske R, et al (2003) Initial clinical experience with the MammoSite breast brachytherapy applicator in women with early-stage breast cancer treated with breast-conserving therapy. Int J Radiat Oncol Biol Phys 55(2):289–293

14. Keisch M, Vicini F, Scroggins T, et al (2005) Thirty-nine month results with the MammoSite brachytherapy applicator: details regarding cosmesis, toxicity and local control in partial breast irradiation. Int J Radiat Oncol Biol Phys 63:56 (abstract)

15. Kirk MC, Hsi WC, Chu J, et al (2004) Dose perturbation induced by radiographic contrast inside brachytherapy balloon applicators. Med Phys 31(5):1219–1224

16. Richards GM, Berson AM, Rescigno J, et al (2004) Acute toxicity of high-dose-rate intracavitary brachytherapy with the MammoSite applicator in patients with early-stage breast cancer. Ann Surg Oncol 11(8):739–746

17. Spurlock JP, Kuske RR, McKinnon WMP, et al (2000) A caprine breast model for testing a novel balloon brachytherapy device. OJVR 4(1):106–123

18. Vicini F, Beitsch P, Quiet C, et al (2005) First analysis of patient demographics, technical repro-
    ducibility, cosmesis, and early toxicity. Cancer 104(6):1138–1148

19. Wazer DE, Lowther D, Boyle T, et al (2001) Clinically evident fat necrosis in women treated
    with high-dose-rate brachytherapy alone for early-stage breast cancer. Int J Radiat Oncol Biol
    Phys 50:107–111

20. Zannis VJ, Walker LC, Barclay-White B, et al (2003) Postoperative ultrasound-guided percuta-
    neous placement of a new breast brachytherapy balloon catheter. Am J Surg 186(4):383–385

3D Conformal External Beam Technique

Yasmin Hasan and Frank A. Vicini

11

Contents

11.1 Introduction

Three-dimensional conformal external beam accelerated partial breast irradiation (3D conformal APBI) allows non-invasive delivery of hypofractionated adjuvant radiation treatment to the region of the breast at highest risk of local recurrence. The potential advantages of a 3D conformal radiation therapy approach to partial breast irradiation (PBI) compared to brachytherapy include improved dose homogeneity within the target volume and, therefore, likely better cosmetic outcome. In addition, elimination of an additional surgical procedure may reduce complication rates and cost. While brachytherapy requires additional training, most radiation facilities already have the technologic tools and experience required to deliver 3D conformal APBI. The primary disadvantage is that the breast represents a moving target, and as a result, potentially larger volumes of normal breast tissue may need to be irradiated to avoid a geographic miss, with uncertain effects on cosmetic outcome.

In developing a partial breast 3D conformal technique, specific objectives include: (1) defining an appropriate clinical target volume (CTV), (2) defining dose-volume constraints for the entire ipsilateral breast, contralateral breast, lung, heart, and skin to assist in treatment plan optimization, (3) developing a relatively standardized beam arrangement (within the geometric couch and gantry angle limitations for the linear accelerator) that can be readily adapted to a majority of patients and that optimizes target coverage and minimizes the dose to normal structures, (4) defining an appropriate CTV-to-PTV (planning target volume) margin accounting for the geometric uncertainty of the CTV location as a result of respiratory motion and daily patient set-up error, (5) verification of accurate dose delivery, and (6) assessing patient tolerance (Baglan et al. 2003). At the present time, the two ways of delivering 3D conformal APBI differ primarily by patient positioning, either supine or prone. The major studies of 3D conformal APBI (Table 11.1), the technique of treatment delivery, and the potential challenges are discussed.

11.2 History

11.2.1 Rationale for External Beam APBI

Data supporting the concept of PBI result from major randomized studies that have evaluated the role of adjuvant radiation therapy in breast conservation (Clark et al. 1996; Liljegren et al. 1994; Veronesi et al. 2001). These studies are reviewed elsewhere in this textbook, but basically demonstrate that ipsilateral breast recurrences largely occur at the original tumor bed and the ipsilateral breast elsewhere failure rate is similar to the contralateral breast new primary rate (1.5–4% at 13 years) (Perera et al. 1995; Vicini et al. 2004). Based on these data, the partial breast target volume comprising the lumpectomy cavity with a margin may be adequate in reducing the risk of local recurrence in women with small, adequately resected tumors. With hypofractionated radiation therapy, reducing the target volume from the whole breast to the cavity with a margin is intended to reduce late toxicity including telangiectasias and fibrosis, which are more prominent when the whole breast is treated with a hypofractionated schedule. APBI is now a potential adjuvant treatment option for patients with early-stage breast cancer who, due to comorbid conditions and/or age, and/or logistics, are not suitable candidates for 6–7 weeks of daily radiation therapy, but would benefit from adjuvant treatment based on life expectancy. However, some patients who are candidates for PBI are not appropriate candidates for brachytherapy applicators such as the MammoSite balloon or interstitial needles (due to the location of the lumpectomy cavity, or size, shape, ratio of breast/cavity volumes), or would rather undergo a non-invasive treatment approach. In such patients, 3D conformal APBI may be most applicable.

Table 11.1 APBI: external beam radiotherapy studies (Rosenstein et al. 2004)

Series	Patients (n)	Age (years)	Tumor size (cm)	Dose fractionation	Median follow-up (months)	Technique	Field arrangement	Tumor bed definition (CTV)	Margin (cm)	Ipsilateral breast recurrence rate (%)
Christie Hospital	353	<70	<4	5 Gy × 8 in 10 days	96	Supine, 10-MeV electrons	Single electron beam	Tumor bed at surgery	0	6 (21/355)
New York University	47	Postmenopausal	<2	6 Gy × 5 in 10 days	17	Prone, 6-MV photons	Two coplanar minitangents	Architectural distortion on CT	1.5–2	0
William Beaumont Hospital	31	50	<3	3.4 Gy × 10 in 5 days or 3.85 Gy × 10 in 5 days	10	Supine, 6-MV, 18-MV photons	Three to five noncoplanar beams	Architectural distortion and surgical clips on CT	1–1.5	–

11.2.2 Prospective Randomized Data Comparing APBI and External Beam APBI to Whole-Breast Radiation Therapy

Polgar et al. reported the 5-year results of a phase I/II study and initial findings of a randomized phase III trial assessing adjuvant brachytherapy alone following breast-conserving therapy for stage I breast cancer (Polgar et al. 2002). Initially, 45 patients with stage I breast cancer were prospectively selected to undergo adjuvant tumor bed radiotherapy (TBRT) via interstitial high dose-rate (HDR) implants used to deliver seven fractions of either 4.33 Gy or 5.2 Gy. With a median follow-up of 57 months, 4.4% local, 6.7% axillary, and 6.7% distant failures, and 4.4% deaths due to breast cancer were observed. The 5-year probability of cancer-specific, relapse-free and local recurrence-free survival was 90%, 85.9%, and 95.6%, respectively. Cosmetic results were excellent in 97.8% of patients and no toxicity greater than grade 2 was observed. Based on the technical feasibility and results of the study, a phase III study was initiated and 126 further patients were randomized to receive 50 Gy WBRT ($n=63$) or TBRT ($n=63$) alone consisting of interstitial HDR brachytherapy delivering 5.2 Gy in seven fractions ($n=46$) or electron beam irradiation used to deliver 50 Gy ($n=17$). At a mean follow-up of 30 months, locoregional control was 100% in both arms and the 3-year probability of cancer-specific and relapse-free survival rates were similar in both arms. Furthermore, radiation-related side effects were also not significantly different between the treatment arms. Based on these 5-year results demonstrating technical feasibility and acceptable cosmetic outcome with short-term follow-up demonstrating similar outcome to WBRT, the authors concluded that TBRT might be an appropriate alternative in appropriately selected patients. To our knowledge, this study represents one of only two phase III trials that have utilized external beam radiotherapy to deliver APBI.

The only other phase III prospective randomized trial comparing external beam APBI to whole-breast irradiation (WBI) was conducted at the Christie Hospital, Manchester, UK (Ribeiro et al. 1990, 1993). The study included 708 patients with clinically palpable breast carcinomas (invasive ductal or lobular) measuring 4 cm or less with no palpable axillary adenopathy. Following lumpectomy (with no sentinel or axillary node dissection), the patients were randomized to receive either limited field (LF) PBI including the tumor bed, or wide field (WF) radiation including the whole breast and regional lymph nodes. Although microscopic margin status was not reported, the primary tumor was reported as grossly completely excised in 80% of cases, incompletely excised in 10% of cases and could not be assessed in 10% of cases. In the LF group, 40 to 42.5 Gy was delivered in eight fractions over 10 days, using 8–14 MeV electrons prescribed to the 100% isodose line (IDL). The average field size was 8×6 cm. Patients in the WF arm were treated via an opposed tangential field arrangement using 4 MV photons to deliver 40 Gy in 15 fractions over 21 days. The anterior supraclavicular/axillary nodal region was treated with a separate field using 4 MV photons.

At 6 years from the first randomization, 96% of the WF group and 92% of the LF group were free of breast recurrence. The actuarial breast recurrence-free survival at 5 years was 94% and 87% for the WF and LF groups, respectively. In the 8-year update, overall survival rates were similar between the groups (73% and 71% for the LF and WF groups, respectively). The actuarial breast recurrence rates were 20% and 11% in the LF and WF arms, respectively ($P=0.0008$). However, when histology was factored into the analysis, invasive lobular histology appeared to account for a significant proportion of the local recurrences in the LF group compared to the WF group (34% and 8%, respectively). The local recurrence with invasive ductal carcinomas was similar in both arms (15% in the LF group, and 11% in the WF group). Extensive intraductal carcinoma in situ was associated with higher recurrence rates in both arms, 21% for the LF arm and 14% for the WF arm, with salvage surgery possible in 86% and 90% of patients in each arm, respectively. Of note, the marginal miss/true recurrence (outside the treated field) of invasive ductal carcinoma in the LF arm was 5.5%. The rate of fibrosis and telangiectasias was higher in the LF arm, with worse cosmetic outcome. However, unlike contemporary 3D conformal APBI, PBI was delivered by electron beams, not unexpectedly resulting in a higher skin dose and therefore a less than optimal cosmetic outcome.

Further differences between patient management in this study and the care provided today include lack of sentinel lymph node biopsy or axillary node dissection, systemic treatment, and evaluation of microscopic margins. Also, most patients did not have pre- or postoperative mammography, and therefore multicentric disease could not be excluded. Furthermore, tumor size was unknown in 42% of patients, extensive ductal carcinoma in situ was not excluded, and all histologies were allowed. The simulation and treatment delivery did not have quality assurance criteria, CT scan evaluation or planning, 3D treatment planning, localization of the lumpectomy cavity borders or depth, daily verification of treatment field, or DVH analysis. Although the authors conclude that limited field irradiation results in a higher recurrence rate, with the current standard of care and the fact that the rate of recurrence with invasive ductal carcinoma was similar between the two arms, 3D conformal APBI appears to have a significant role in the adjuvant treatment of early-stage breast cancer.

11.3 Physics and Techniques

11.3.1 Prone 3D Conformal APBI

Patients who may benefit from the displacement of the lumpectomy cavity away from the chest wall, and thus, the heart and lungs, with the prone treatment technique are those who are physically able to tolerate lying prone during simulation and treatment. Patient positioning during treatment delivery is geared toward optimizing daily reproducibility, limiting normal surrounding tissue dose, and ensuring appropriate dose coverage to the

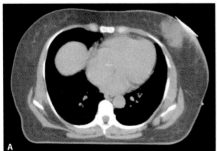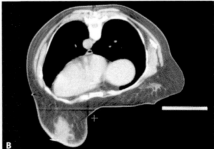

Fig. 11.1 Supine (**A**) and prone (**B**) patient positioning (Formenti 2005)

target structure. In the case of PBI, the respiratory and cardiac motion may potentially result in movement of breast tissues and thus the target area during treatment delivery. The prone treatment position has been used to reduce breast tissue motion resulting from cardiac systole and respiratory movement (el Fallah et al. 1997). In such a position, excursion of the chest wall can be reduced to 5 mm (Jozsef et al. 2000), minimizing breast tissue motion and therefore target motion. Also, if the breast is allowed to hang through an opening in the table, this may allow the cavity to fall away from the chest wall due to gravity (Formenti 2005) (Fig. 11.1) resulting in exclusion of the heart and lung from the treatment field (Griem et al. 2003).

11.3.2 Dose Fractionation Scheme for Postoperative Supine and Prone External Beam APBI

Baillet et al. completed a prospective study of 230 elderly patients who were randomized to receive hypofractionated postoperative WBI therapy to 23 Gy in four fractions over 17 days versus 45 Gy in 25 fractions over 33 days, which resulted in equivalent local control at 4 years (7% versus 5%, respectively), although the cosmetic outcome was inferior in the hypofractionated treatment arm (Baillet et al. 1990). The fibrosis rate was 18% in the group randomized to hypofractionated radiation treatment compared to 9% in the standard fractionation group. As surrounding normal structures, such as heart and lung, do not significantly restrict the target volume coverage for patients treated in the prone position, hypofractionated PBI doses were safely explored. The linear-quadratic cell survival model with an alpha-beta value of 4 for breast carcinoma was used to develop fractionation schedules including a dose of 30 Gy in five fractions over 10 days, which is biologically equivalent to delivering 50 Gy in 25 fractions of 2 Gy per fraction over 5 weeks (Barendsen 1982; Steel et al. 1987; Yamada et al. 1999). With respect to cosmesis, the late tissue complications were similar to those observed with 5 weeks of standard WBI followed by a boost to 60 Gy to the tumor bed, which results in an acceptable cosmetic outcome (Archambeau et al. 1995; de la Rochefordiere et al. 1992).

Biologically equivalent doses of different fractionation schemes are listed in Table 11.2.

11.4 Clinical Results

11.4.1 Pilot Phase I Dose-Escalation Trial

Formenti et al. initially conducted a study at the University of Southern California using two "radiosurgical" approaches originally intended to substitute surgical excision for patients with breast cancers ≤5 mm (Formenti 2005; Jozsef et al. 2000). The treatment techniques used included using 4 MV photons to deliver 15, 18, and 20 Gy (with a 32 mm diameter collimator) via (1) seven fixed horizontal beams or (2) six 45° arcs and a 90° sagittal arc, with minimum target dose at 83% and 86% of the dose maximum, respectively. Post-treatment target area excisions of the first three patients demonstrated viable tumor 8–10 weeks after therapy. Therefore, the research focus was modified to treat the post-lumpectomy cavity with margin.

Table 11.2 Biologically equivalent doses of different fractionation schemes (Formenti 2005)

Endpoint	α/β	50 Gy/25 fractions	30 Gy/5 fractions	60 Gy/30 fractions	34 Gy/10 fractions
Erythema	8[b]	63 Gy$_8$	53 Gy$_8$	75 Gy$_8$	48 Gy$_8$
Desquamation	11[b]	59 Gy$_{11}$	6 Gy$_{11}$	71 Gy$_{11}$	45 Gy$_{11}$
Telangiectasia	4[b]	75 Gy$_4$	75 Gy$_4$	90 Gy$_4$	63 Gy$_4$
Fibrosis	2[b]	100 Gy$_2$	120 Gy$_2$	120 Gy$_2$	92 Gy$_2$
Tumor control	4	75 Gy$_4$	75 Gy$_4$	90 Gy$_4$	63 Gy$_4$
Tumor control[a]	4	72 Gy$_4$	75 Gy$_4$	86 Gy$_4$	63 Gy$_4$

[a] Taking into account cell proliferation during the course of treatment (Barendsen 1982; Steel et al. 1987; Yamada et al. 1999)
[b] Data from Archambeau et al. 1995

Subsequently, Formenti et al. conducted a pilot dose escalation study to evaluate the feasibility of hypofractionated conformal PBI therapy in the prone position (Formenti et al. 2002). Eligibility criteria included postmenopausal status, nonpalpable pT1 invasive breast cancer, estrogen receptor-positive tumors, lack of extensive intraductal component, negative surgical margins by at least 2 mm, and patient refusal to undergo 6 weeks of radiation therapy. All nine patients who underwent treatment received five fractions over 10 days, with total doses ranging from 25 to 30 Gy. Patients were treated in the prone position on a table with an aperture with variable diameter settings, which allows the breast to hang. Daily set-up was based upon external markings on the patient's skin and also radiopaque markers in the lumpectomy cavity (clips) if present. Set-up accuracy was verified with orthogonal post films prior to each fraction and at least two fields were ported as well. Target definition was accomplished by CT contours of the lumpectomy cavity and a 2-cm margin. The prescription dose was defined as the minimum dose encompassing 95% of the PTV. The maximum dose was not to exceed the prescription dose by more than 10% (Fig. 11.2). In most cases, the treatment fields were five to seven horizontal fixed beams in a coronal plane (Fig. 11.3). Out of a total of nine randomized and treated patients, three received 5 Gy per fraction, four received 5.5 Gy per fraction, and two received 6 Gy per fraction. Two of the nine patients did not undergo lymph node sampling. Follow-up ranged from 36 to 53 months, and cosmetic results were good to excellent in all patients.

11.4.2 Phase I/II Trial of Prone 3D Conformal APBI – New York University

On the basis of the results of the pilot study, Formenti et al. conducted a study of 47 postmenopausal women with stage I T1N0 breast cancer, who refused to undergo 6 weeks of WBI, treated to 30 Gy in five 6-Gy fractions over 10 days (Monday, Wednesday, Friday, Monday, and Wednesday) (Formenti et al. 2004). Other eligibility criteria included

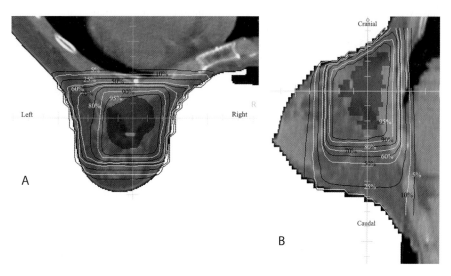

Fig. 11.2 A PTV and isodose distributions (left–right). **B** PTV and isodose distributions (cranial–caudal). New York University (Formenti et al. 2002)

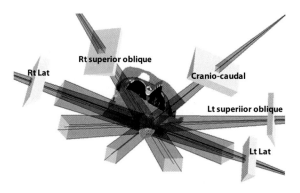

Fig. 11.3 3D graphic reconstruction of five beam eye views for prone 3D conformal APBI (Formenti et al. 2002)

negative margins by at least 5 mm. The patients were treated in the prone position and the PTV was defined as the lumpectomy cavity with a 1.5-cm margin, limited anteriorly by skin and posteriorly by the chest wall. CT-defined target volumes were treated with opposed minitangents with wedges (Fig. 11.4). The dose was normalized to 100% at the isocenter before an isodose was selected that encompassed the PTV, 95% IDL. Dose inhomogeneity was less than 110%. Of the ipsilateral breast volume, 50% received less than 50% of the prescribed dose (Fig. 11.5). The contralateral breast and ipsilateral heart and lung were avoided completely in the beam arrangement. Of 47 patients entering treatment, 46 completed. Most of the patients were treated in the prone position (four were treated supine due to patient intolerance of the prone position or because the lumpectomy cavity was located in the axillary tail). The median follow-up was 18 months. The most common acute toxicity was erythema which was seen in 60% of patients at grade 1–2. Late toxicity, totaling 21 in 14 patients, was primarily grade 1 and cosmetic results were mostly "good" to "excellent". Only two patients had "fair" cosmetic results and no patients had a worse score after radiation than their postoperative baseline score. At this short follow-up, no patients had local recurrence. The mean and median lumpectomy cavity or CTV was 52 cm^3 and 34 cm^3, respectively (range 7–379 cm^3). The mean and median PTV was 228 cm^3 and 192 cm^3, respectively (range 57–1118 cm^3). The mean and median ipsilateral breast volumes were 1102 cm^3 and 1006 cm^3, respectively (range 258–346 cm^3). The coverage of the PTV by the 30 Gy IDL was 100% (both mean and median). The ipsilateral breast volume receiving 100% of the prescribed dose ranged from 10% to 45% (mean and median, 26% and 27%, respectively). In 25% of patients, >50% of the ipsilateral breast volume was treated to >50% of the prescribed dose in order to cover the PTV adequately (Table 11.3). The mean percentages of lung volume and heart volume receiving 20, 10, and 5 Gy were 0% and 0%, respectively, in the patients treated in the prone position. In the four patients treated in the supine position, the median doses to the lung receiving 20, 10, and 5 Gy were 2%, 4%, and 6%, respectively.

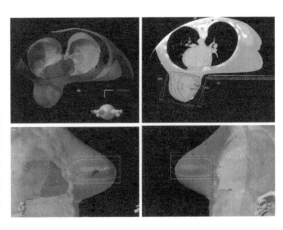

Fig. 11.4 *Upper*: Example of relationship of tumor bed to PTV (*red wash* tumor bed, *blue* PTV, *pink* heart, *light green* lung). The PTV is represented by a 1.5-cm margin on the tumor bed. *Lower*: Digital reconstructed radiographs, right anterior oblique and left posterior oblique portals for left-sided breast cancer (Formenti et al. 2004)

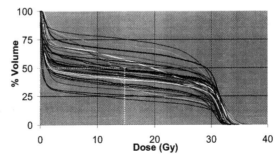

Fig. 11.5 Dose–volume histogram of ipsilateral breast of 47 patients (Formenti et al. 2004)

Table 11.3 Dosimetric findings: CTV, PTV, and ipsilateral breast tissue volume (*IBV*). New York University (Formenti et al. 2004)

Dosimetric characteristics	Mean	Median	Range
IBV (cm³)	1102	1006	258–3468
CTV (cm³)	52	34	7–379
PTV (cm³)	228	192	57–1118
Maximal dose (% of prescribed dose)	110	108	105–117
PTV coverage by 95% isodose surface (%)	100	100	–
Ipsilateral breast coverage (% IBV encompassed by % of PD)			
100% of prescribed dose	26	27	10–45
75% of prescribed dose	41	40	20–68
50% of prescribed dose	47	46	23–75
25% of prescribed dose	53	53	27–82
CTV/IBV (%)	5	4	1–22
PTV/IBV (%)	22	20	10–55
CTV/PTV (%)	20	20	6–46

11.4.3 The William Beaumont Hospital Experience – 3D Conformal APBI in Supine Position

Initial clinical experience at William Beaumont Hospital in utilizing 3D conformal radiation therapy to deliver PBI in patients with early-stage breast cancer treated with breast-conserving therapy supported the technical feasibility of such treatment delivery (Baglan et al. 2003; Vicini et al. 2003a, 2003b). In this phase I/II study, 23 patients were prospectively enrolled between August 2000 and December 2002. An additional 5 patients were treated according to the guidelines of the protocol for compassionate purposes. Eligibility for the protocol included patient age ≥50 years, tumor size ≤3 cm, invasive ductal histology, lumpectomy with negative surgical margins by at least 2 mm, negative axillary lymph nodes with a minimum of six sampled (or negative sentinel lymph node biopsy), no extensive intraductal component or skin involvement, and no Paget's disease of the nipple. The details of the simulation and treatment planning are as follows. All patients initially underwent virtual CT breast simulation with alpha-cradle immobilization and delineation of the breast borders with physician-placed radiopaque catheters. The CTV was defined as the lumpectomy cavity uniformly expanded by 10–15 mm, limited by 5 mm from the skin surface and lung–chest wall interface. PTV was defined by adding to the CTV 5 mm for breathing motion and another 5 mm for set-up error. The beam arrangement included three, four, five, or seven noncoplanar beams with 6 MV photons alone in 21 patients, combined 6 and 18 MV photons in four patients, a combination of photons and electrons in two patients and electrons alone in one patient. Field arrangements were designed with the isocenter placed in the center of the PTV and approximated breast tangents with a 10–20° steeper gantry angle for the medial beams for maximal breast tissue sparing and a couch angle of 15–70°.

The procedure used to set up the four-field technique, consisting of a left anterior superior-to-inferior oblique (Lt ASIO), left anterior inferior-to-superior oblique (Lt AISO), right anterior inferior-to-superior oblique (Rt AISO), and right posterior superior-to-inferior oblique (Rt PSIO) for a right breast lesion, was as follows (Fig. 11.6). First, three medial tangents (couch angle of 0° for two and 180° for one of the beams) and one lateral tangent (couch angle of 0°) were constructed. Typically, the medial tangents had a 10–20° steeper gantry angle than whole breast tangents to spare more breast tissue. The lateral tangent could also have a slightly shallower gantry angle to spare breast tissue, provided that it did not exit through the contralateral breast. Next, couch angles were applied to each beam. Typical couch angles for the three anterior oblique fields were 35–45° from a transverse plane. However, for the Rt AISO beam, particular care was taken to ensure that the field exited superior to the heart. The couch angle used for the posterior oblique field was usually only 10–20° to avoid entry through the ipsilateral arm and collision problems with the gantry head and treatment couch.

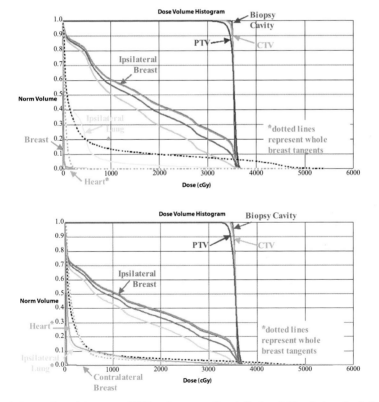

Fig. 11.6 Dose volume histograms (William Beaumont Hospital): four-field technique (*top*), five-field technique (*bottom*)

The five-field technique was initially used for left-sided lesions and consisted of Rt ASIO, Rt Lateral, Rt AISO, Lt PSIO, and Lt PISO beams. The primary differences which make this technique better suited to left-sided lesions was the elimination of the Lt AISO beam which would exit through the heart. The trade-off was a larger volume of normal breast tissue irradiated (Fig. 11.7). With additional experience, only three- and four-beam combinations were employed. It should be noted that these beam arrangements may not be possible with linear accelerators which have larger gantry heads than the Elekta SL20. Each field had a universal 60° wedge in place for part of the treatment time. The heel of the wedge was directed anteriorly for all fields and its direction manually optimized if necessary. The field edge was 5–7 mm beyond the PTV to allow for penumbra. Beam weights were manually optimized such that the CTV was completely encompassed by the 100% IDL and the PTV by the 95% IDL, while maintaining a hot spot of <110%. The initial dose fractionation schedule was 34 Gy delivered in ten fractions of 3.4 Gy administered twice daily over five consecutive days with at least a 6-hour interfraction interval, which is identical to the RTOG 95-17 brachytherapy dose schedule. After treating six patients, the fraction size was increased to 3.85 Gy, giving a total dose to 38.5 Gy. This corresponds to a radiobiological dose of approximately 45 Gy given in 25 fractions using WBI and assuming an α/β ratio of 10.

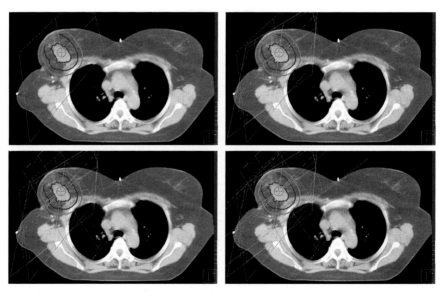

Fig. 11.7 Consecutive addition of Lt ASIO, Lt AISO, Rt AISO, Rt PO beams (William Beaumont Hospital)

Additional normal tissue dose guidelines were used during beam weight optimization. These included limiting 50–60% of the ipsilateral breast volume to ≤50% of the prescribed dose and 25–35% of the ipsilateral breast volume to ≤100% of the prescribed dose. In addition, the heart and lung dose–volume histograms (DVHs) were below that for whole breast tangents for left-sided lesions. In all patients, a comparison was made

Table 11.4 Dosimetric findings: CTV, PTV, and ipsilateral breast (protocol patients, $n=26$). William Beaumont Hospital

Dosimetric characteristics	Mean	Median	Range
Maximum dose (% of prescribed dose)	109	109	100–112
CTV coverage (%)			
100% IDL	98	100	54–100
95% IDL	100	100	99–100
PTV coverage (%)			
95% IDL	100	100	97–100
Ipsilateral breast coverage			
100% IDL	23	21	14–39
75% IDL	36	35	26–53
50% IDL	47	46	34–60
25% IDL	60	60	39–92
PTV/total breast volume (%)	17	17	11–22

Table 11.5 Dosimetric findings and normal tissue doses ($n=26$). Tangents versus APBI. William Beaumont Hospital

Dosimetric character-istics	Mean		Median		Range	
	Tangents	PBI	Tangents	PBI	Tangents	PBI
Cardiac doses						
V30	1%	0%	0%	0%	0–9%	0–1%
V20	2%	0%	0%	0%	0–12%	0–3%
V10	2%	0%	0%	0%	0–16%	0–7%
Lung doses						
V20	10%	4%	11%	4%	2–19%	0–8%
V10	14%	9%	14%	9%	4–23%	0–34%
V5	18%	16%	19%	16%	8–30%	0–37%

in the doses delivered to normal tissues between the 3D conformal APBI plan and standard tangents. The goals were to accept plans that matched or preferably reduced doses to the heart and lung. Mean and median values (as well as ranges) for doses to the CTV, PTV, heart, and lung with the 3D conformal APBI plans were calculated on the protocol patients only. It should be noted also that serial CT scans were performed to determine the lumpectomy cavity changes over time in 18 patients. In 72% of the patients, the cavity decreased by a mean of 49% and a median of 45%, with mean and median times between CT scans of 7 and 11 days, respectively. In 22% of patients, the cavity increased in volume by a mean of 61% and median of 50% (range 27–116%). The mean and median times between the CT scans was 22 and 17 days, respectively. Dosimetric findings are given in Table 11.4.

The mean and median size of the lumpectomy cavity at the time of dosimetric treatment planning was 22 cm^3 and 14 cm^3, respectively (range 3–70 cm^3). The mean and median volumes of the CTV were 118 cm^3 and 112 cm^3, respectively (range 28–231 cm^3). The mean and median coverages of the CTV by the 100% IDL were 97% and 100%, respectively. The mean and median coverages of the CTV by the 95% IDL were both 100%. The mean and median coverages of the PTV by the 95% IDL were both 100%. The mean and median volumes of the ipsilateral breast receiving 100% of the prescribed dose were 23% and 21%, respectively. The mean and median volumes receiving 50% of the prescribed dose were 47% and 46%, respectively. The mean and median volumes of the heart receiving 10%, 20% and 30% of the prescribed dose were compared between the 3D conformal APBI technique and standard WBI, and are presented in Table 11.5. For all parameters examined, unnecessary doses to the heart delivered with the APBI technique were less than or equal to those delivered with standard WBI. Likewise, the mean and median volumes of the lung receiving 5%, 10%, and 20% of the prescribed dose were compared between the 3D conformal APBI technique and standard WBI, and are also presented in Table 11.5. Again, for all parameters examined, unnecessary doses to the lung delivered with the PBI technique were less than or equal to those delivered with standard WBI.

Patients were initially seen in follow-up 4–6 weeks after completing treatment and then at 3-month intervals. The median follow-up duration was 8 months (range 1–24 months) and cosmetic results and acute toxicity were assessed for protocol patients only. Of the 28 patients, 19 (68%) experienced grade 1 toxicity and 11% (three patients) had grade 2 toxicity in the first 6 weeks of follow-up. Cosmetic results were rated as good/excellent in all evaluable patients at 6 months ($n=2$), 12 months ($n=3$), 18 months ($n=4$), and in the three evaluable patients at >18 months after treatment. Six-month follow-up mammograms were negative in all evaluable patients ($n=12$).

11.4.4 Ongoing William Beaumont Hospital Experience

The ongoing experience at William Beaumont Hospital was reported by Vicini et al. regarding 31 patients treated with 3D conformal APBI (Vicini et al. 2003b). Of these 31 patients, 94% had surgical clips outlining the lumpectomy cavity (mean six clips). The CTV consisted of the lumpectomy cavity plus a 10-mm margin in 9 patients and a 15-mm margin in 22 patients (median 15 mm). The PTV consisted of the CTV plus a 10-mm margin for breathing motion and treatment set-up uncertainties. The prescribed dose was 34 or 38.5 Gy (6 patients and 25 patients, respectively) in ten fractions twice daily separated by 6 hours and delivered on five consecutive days. Patients were treated in the supine position with three to five beams (mean four) designed to irradiate the CTV with <10% inhomogeneity and a comparable or lower dose to the heart, lung, and contralateral breast compared with standard whole-breast tangents. The mean coverage of the CTV by the 100% IDL was 98% (range 54–100%, median 100%) and by the 95% IDL, 100% (range 99–100%). The mean coverage of the PTV by the 95% IDL was 100% (range 97–100%). The mean percentage of the breast receiving 100% of the prescribed dose was 23% (range 14–39%). The mean percentage of the breast receiving 50% of the prescribed dose was 47% (range 34–60%). The data are summarized in Table 11.4.

The median follow-up duration was 10 months (range 1–30 months). Four patients were followed >2 years, 6 for >1.5 years, and 5 for >1 year. The remaining 16 patients had been followed for <12 months. While all patients had none to minimal skin changes during treatment, at the initial 6-week follow-up, 61% had grade 1 toxicity and 10% had grade 2 toxicity. The remaining 29% of patients had no observable side effects and no grade 3 toxicities were observed. Cosmetic results were rated as good/excellent in all evaluable patients at 6 months (*n*=3), 12 months (*n*=5), 18 months (*n*=6), and in the four evaluable patients at >2 years after treatment. Based on these results, further studies were conducted, including RTOG 0319.

11.4.5 RTOG 0319 – Preliminary Results

Activated in August of 2003, the RTOG 0319 study was based upon the William Beaumont Hospital experience. The same eligibility criteria and treatment technique, doses and fractionation schedule in RTOG 95-13 were employed in this study. The accrual goal was 42 patients and a total of 52 were treated by the completion of accrual in April 2004. Only 4 of the first 42 evaluable treatments were scored as unacceptable and the treatment technique was shown to be reproducible, as presented at the 2004 San Antonio Breast Cancer Symposium.

11.4.6 Massachusetts General Hospital Experience

The initial clinical data acquired from the first 22 patients who underwent treatment reported by Taghian et al. at a follow-up of 1–6 months supports the feasibility and minimal acute toxicity of 3D conformal APBI demonstrated in other studies. The eligibility criteria included histology of invasive ductal carcinoma ≤ 2 cm, negative lymph nodes, negative margins by at least 2 mm, and no lymphovascular space invasion or extensive intraductal component. The prescribed dose was 32 Gy in eight fractions twice daily separated by 6 hours, delivered over 4–5 days. The PTV consisted of the lumpectomy cavity with a margin of 15–20 mm. The dose inhomogeneity was less than 10% across the PTV. The patients were treated in the supine position with three or four beams of mostly mixed photons and electrons (one patient was treated with only photons). The mean and median tumor sizes were 0.86 cm and 0.9 cm, respectively, with mean and median lumpectomy volumes of 42.9 cm^3 and 34.0 cm^3, respectively. The mean and median PTVs were 178.1 cm^3 and 151 cm^3, respectively. The mean doses received by 20% (V20), 10% (V10), and 5% (V5) of the ipsilateral lung volumes were 2.3 Gy, 4.5 Gy and 6.7 Gy, respectively. The mean V20, V10, and V5 of the heart for left sided lesions were 1.5 Gy, 2.2 Gy, and 3.2 Gy, respectively. Of the non-target breast volume, 50% was an average of 6.7 Gy. At the initial follow-up, 41% of patients had mild erythema and 9% had moderate erythema, with no patients having moist desquamation. Cosmetic results were good to excellent in all patients.

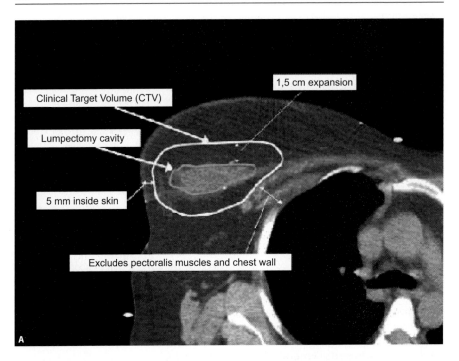

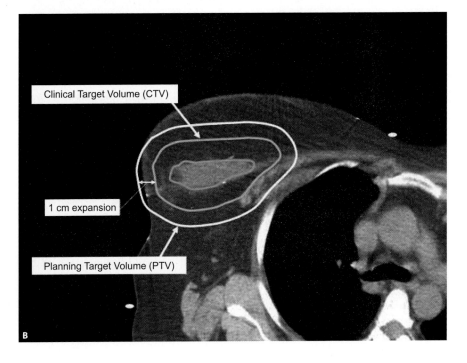

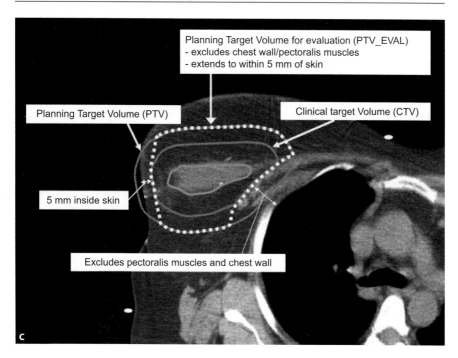

Planning Target Volume for evaluation (PTV_EVAL)
- excludes chest wall/pectoralis muscles
- extends to within 5 mm of skin

Planning Target Volume (PTV)

Clinical target Volume (CTV)

5 mm inside skin

Excludes pectoralis muscles and chest wall

◄ ▲ **Fig. 11.8**   Phase III NSABP-B39/RTOG 0413 3D conformal APBI: **A** cavity and CTV; **B** cavity, CTV, and PTV; **C** cavity, CTV, PTV, and PTV_EVAL

11.5 Challenges and Limiting Factors in the Application of 3D Conformal APBI

A primary potential disadvantage of 3D conformal APBI relates to organ motion effects and patient set-up, which can necessitate a larger target volume in order to avoid a geographic miss. Based on previously published data (Frazier et al. 2004), a 5 mm CTV to PTV expansion should account for normal breathing (Baglan et al. 2003) and the use of 10 mm CTV–PTV margin also allows for random and systematic components of set-up error. The final component of geometric uncertainty is the potential for the lumpectomy cavity to change shape and/or position independently of the surrounding breast tissue. A potential method of accounting for this motion involves online image guidance, which may employ the use of surgical clips to serve as a surrogate for the lumpectomy cavity (Weed et al. 2004) during the abbreviated course of treatment.

The William Beaumont Hospital data were analyzed to determine if certain variables could be identified to predict whether a patient was technically suitable for the 3D conformal quadrant technique (Vicini et al. 2003b). Based on previously published PBI brachytherapy data, a "borderline acceptable" plan was determined to have >50–60% of the breast volume covered by the 50% IDL. Based on this endpoint, several factors were analyzed for their association with the probability of a particular case being appropriate for 3D conformal APBI, including cavity volume, CTV, PTV, breast volume (BV), CTV:

Table 11.6 Dosimetric comparison of 3D conformal APBI techniques (Rosenstein et al. 2004) (*TBV* total breast volume)

Series	PTV (cm³)	PTV/TBV (%)	Ipsilateral breast coverage			
			100%	75%	50%	25%
New York University						
Median	192	22	27	40	46	53
Range	57–118	10–55	10–45	20–68	23–75	27–82
William Beaumont Hospital						
Median	240	17	21	35	46	60
Range	82–482	11–22	14–39	26–53	34–60	39–92

BV ratio, PTV:BV ratio (Table 11.6), tumor location, etc. The factor found to have the highest correlation with the ability to meet the dose–volume constraints was the PTV: BV ratio, with ratios >0.2 unlikely to meet the requirements of the protocol.

Finally, as with the delivery of any form of irradiation, the issue of verification of treatment delivery, when the uncertainty factors have been accounted for in planning, must also be addressed. This is especially important during external beam APBI as small inaccuracies may be more clinically significant resulting in a potential geographic miss. As described previously, surgical clips have been used to delineate the lumpectomy cavity and this may be assessed at some institutions via CT scanning.

11.6 Future Directions

To determine whether PBI limited to the region of the tumor bed following lumpectomy provides equivalent local tumor control in the breast compared to conventional WBI in the local management of early-stage breast cancer, the first phase III randomized study of conventional WBI versus PBI opened in March 2005. This study includes patients with stage 0, I, or II breast cancer resected by lumpectomy with tumor size ≤3 cm and no more than three histologically positive axillary lymph nodes. The stratification of patients is based upon disease stage (DCIS only, invasive and node negative, invasive with one to three lymph nodes involved), menopausal status, hormone receptor status, and intention to receive chemotherapy. Randomization is completed after the patient is determined to be an appropriate candidate for possible APBI based on CT criteria including lumpectomy cavity shape, absolute volume, volume in reference to the whole breast volume, location, and distance from the skin surface. If the patient is determined to be an appropriate candidate, randomization places her into either group 1 (WBI) or group 2 (PBI). WBI involves the delivery of 45–50 Gy in 25 fractions of 1.8–2.0 Gy per fraction to the whole breast followed by an optional boost to ≥60 Gy. If the patient is randomized to group 2, she will receive, as determined by her physicians in addition to patient preference, APBI via one of three modalities. The first two methods involve delivery of 34 Gy in 3.4 Gy fractions twice daily over 5–10 days using multicatheter brachytherapy or the

MammoSite balloon applicator. The third method of APBI delivery is via 3D conformal external beam irradiation in which 38.5 Gy is delivered twice daily over 5–10 days in 3.85 Gy fractions. The interfraction time for all treatments is at least 6 hours (Fig. 11.8). The results of this study will determine future directions in the treatment of early-stage breast cancer.

References

1. Archambeau JO, Pezner R, Wasserman T (1995) Pathophysiology of irradiated skin and breast. Int J Radiat Oncol Biol Phys 31:1171–1185

2. Baglan KL, Sharpe MB, Jaffray D, et al (2003) Accelerated partial breast irradiation using 3D conformal radiation therapy (3D-CRT). Int J Radiat Oncol Biol Phys 55:302–311

3. Baillet F, Housset M, Maylin C, et al (1990) The use of a specific hypofractionated radiation therapy regimen versus classical fractionation in the treatment of breast cancer: a randomized study of 230 patients. Int J Radiat Oncol Biol Phys 19:1131–1133

4. Barendsen GW (1982) Dose fractionation, dose rate and iso-effect relationships for normal tissue responses. Int J Radiat Oncol Biol Phys 8:1981–1997

5. Clark RM, Whelan T, Levine M, et al (1996) Randomized clinical trial of breast irradiation following lumpectomy and axillary dissection for node-negative breast cancer: an update. Ontario Clinical Oncology Group. J Natl Cancer Inst 88:1659–1664

6. de la Rochefordiere A, Abner AL, Silver B, Vicini F, Recht A, Harris JR (1992) Are cosmetic results following conservative surgery and radiation therapy for early breast cancer dependent on technique? Int J Radiat Oncol Biol Phys 23:925–931

7. el Fallah AI, Plantec MB, Ferrara KW (1997) Ultrasonic measurement of breast tissue motion and the implications for velocity estimation. Ultrasound Med Biol 23:1047–1057

8. Formenti SC (2005) External-beam partial-breast irradiation. Semin Radiat Oncol 15:92–99

9. Formenti SC, Rosenstein B, Skinner KA, Jozsef G (2002) T1 stage breast cancer: adjuvant hypofractionated conformal radiation therapy to tumor bed in selected postmenopausal breast cancer patients—pilot feasibility study. Radiology 222:171–178

10. Formenti SC, Truong MT, Goldberg JD, et al (2004) Prone accelerated partial breast irradiation after breast-conserving surgery: preliminary clinical results and dose-volume histogram analysis. Int J Radiat Oncol Biol Phys 60:493–504

11. Frazier RC, Vicini FA, Sharpe MB, et al (2004) Impact of breathing motion on whole breast radiotherapy: a dosimetric analysis using active breathing control. Int J Radiat Oncol Biol Phys 58:1041–1047

12. Griem KL, Fetherston P, Kuznetsova M, Foster GS, Shott S, Chu J (2003) Three-dimensional photon dosimetry: a comparison of treatment of the intact breast in the supine and prone position. Int J Radiat Oncol Biol Phys 57:891–899

13. Jozsef G, Luxton G, Formenti SC (2000) Application of radiosurgery principles to a target in the breast: a dosimetric study. Med Phys 27:1005–1010

14. Liljegren G, Holmberg L, Adami HO, Westman G, Graffman S, Bergh J (1994) Sector resection with or without postoperative radiotherapy for stage I breast cancer: five-year results of a randomized trial. Uppsala-Orebro Breast Cancer Study Group. J Natl Cancer Inst 86:717–722

15. Perera F, Chisela F, Engel J, Venkatesan V (1995) Method of localization and implantation of the lumpectomy site for high dose rate brachytherapy after conservative surgery for T1 and T2 breast cancer. Int J Radiat Oncol Biol Phys 31:959–965

16. Polgar C, Sulyok Z, Fodor J, et al (2002) Sole brachytherapy of the tumor bed after conservative surgery for T1 breast cancer: five-year results of a phase I-II study and initial findings of a randomized phase III trial. J Surg Oncol 80:121–128

17. Ribeiro GG, Dunn G, Swindell R, Harris M, Banerjee SS (1990) Conservation of the breast using two different radiotherapy techniques: interim report of a clinical trial. Clin Oncol (R Coll Radiol) 2:27–34

18. Ribeiro GG, Magee B, Swindell R, Harris M, Banerjee SS (1993) The Christie Hospital breast conservation trial: an update at 8 years from inception. Clin Oncol (R Coll Radiol) 5:278–283

19. Rosenstein BS, Lymberis SC, Formenti SC (2004) Biologic comparison of partial breast irradiation protocols. Int J Radiat Oncol Biol Phys 60:1393–1404

20. Steel GG, Deacon JM, Duchesne GM, Horwich A, Kelland LR, Peacock JH (1987) The dose-rate effect in human tumour cells. Radiother Oncol 9:299–310

21. Veronesi U, Marubini E, Mariani L, et al (2001) Radiotherapy after breast-conserving surgery in small breast carcinoma: long-term results of a randomized trial. Ann Oncol 12:997–1003

22. Vicini F, Arthur D, Polgar C, Kuske R (2003a) Defining the efficacy of accelerated partial breast irradiation: the importance of proper patient selection, optimal quality assurance, and common sense. Int J Radiat Oncol Biol Phys 57:1210–1213

23. Vicini FA, Remouchamps V, Wallace M, et al (2003b) Ongoing clinical experience utilizing 3D conformal external beam radiotherapy to deliver partial-breast irradiation in patients with early-stage breast cancer treated with breast-conserving therapy. Int J Radiat Oncol Biol Phys 57:1247–1253

24. Vicini FA, Kestin LL, Goldstein NS (2004) Defining the clinical target volume for patients with early-stage breast cancer treated with lumpectomy and accelerated partial breast irradiation: a pathologic analysis. Int J Radiat Oncol Biol Phys 60:722–730

25. Weed DW, Yan D, Martinez AA, Vicini FA, Wilkinson TJ, Wong J (2004) The validity of surgical clips as a radiographic surrogate for the lumpectomy cavity in image-guided accelerated partial breast irradiation. Int J Radiat Oncol Biol Phys 60:484–492

26. Yamada Y, Ackerman I, Franssen E, MacKenzie RG, Thomas G (1999) Does the dose fractionation schedule influence local control of adjuvant radiotherapy for early stage breast cancer? Int J Radiat Oncol Biol Phys 44:99–104

Intraoperative Radiotherapy: a Precise Approach for Partial Breast Irradiation

12

Jayant S. Vaidya

Contents

12.1 The "New" Thinking that Became the New Dogma

It took the mammoth effort of a meta-analysis of 26,000 women in 36 randomized trials (Early Breast Cancer Trialists' Collaborative Group 1995, 2000) to make the move from radical mastectomy described by William Halsted more than 100 years ago (Halsted 1894) to breast-conserving therapy that is considered the norm today. As we stand on these giants' shoulders, the next step—the real paradigm shift—to a local therapy truly localized to the tumor and its environs might be easier.

The preceding chapters deal with the rationale of using partial breast irradiation. In this chapter, I give a synopsis of this rationale followed by details about the intraoperative approach of delivering partial breast radiotherapy.

The dogma that 4–6 weeks of postoperative radiotherapy after breast-conserving surgery is necessary for all patients is one of the main obstacles to the widespread utilization of breast-conserving surgery. The radiotherapy schedule is inconvenient for patients and contributes substantially to the unacceptable waiting lists in many oncology departments worldwide. In making decisions about which operation to choose, recurrence, radiation therapy and quick recovery are the main factors women are concerned about (Katz et al. 2005). Consequently, if radiation can be completed at the time of the surgery then two large concerns will be taken care of, and perhaps fewer women will feel obliged to choose mastectomy just because they live far away from a radiotherapy facility

(Athas et al. 2000) or to avoid prolonging their treatment. A delay in delivery of radiotherapy either because of long waiting time or because chemotherapy is given first, may jeopardize its effectiveness (Mikeljevic et al. 2004; Wyatt et al. 2003) and the window of opportunity to sterilize the target tissues of tumor cells/potential tumor cells may be lost. Furthermore, It has been estimated that the externally delivered boost dose misses target volume in 24% to 88% of cases (Machtay et al. 1994; Sedlmayer et al. 1996). Thus a large proportion of local recurrences could be attributed to this geographical miss. Finally, whole-breast irradiation carries the risks of acute and long-term complications such as erythema, fatigue, prolonged discomfort, radiation pneumonitis, rib fracture, cardiovascular effects, and carcinogenesis that could compromise the long-term benefit from postoperative radiotherapy (Early Breast Cancer Trialists' Collaborative Group 2000; Rutqvist and Johansson 1990).

Recent data suggest that local recurrence may be facilitated by a local field defect. The morphologically normal cells surrounding breast cancer demonstrate a loss of heterozygosity, which is often identical to that of the primary tumor (Deng et al. 1996). In addition, aromatase activity in the index quadrant is higher than in other quadrants (O'Neill et al. 1988) and via estrogen has the potential to stimulate mutagenesis, growth and angiogenesis (Lu et al. 1996; Nakamura et al. 1996). Patients with ipsilateral breast tumor recurrence (IBTR) have an increased risk of carrying the mutant p53 gene (23% vs. 1%) (Turner et al. 2000) and young patients (<40 years) with IBTR have a disproportionately increased risk (40%) of carrying a deleterious BRCA1/2 gene mutation (Turner et al. 1999). This suggests that local recurrence is probably related more to background genetic instability than to a different tumor biology at younger age. It appears that a dynamic interaction between the local factors (such as aromatase) present in the breast parenchyma, the systemic hormonal milieu and genetic instability will determine the risk of local recurrence, in addition to the biology of the excised primary tumor.

The location of recurrence in the breast with respect to site of the primary tumor shows an interesting distribution. Between 80% and 100% of early breast recurrences occur in the quadrant that harbored the primary tumor which is in contrast to the findings of 3D analysis of mastectomy specimens (Vaidya et al. 1996) which reveals that 63% of breasts harbor occult cancer foci and 80% of these are situated remote from the index quadrant. It therefore appears that these widespread and occult multifocal/multicentric cancers in other quadrants of the breast remain dormant for a long time and have a low risk of causing clinical tumors. This is corroborated by the fact that although there is a high frequency [20% in young women (median age 39 years) and 33% in women between 50 and 55 years] of tumors in breasts at autopsy (Nielsen et al. 1987), the frequency of clinical breast cancer in the population is considerably lower.

Arguably, in the EORTC study (Bartelink et al. 2001) only 56% of local recurrences were reported to have occurred in the original tumor bed. In fact, a further 27% recurred diffusely throughout the breast including the tumor bed, leaving 29% recurrences outside the index quadrant. However, patients in this study received intensive mammographic follow-up which might have unearthed subclinical occult tumors in other quadrants of unproven clinical significance.

It appears that local recurrence occurs in the index quadrant, whether or not radiotherapy is given (Clark et al. 1982, 1992; McCulloch and MacIntyre 1993) and irrespective of clear margins. Of the breast conserving trials that have tested the effect of radiotherapy, the NSABP-B06 (Fisher et al. 1995), Ontario (Clark et al. 1996), Swedish

(Liljegren et al. 1999) and Scottish (Forrest et al. 1996) trials had less extensive surgery compared with the Milan III trial (Veronesi et al. 1993). The recurrence rate in the control arm of the Milan III trial, in which the tumors were smaller and excision was considerably wider, was low (8.8% vs. 24–27% in other trials) albeit at the cost of cosmesis. Nevertheless, radiotherapy reduced it even further and at the same proportional rate as in other trials. If local recurrence were caused by residual disease only, then radiotherapy should have led to a much larger proportional reduction in those patients with positive margins or less extensive surgery, but radiotherapy is as effective in patients with negative margins suggesting that radiotherapy may have an effect on the soil rather than the seed (Vaidya et al. 2004b).

Thus, radiotherapy may have the dual effect of inhibiting the growth of genetically unstable cells around the primary tumor and of making the whole breast tissue less conducive to growth (Vaidya et al. 2004b). Systemic therapies such as aromatase inhibitors or ovarian suppression may achieve the latter effect through reduction of estrogen concentration in the breast and may have a synergistic effect with radiotherapy (Azria et al. 2005). Thus, with increasing use of systemic therapy, radiotherapy to the tissues surrounding the primary tumor might be all that is necessary, and such an approach may solve many of the problems of postoperative radiotherapy discussed earlier and may allow many more women with breast cancer to conserve their breast.

For many patients, especially those in the postmenopausal age group with small, low grade, hormone receptor-positive, lymph node-negative tumors, the necessity for a lengthy and sometimes damaging course of radiation therapy is questionable.

In this chapter we talk about a way in which partial breast irradiation could be delivered as a single fraction in the operating room, usually at the time of primary surgery.

12.2 Intraoperative Radiotherapy: an Elegant Method of Partial Breast Irradiation

Modern intraoperative radiotherapy (IORT) devices have benefited from miniaturization technology. No longer do we need to transport the patient to a purposed-built radiotherapy suite—the (mini)radiotherapy suite comes to the patient right in the operating room! The first such device to be used for IORT was the Intrabeam (Photoelectron Corporation, Lexington, MA, USA) (Vaidya et al. 1999, 2001), which is now manufactured by Carl Zeiss (Oberkochen , Germany) (Fig. 12.1). The two other mobile linear accelerator systems are the Mobetron system (Oncology Care Systems Group of Siemens Medical Systems, Intraop Medical, Santa Clara CA, USA) and the Novac7 system (Hitesys, Italy). Some of the characteristics of these machines are given below (Table 12.1).

12.3 Radiobiology of Intraoperative Radiotherapy

The main basis of IORT is that a single dose of IORT could have a biological effect on tissue that is equivalent to a full course of fractionated external beam radiotherapy (EBRT). This is therefore being tested in randomized trials. There is already some evidence suggesting the safety and effectiveness of a single dose of radiotherapy in achieving tumor cell kill (Vaidya et al. 2004b, 2005b). The theoretical basis for calculation of the biological effects of a given dose of radiation is the linear-quadratic model. This model is based on the different shapes of cell survival curves of acute and late-reacting tissues. It is assumed that large single doses of radiation are more effective on late-responding tissues as compared to acute-reacting tissues. However, the LQ model is reliable for single doses up to 6–8 Gy only and may therefore not be appropriate for modeling the effects of higher single doses (20–25 Gy) which are used in IORT or radiosurgery. There is now abundant clinical information about the effects and side effects of high single doses. Radiosurgery doses of 20–25 Gy are sufficient to sterilize macroscopic brain metastases with a very low risk of causing brain necrosis or functional damage when the dose is given to a small volume (Flickinger et al. 1995, 2003; Wenz et al. 1998). Long-term follow-up of large Swedish (Swedish Rectal Cancer Trial 1997) and Dutch (Kapiteijn et al. 2001) rectal cancer trials in which 25 Gy given in five fractions was prescribed to the pelvis has not shown unacceptable toxicity. Thus, severe long-term side effects would not be expected after administration of 5–7 Gy to 1 cm of breast tissue surrounding an excision cavity, although caution should be exercised when giving high single doses to skin and ribs (Reitsamer et al. 2004).

A detailed analysis of the radiobiological aspects specific to the Intrabeam system requires consideration of the increased relative biological efficiency (RBE) of the low-energy x-rays, a steep dose-dependency of RBE, and the rate of damage repair during radiotherapy delivery (30–50 minutes). Brenner et al. (1999) have estimated an RBE of about 1.5 for this type of low-energy x-rays. For a complete modeling of RBE, the introduction of the Lea-Catchside time factor (Herskind et al. 2005) is important. Using this equation, an RBE of 1.0 at the applicator surface, of 1.5 at 10 mm, and about 2.0 at 25 mm can be estimated, with the exact value depending on the size of the applicator. The risk of side effects can also calculated, although there are insufficient data as to the impact of the volume of treatment to include this as a factor. (However, since the treatment volume is small for IORT, the risk of side effects will probably be lower than that calculated from this model.) Since the $TD_{50}/_5$ for pneumonitis is about 9–10 Gy, the thickness of the chest wall should ensure that there is virtually no risk of pneumonitis. The same is true for the heart. Since the dose to the heart and lungs during IORT is

Table 12.1 Some characteristics of intraoperative radiotherapy systems (from Vaidya et al. 2004b)

Device	Company	Radiation type	Dose	Weight of treatment device (kg)
Intrabeam	Carl Zeiss, Oberkochen, Germany	Soft x-rays at 50 kV	Physical dose of 20 Gy next to the applicator (with a quick attenuation) over 25–30 minutes. Setting up time about 10–12 minutes	1.8
Mobitron	Intraop Medical, Santa Clara, CA, USA	Electrons at 4–12 MeV	20 Gy physical dose in 3–5 minutes. Setting up time about 20 minutes	1275
Novac7	Hitesys, Latina, Italy	Electrons at 4–12 MeV	20 Gy physical dose in 3–5 minutes Setting up time about 20 minutes	650

almost negligible, the mortality from cardiac ischemia that has been observed in some trials using conventional radiation therapy (Bates and Evans 1995; Lind et al. 1997; Meinardi et al. 2001; Rutqvist and Johansson 1990) should not be seen. The $TD_{50/5}$ for subcutaneous fibrosis is in the range of 13 Gy. The risk of fibrosis shows a steep decrease with increasing distance from the applicator, reaching nearly zero at about 5 mm tissue depth. The calculated low risk of toxicity is in good agreement with the available clinical data in 13 patients with a maximum follow-up of 4 years (Vaidya et al. 2003).

The single-dose radiation using Intrabeam [called Targeted Intraoperative Radiotherapy, TARGIT (Vaidya et al. 1999)] is administered over 15–35 minutes. Since normal tissues can repair their DNA within a few minutes, a large proportion of radiation-induced DNA damage is repaired in normal tissues during this long duration of IORT. On the other hand, cancer cells or precancerous cells with a poor DNA-repair machinery are unable to do so. Thus radiation using Intrabeam administered over 25–35 minutes would have a high therapeutic index, and would induce less damage to normal tissue than similar doses given over 2–3 minutes. Specific laboratory experiments to test this concept are already underway.

We have developed a mathematical model (Enderling et al. 2005) to estimate the effect of a single dose of radiotherapy as given with Intrabeam in the TARGIT trial. We believe that the therapeutic effectiveness or not of radiotherapy is influenced by the fact that breast cancers are surrounded by morphologically normal cells that already have loss of heterozygosity in critical genes (Deng et al. 1994, 1996). These cells would be able to repair their DNA in response to fractionated radiotherapy just like normal cells. Continuing survival and subsequent transformation of these cells may be a large factor in development of local recurrence. This mathematical model is the first to offer an explanation for the fact that conventional radiotherapy is effective in only two-thirds of cases of early breast cancers. This proportional reduction in recurrence by conventional radiotherapy (of 66%) is constant across tumor sizes, and excision extents! However, when subjected to a single large dose of radiotherapy as in TARGIT, these cells would succumb, and thus the source of local recurrence would be eliminated.

The method of delivery of IORT ensures that the volume of tissues radiated is small so that the early and late side effects is minimal. Furthermore, the radiobiological effect of a single fraction of radiotherapy may actually be paradoxically higher at greater depth (Astor et al. 2000).

The radiation produced by Intrabeam (the x-ray source is called PRS – Photon Radiosurgery System) has been found to induce both necrotic and apoptotic cell death in addition to rapid cell death through non-apoptotic pathways (Kurita et al. 2000). Animal experiments have demonstrated that PRS can induce well-demarcated ablation in canine liver and kidney (Chan et al. 2000; Koniaris et al. 2000; Solomon et al. 2001). As a demonstration of its efficacy in ablating tumor tissue a series of three breast cancer patients (T=1–2.5 cm) have been treated with a PRS 400 (bare probe only—i.e., without the applicators, but with the same Intrabeam machine that is used for IORT—shown in the left upper part of Fig. 12.2). These patients were too frail to have surgery. The tumor was localized on the Mammotest, a digital stereotactic prone mammography table. The tip of the probe was placed in the center of the tumor and radiation delivered in about 6–12 minutes. The tumors, ranging in size from 1 to 2.5 cm, were ablated with a single dose of radiotherapy as demonstrated on biopsy and serial contrast-enhanced MRI (Vaidya et al. 2002c).

Another radiobiological question of importance is whether the tolerable dose is sufficient to prevent local recurrence. We have previously discussed how a single IORT treatment of 20 Gy compares to a course of fractionated EBRT of about 50 Gy (Vaidya et al. 2004a). One advantage of IORT is that there is no delay between tumor excision and treatment, so there is no loss of efficacy due to tumor cell proliferation before starting EBRT or during the EBRT course. The RBE of low-energy x-rays for early-reacting tissues and tumor cells (α/β ratio of 3 Gy) is higher than for late-reacting tissues (α/β ratio of 10 Gy). As noted above, the RBE increases with distance from the applicator (Herskind et al. 2005). Thus, the surviving fraction of tumor cells at the applicator surface will be 10^{-12}; 99% of the tumor cells 10 mm from the applicator surface should be sterilized. Thus the tissues immediately next to the applicator would receive a high physical dose (with a low therapeutic ratio), and those further away from the applicator would receive a lower physical dose but with a high therapeutic ratio (Astor et al. 2000). This is an advantage of Intrabeam over the systems using electrons to deliver a uniform dose of radiation because its small high (physical) dose region would be expected to increase tumor cell killing while reducing normal tissue damage and long-term toxicity. In contrast, EBRT has a homogeneous dose distribution, and therefore the spatial distribution of the risk of recurrence depends only on the tumor cell density (which is highest close to the excision cavity). One may therefore expect that there is a "sphere of equivalence" around the excision cavity in which the risk of recurrence for IORT is equivalent to that of EBRT (Early Breast Cancer Trialists' Collaborative Group 2000). The radius of this sphere depends on the applicator size and is about 15 mm for the most-often used applicators.

There is yet another theoretical advantage of IORT as opposed to other methods of radiotherapy: the temporal immediacy. The radiotherapy delivered by TARGIT is at the crucial time—immediately after surgery and before wound healing begins when several chemokines and growth factors will start working on the tumor bed and any residual potentially malignant cells, and TARGIT may favorably alter the microenvironment

As yet, there is no firmly established standardized IORT dose or dose rate for use in early breast cancer. IORT doses investigated for use in early breast cancer have ranged from 5 Gy to 22 Gy using a variety of different IORT systems. The Intrabeam IORT system delivers a physical dose of 18–20 Gy administered to the tumor bed and about 5–7 Gy at a distance of 1.0 cm from the breast tumor cavity for a period of 20–25 minutes. Using their Novac7 IORT technology, Veronesi et al. have estimated that an external beam dose of 60 Gy delivered in 30 fractions at 2 Gy/fraction is equivalent to a single IORT fraction of 20–22 Gy (using an α/β ratio at 10 Gy, typical for tumors and acute-reacting tissues). The doses delivered by other methods of partial breast irradiation such as intraoperative systems such as Novac7 have been criticized as being large (Pawlik and Kuerer 2005) and the dose delivered in TARGIT may be the optimal dose. However, the randomized trials TARGIT and ELIOT will provide the answer as to which dose is adequate without compromising cosmetic outcome.

12.4 The Intrabeam Machine and Surgical Technique

The Intrabeam machine contains a miniature electron gun and electron accelerator contained in an x-ray tube which are powered by a 12 V power supply. "Soft" x-rays (50 kVp) are emitted from the point source. Tissue is kept at a distance from the source by spheri-

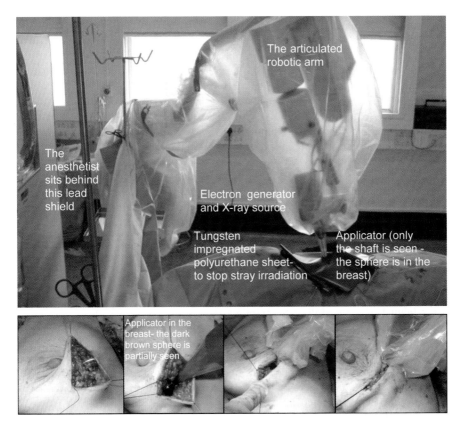

Fig. 12.1 *Top* The Intrabeam system – with the x-ray source in the breast wound – and the electron generator and accelerator held by the articulated arm. *Bottom* The target breast tissue wraps around the applicator giving true conformal brachytherapy

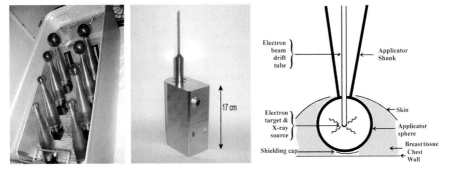

Fig. 12.2 The Intrabeam x-ray source (*middle*) and applicators (*left*). The schematic diagram (*right*) shows how the target tissues are irradiated from within the breast and how the intrathoracic structures are protected with a thin shield

cal applicators to give a uniform dose. Depending upon the size of the surgical cavity, various sizes of applicator spheres are available. The precise dose rate depends on the diameter of the applicator and the energy of the beam, both of which may be varied to optimize the radiation treatment. For example, a dose of 18–20 Gy at the applicator surface, i.e., the tumor bed, can be delivered in about 20 minutes with a 3.5-cm applicator. The quick attenuation of the radiation minimizes the need for radiation protection to the operating personnel. Usually the operating team leaves the room, but the anesthetist (and anyone else interested in observing the procedure) sits behind a mobile lead shield which prevents exposure. The technique has been previously described in detail (Vaidya et al. 2002a), and an operative video is available from the authors via the internet.

In the operating room, wide local excision of the primary tumor is carried out in the usual manner, with a margin of normal breast tissue. After the lumpectomy, it is important to achieve complete hemostasis, because even a small amount of bleeding in the 20–25 minutes during which radiotherapy is being delivered can distort the cavity enough to considerably change the dosimetry. Different size applicators are tried until one is found that fits snugly within the cavity. A purse string suture needs to be skillfully placed. It must pass through the breast parenchyma and appose it to the applicator surface. It is important to protect the dermis, which should not be brought within 1 cm of the applicator surface. Fine prolene sutures can be used to slightly retract the skin edge away from the applicator are useful. However, complete eversion of the skin or using self-retaining retractors will increase the separation from the applicator so much that it would jeopardize the radiation dose and risk under-treatment. For skin further away from the edge that cannot be effectively retracted for fear of reducing the dose to target tissues, a customized piece of surgical gauze soaked in saline, 0.5 to 0.9 cm thick, can be inserted deep to the skin—this allows the dermis to be lifted off the applicator, while allowing the breast tissue just deep to it still to receive radiotherapy. If necessary, the chest wall and skin can be protected by radioopaque tungsten-filled polyurethane material. These thin rubber-like sheets are supplied as caps that fit on the applicator or as a larger flat sheet that can be cut to size on the operating table to fit the area of pectoralis muscle that is exposed and does not need to be irradiated. These provide effective (95% shielding) protection to intrathoracic structures.

In patients undergoing sentinel node sampling with immediate cytological or histological evaluation (so that complete axillary clearance can be carried out at the same sitting), TARGIT can often be delivered while the surgical team waits for this result without wasting operating room time. With this elegant approach the pliable breast tissue around the cavity of surgical excision wraps around the radiotherapy source, i.e. the target is "conformed" to the source. This simple, effective technique avoids the unnecessarily complex and sophisticated techniques of using interstitial implantation of radioactive wires or the even more complex techniques necessary for conformal radiotherapy by external beams with multileaf collimators from a linear accelerator. It eliminates geographical miss and delivers radiotherapy at the earliest possible time after surgery. The quick attenuation of the radiation dose protects normal tissues and allows the treatment to be carried out in unmodified operating theatres. Thus in theory, the biological effect and cosmetic outcome could be improved.

12.5 The Novac7 System

The Milan group is also testing the same approach (Intra et al. 2002; Veronesi et al. 2001) using a mobile linear accelerator (Novac7; see Fig. 12.3) in a randomized trial (ELIOT). Novac7 (Hitesys, Italy) is a mobile dedicated linear accelerator. Its radiating head can be moved by an articulated arm which can work in an existing operating room. It delivers electron beams at four different nominal energies: 3, 5, 7, 9 MeV radiation. The beams are collimated by means of a hard-docking system, consisting of cylindrical Perspex applicators available in various diameters. The source to surface distance is between 80 and 100 cm. For radiation protection reasons, a primary beam stopper, consisting of a lead shield 15 cm thick, mounted on a trolley and three mobile barriers (100 cm long, 150 cm high, 1.5 cm lead thickness) are provided. Electron beams that are delivered by Novac7 have very high dose/pulse values compared with conventional linear accelerators.

Once the local resection has been performed, the breast is mobilized off the pectoral muscle for 5–10 cm around the tumor bed and separated from the skin for 3–5 cm in all directions. In order to minimize the irradiation to the thoracic wall, dedicated aluminum–lead disks (4 mm aluminum + 5 mm lead) of various diameters (4 to 10 cm) are placed between the deep face of the residual breast and the pectoralis muscle. The breast is now sutured so as to obliterate the tumor bed and to bring the target tissues together.

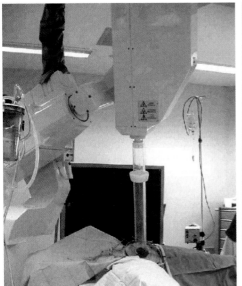
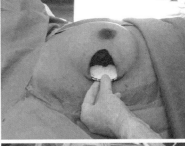
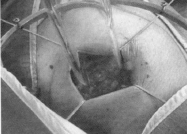

Fig. 12.3 The Novac7 system. The arm of the mobile linear accelerator (*left*) is attached to a Perspex cylinder that is introduced into the breast wound (*lower right*). The breast tissue is mobilized from the chest wall and overlying skin and apposed in the wound after placing a lead shield between the breast and pectoralis muscle (*upper right*). Images from Veronesi et al. 2001, with the kind permission of Prof. Umberto Veronesi

The thickness of the target volume is measured by a needle and a ruler in at least three points and averaged. The skin margins are stretched out of the radiation field using a device consisting of a metallic ring furnished with four hooks. The cylindrical applicator (4–10 cm diameter) is placed through the skin incision and the source cylinder is "docked" onto the upper end of the applicator. Four barriers are placed to shield stray radiation and all the personnel leave the operating room. Once the radiotherapy is finished the wound is closed in the usual manner.

The dose delivered by this technique is much higher than that delivered by the Intrabeam system. Only the results of clinical trials will tell us which dose achieves the best balance between cosmetic outcome and local control of disease.

12.6 Results of Clinical Trials with the Intrabeam System

Based on the hypothesis that index quadrant irradiation is sufficient, in July 1998 we introduced the technique of TARGIT (Vaidya 2002; Vaidya et al. 2001, 2002b, 2004b) radiotherapy delivered as a single dose using low-energy x-rays targeted to the peritumoral tissues from within the breast using the Intrabeam device. In patients with small well-differentiated breast cancers, which are now the majority, this could be the sole radiotherapy treatment. In those with a high risk of local recurrence elsewhere in the breast (e.g. lobular carcinoma and those with an extensive intraductal component, EIC), it would avoid any geographical miss, and in combination with EBRT, may even reduce local recurrence.

In the pilot studies in the United Kingdom, the United States, Australia, Germany, and Italy testing the feasibility and safety of the technique, 301 patients (302 Cancers) underwent TARGIT as a boost dose (Vaidya et al. 2005a) and also received whole-breast EBRT. The median follow-up at the time of writing was 27 months, but the first patient was treated in July 1998 and the longest follow-up was 80 months). Amongst these patients, four have had local recurrence. These included one with diffuse recurrence at 10 months, one with a focus of DCIS in the scar at 32 months and two with a new primary outside the index quadrant at 40 and 77 months. It appears that given as a boost, TARGIT yields very low recurrence rates (actuarial rate = 2.6% at 5 years).

In addition, during this pilot phase, 22 patients (Vaidya et al. 2005b) received TARGIT as the sole modality of radiotherapy. For these patients, the median follow-up at the time of writing was 26 months for these patients and one patient had a local recurrence after 5 years.

Apart from two patients treated early in these studies, wound healing has been excellent. The cosmetic outcome was assessed formally in available patients treated in the United Kingdom at a median follow-up of 42 months by a surgeon and a nurse not involved in the trial (Vaidya et al. 2003). On a scale of 1–5 (with 5 being the best), the mean scores for appearance, texture and comfort of the breast given by these observers were 3.5, 2.7 and 3.7. The corresponding scores given by the patient herself were 4, 3.1 and 3.5.

The multicenter randomized trial TARGIT (Vaidya 2002; Vaidya et al. 1999, 2002d, 2004b) using the Intrabeam system is now recruiting patients in the United Kingdom, Germany, Italy, the United States, and Australia. This is a randomized trial in which patients are enrolled prior to tumor excision to receive either IORT or conventional whole-breast radiotherapy. However, each center may decide that patients randomized to IORT who are found to have certain pathological findings (e.g. lobular carcinoma or an EIC) may subsequently receive whole-breast irradiation in addition. This facility allows pragmatic management of patients with an equipoise that can be decided by every individual center. Furthermore, the trial allows the radiotherapy to be delivered at a second procedure, after the final histopathology is available and eligibility criteria are met satisfactorily. Initially, at University College London we were exclusively delivering IORT at the time of the primary operation. The Australian group found that it is if it is given at a second procedure, it is easier to manage clinically and logistically. At Dundee, we are using both approaches which allow us to recruit patients from another hospital that is part of the same National Health Service trust, but is situated some distance away in Perth.

The first patient was randomized in the TARGIT trial in March 2000. At the time of writing, 8 centers are recruiting in this trial and in the last year the accrual had picked up significantly—over 425 patients had been randomized. The final goal is just over 2232. The outcome measures are local recurrence, cosmetic outcome, patient satisfaction and cost analysis., and it is expected that the first results of this trial will be available in 2007.

It is well recognized as in every adjuvant situation that postoperative whole-breast radiotherapy is an over-treatment 60–70% of times since only 30–40% of patients will ever get a local recurrence after surgery alone. Our approach using IORT intends to refine the treatment of breast cancer patients by introducing a risk-adapted strategy: the elderly patient with a T1G1a tumor should perhaps be treated with a different kind of therapy such as TARGIT only, as compared to the young patient with a T2G3 tumor who would have a more accurate boost with TARGIT in addition to whole-breast radiotherapy. The TARGIT trial is testing exactly such a strategy. Hence, the TARGIT trial should not be mistaken for a trial solely designed to compare IORT with postoperative radiotherapy, when actually, it is testing two different treatment approaches—the conventional blanket approach versus the new approach of tailored treatment.

The Milan trial (ELIOT) using the Novac7 has also been recruiting since November 2000 at a fast rate and their preliminary results are encouraging. In their pilot studies (Veronesi et al. 2005), 590 patients affected by unifocal breast carcinoma up to a diameter of 2.5 cm received wide resection of the breast followed by IORT with electrons (ELIOT). Most patients received 21 Gy intraoperatively, biologically equivalent to 58–60 Gy in standard fractionation. After a median follow-up of 20 months, 19 patients (3.2%) had developed breast fibrosis and 3 patients (0.5%) local recurrences, 3 patients ipsilateral carcinomas in other quadrants, and another 5 patients contralateral breast carcinoma. One patient (0.2%) died of distant metastases.

12.7 Health Economics

Delivering IORT with the Intrabeam prolongs the primary operation by 5–45 minutes (the extra time is less when it is performed in conjunction with immediate analysis of the sentinel lymph node). In addition, approximately 1 hour of a radiotherapy physicist's time is needed to prepare the device. EBRT requires about 9 man-hours of planning, 6 hours of radiotherapy-room time, and 30–60 hours of patient time. If the cost of conventional radiotherapy were £2400 (US $1360), using the most conservative estimates, then considering only the 66% saving of man-hours this novel technique would save £1800 (US $1020) per patient. If we assume that 25% of the 27,000 breast cancer patients diagnosed every year in the United Kingdom might be treated by breast-conserving surgery and IORT instead of conventional EBRT, the yearly savings for the National Health Service would be £12,150,000 (US $6,880,000). This does not include the substantial saving of expensive time on the linear accelerators, which would allow reduced waiting lists and, most importantly, the saving of time, effort, and inconvenience for patients. Thus, unlike most other "new" treatments, this one may be actually be less expensive than the current standard!

As we have stated before (Vaidya et al. 2004a, 2004b), mere novelty and the convenience of the this new technology should not come in the way of its proper scientific assessment before it is used for standard care. Randomized clinical trials are essential to test this revolutionary approach. We believe that the future for local treatment of breast cancer could be tailored to the needs of the patient and the tumor. The patient, the surgeon and the radiation oncologist will be able to choose from several well-tested approaches. This may mean not just wider availability of breast-conserving therapy, but also that small incremental benefits from targeted and tailored treatment may reduce morbidity and even mortality.

References

1. Astor MB, Hilaris BS, Gruerio A, Varricchione T, Smith D (2000) Preclinical studies with the photon radiosurgery system (PRS). Int J Radiat Oncol Biol Phys 47:809–813
2. Athas WF, Adams-Cameron M, Hunt WC, Amir-Fazli A, Key CR (2000) Travel distance to radiation therapy and receipt of radiotherapy following breast-conserving surgery. J Natl Cancer Inst 92:269–271
3. Azria D, Larbouret C, Cunat S, Ozsahin M, Gourgou S, Martineau P, Evans DB, Romieu G, Pujol P, Pelegrin A (2005) Letrozole sensitizes breast cancer cells to ionizing radiation. Breast Cancer Res 7:R156–R163
4. Bartelink H, Horiot JC, Poortmans P, Struikmans H, Van den Bogaert W, Barillot I, Fourquet A, Borger J, Jager J, Hoogenraad W, Collette L, Pierart M; the European Organization for Research and Treatment of Cancer Radiotherapy and Breast Cancer Groups (2001) Recurrence rates after treatment of breast cancer with standard radiotherapy with or without additional radiation. N Engl J Med 345:1378–1387
5. Bates T, Evans RG (1995) Audit of brachial plexus neuropathy following radiotherapy. Clin Oncol (R Coll Radiol) 7:236
6. Brenner DJ, Leu CS, Beatty JF, Shefer RE (1999) Clinical relative biological effectiveness of low-energy x-rays emitted by miniature x-ray devices. Phys Med Biol 44:323–333
7. Chan DY, Koniaris L, Magee C, Ferrell M, Solomon S, Lee BR, Anderson JH, Smith DO, Czapski J, Deweese T, Choti MA, Kavoussi LR (2000) Feasibility of ablating normal renal parenchyma by interstitial photon radiation energy: study in a canine model. J Endourol 14:111–116
8. Clark RM, Wilkinson RH, Mahoney LJ, Reid JG, MacDonald WD (1982) Breast cancer: a 21 year experience with conservative surgery and radiation. Int J Radiat Oncol Biol Phys 8:967–979

9. Clark RM, McCulloch PB, Levine MN, Lipa M, Wilkinson RH, Mahoney LJ, Basrur VR, Nair BD, McDermot RS, Wong CS (1992) Randomized clinical trial to assess the effectiveness of breast irradiation following lumpectomy and axillary dissection for node-negative breast cancer. J Natl Cancer Inst 84:683–689

10. Clark RM, Whelan T, Levine M, Roberts R, Willan A, McCulloch P, Lipa M, Wilkinson RH, Mahoney LJ (1996) Randomized clinical trial of breast irradiation following lumpectomy and axillary dissection for node-negative breast cancer: an update. Ontario Clinical Oncology Group. J Natl Cancer Inst 88:1659–1664

11. Deng G, Chen LC, Schott DR, Thor A, Bhargava V, Ljung BM, Chew K, Smith HS (1994) Loss of heterozygosity and p53 gene mutations in breast cancer. Cancer Res 54:499–505

12. Deng G, Lu Y, Zlotnikov G, Thor AD, Smith HS (1996) Loss of heterozygosity in normal tissue adjacent to breast carcinomas. Science 274:2057–2059

13. Early Breast Cancer Trialists' Collaborative Group (1995) Effects of radiotherapy and surgery in early breast cancer. An overview of the randomized trials. N Engl J Med 333:1444–1455

14. Early Breast Cancer Trialists' Collaborative Group (2000) Favourable and unfavourable effects on long-term survival of radiotherapy for early breast cancer: an overview of the randomised trials [see comments]. Lancet 355:1757–1770

15. Enderling H, Anderson AR, Chaplain MA, Munro AJ, Vaidya JS (2005) Mathematical modelling of radiotherapy strategies for early breast cancer. J Theor Biol doi:10.1016/j.jtbi.2005.11.015

16. Fisher B, Anderson S, Redmond CK, Wolmark N, Wickerham DL, Cronin WM (1995) Re-analysis and results after 12 years of follow-up in a randomized clinical trial comparing total mastectomy with lumpectomy with or without irradiation in the treatment of breast cancer [see comments]. N Engl J Med 333:1456–1461

17. Flickinger JC, Kondziolka D, Lunsford LD (1995) Radiosurgery of benign lesions. Semin Radiat Oncol 5:220–224

18. Flickinger JC, Kondziolka D, Lunsford LD (2003) Radiobiological analysis of tissue responses following radiosurgery. Technol Cancer Res Treat 2:87–92

19. Forrest AP, Stewart HJ, Everington D, Prescott RJ, McArdle CS, Harnett AN, Smith DC, George WD (1996) Randomised controlled trial of conservation therapy for breast cancer: 6-year analysis of the Scottish trial. Scottish Cancer Trials Breast Group [see comments]. Lancet 348:708–713

20. Halsted WS (1894) The results of operations for the cure of cancer of the breast performed at The Johns Hopkins Hospital from June 1889 to January 1894. Johns Hopkins Hospital Rep 4:297–350

21. Herskind C, Steil V, Kraus-Tiefenbacher U, Wenz F (2005) Radiobiological aspects of intraoperative radiotherapy (IORT) with isotropic low-energy X-rays for early-stage breast cancer. Radiat Res 163:208–215.

22. Intra M, Gatti G, Luini A, Galimberti V, Veronesi P, Zurrida S, Frasson A, Ciocca M, Orecchia R, Veronesi U (2002) Surgical technique of intraoperative radiotherapy in conservative treatment of limited-stage breast cancer. Arch Surg 137:737–740

23. Kapiteijn E, Marijnen CA, Nagtegaal ID, Putter H, Steup WH, Wiggers T, Rutten HJ, Pahlman L, Glimelius B, van Krieken JH, Leer JW, van de Velde CJ (2001) Preoperative radiotherapy combined with total mesorectal excision for resectable rectal cancer. N Engl J Med 345:638–646

24. Katz SJ, Lantz PM, Janz NK, Fagerlin A, Schwartz K, Liu L, Deapen D, Salem B, Lakhani I, Morrow M (2005) Patient involvement in surgery treatment decisions for breast cancer. J Clin Oncol 23:5526–5533

25. Koniaris LG, Chan DY, Magee C, Solomon SB, Anderson JH, Smith DO, De Weese T, Kavoussi LR, Choti MA (2000) Focal hepatic ablation using interstitial photon radiation energy. J Am Coll Surg 191:164–174

26. Kurita H, Ostertag CB, Baumer B, Kopitzki K, Warnke PC (2000) Early effects of PRS-irradiation for 9L gliosarcoma: characterization of interphase cell death. Minim Invasive Neurosurg 43:197–200

27. Liljegren G, Holmberg L, Bergh J, Lindgren A, Tabar L, Nordgren H, Adami HO (1999) 10-Year results after sector resection with or without postoperative radiotherapy for stage I breast cancer: a randomized trial [see comments]. J Clin Oncol 17:2326–2333

28. Lind DS, Kontaridis MI, Edwards PD, Josephs MD, Moldawer LL, Copeland EM3 (1997) Nitric oxide contributes to adriamycin's antitumor effect. J Surg Res 69:283–287

29. Lu Q, Nakmura J, Savinov A, Yue W, Weisz J, Dabbs DJ, Wolz G, Brodie A (1996) Expression of aromatase protein and messenger ribonucleic acid in tumor epithelial cells and evidence of functional significance of locally produced estrogen in human breast cancers. Endocrinology 137:3061–3068

30. Machtay M, Lanciano R, Hoffman J, Hanks GE (1994) Inaccuracies in using the lumpectomy scar for planning electron boosts in primary breast carcinoma. Int J Radiat Oncol Biol Phys 30:43–48

31. McCulloch PG, MacIntyre A (1993) Effects of surgery on the generation of lymphokine-activated killer cells in patients with breast cancer. Br J Surg 80:1005–1007

32. Meinardi MT, Van Veldhuisen DJ, Gietema JA, Dolsma WV, Boomsma F, Van Den Berg MP, Volkers C, Haaksma J, De Vries EG, Sleijfer DT, Van Der Graaf WT (2001) Prospective evaluation of early cardiac damage induced by epirubicin-containing adjuvant chemotherapy and locoregional radiotherapy in breast cancer patients. J Clin Oncol 19:2746–2753

33. Mikeljevic JS, Haward R, Johnston C, Crellin A, Dodwell D, Jones A, Pisani P, Forman D (2004) Trends in postoperative radiotherapy delay and the effect on survival in breast cancer patients treated with conservation surgery. Br J Cancer 90:1343–1348

34. Nakamura J, Savinov A, Lu Q, Brodie A (1996) Estrogen regulates vascular endothelial growth/permeability factor expression in 7,12-dimethylbenz(a)anthracene-induced rat mammary tumors. Endocrinology 137:5589–5596

35. Nielsen M, Thomsen JL, Primdahl S, Dyreborg U, Andersen JA (1987) Breast cancer and atypia among young and middle-aged women: a study of 110 medicolegal autopsies. Br J Cancer 56:814–819

36. O'Neill JS, Elton RA, Miller WR (1988) Aromatase activity in adipose tissue from breast quadrants: a link with tumour site. BMJ 296:741–743

37. Pawlik TM, Kuerer HM (2005) Accelerated partial breast irradiation as an alternative to whole breast irradiation in breast-conserving therapy for early-stage breast cancer. Womens Health 1:59–71

38. Reitsamer R, Peintinger F, Kopp M, Menzel C, Kogelnik HD, Sedlmayer F (2004) Local recurrence rates in breast cancer patients treated with intraoperative electron-boost radiotherapy versus postoperative external-beam electron-boost irradiation. A sequential intervention study. Strahlenther Onkol 180:38–44

39. Rutqvist LE, Johansson H (1990) Mortality by laterality of the primary tumour among 55,000 breast cancer patients from the Swedish Cancer Registry. Br J Cancer 61:866–868

40. Sedlmayer F, Rahim HB, Kogelnik HD, Menzel C, Merz F, Deutschmann H, Kranzinger M (1996) Quality assurance in breast cancer brachytherapy: geographic miss in the interstitial boost treatment of the tumor bed. Int J Radiat Oncol Biol Phys 34:1133–1139

41. Solomon SB, Koniaris LG, Chan DY, Magee CA, DeWeese TL, Kavoussi LR, Choti MA (2001) Temporal CT changes after hepatic and renal interstitial radiotherapy in a canine model. J Comput Assist Tomogr 25:74–80

42. Swedish Rectal Cancer Trial (1997) Improved survival with preoperative radiotherapy in resectable rectal cancer. Swedish Rectal Cancer Trial. N Engl J Med 336:980–987

43. Turner BC, Harrold E, Matloff E, Smith T, Gumbs AA, Beinfield M, Ward B, Skolnick M, Glazer PM, Thomas A, Haffty BG (1999) BRCA1/BRCA2 germline mutations in locally recurrent breast cancer patients after lumpectomy and radiation therapy: implications for breast-conserving management in patients with BRCA1/BRCA2 mutations [see comments]. J Clin Oncol 17:3017–3024

44. Turner BC, Gumbs AA, Carbone CJ, Carter D, Glazer PM, Haffty BG (2000) Mutant p53 protein overexpression in women with ipsilateral breast tumor recurrence following lumpectomy and radiation therapy. Cancer 88:1091–1098

45. Vaidya JS (2002) A novel approach for local treatment of early breast cancer. PhD Thesis, University of London

46. Vaidya JS, Vyas JJ, Chinoy RF, Merchant N, Sharma OP, Mittra I (1996) Multicentricity of breast cancer: whole-organ analysis and clinical implications. Br J Cancer 74:820–824

47. Vaidya JS, Baum M, Tobias JS, Houghton J (1999) Targeted Intraoperative Radiotherapy (TARGIT) – trial protocol. Lancet http://www.thelancet.com/journals/lancet/misc/protocol/99PRT-47

48. Vaidya JS, Baum M, Tobias JS, D'Souza DP, Naidu SV, Morgan S, Metaxas M, Harte KJ, Sliski AP, Thomson E (2001) Targeted intra-operative radiotherapy (Targit): an innovative method of treatment for early breast cancer. Ann Oncol 12:1075–1080

49. Vaidya JS, Baum M, Tobias JS, Morgan S, D'Souza D (2002a) The novel technique of delivering targeted intraoperative radiotherapy (Targit) for early breast cancer. Eur J Surg Oncol 28:447–454

50. Vaidya JS, Baum M, Tobias JS, Morgan S, D'Souza D (2002b) The novel technique of delivering targeted intraoperative radiotherapy (Targit) for early breast cancer. Eur J Surg Oncol 28:447–454

51. Vaidya JS, Hall-Craggs M, Baum M, Tobias JS, Falzon M, D'Souza DP, Morgan S (2002c) Percutaneous minimally invasive stereotactic primary radiotherapy for breast cancer. Lancet Oncol 3:252–253

52. Vaidya JS, Joseph D, Hilaris BS, Tobias JS, Houghton J, Keshtgar M, Sainsbury R, Taylor I (2002d) Targeted intraoperative radiotherapy for breast cancer: an international trial. Abstract book of ESTRO-21, Prague 2002. 21:135

53. Vaidya JS, Wilson AJ, Houghton J, Tobias JS, Joseph D, Wenz F, Hilaris B, Massarut S, Keshtgar M, Sainsbury R, Taylor I, D'Souza D, Saunders CS, Corica T, Ezio C, Mauro A, Baum M (2003) Cosmetic outcome after targeted intraoperative radiotherapy (Targit) for early breast cancer. 26th Annual San Antonio Breast Cancer Symposium. Abstract 1039

54. Vaidya JS, Tobias J, Baum M, Keshtgar M, Houghton J, Wenz F, Corica T, Joseph D (2004a) Intraoperative radiotherapy: the debate continues. Lancet Oncol 5:339–340

55. Vaidya JS, Tobias JS, Baum M, Keshtgar M, Joseph D, Wenz F, Houghton J, Saunders C, Corica T, D'Souza D, Sainsbury R, Massarut S, Taylor I, Hilaris B (2004b) Intraoperative radiotherapy for breast cancer. Lancet Oncol 5:165–173

56. Vaidya JS, Baum M, Tobias JS, et al (2005a) Targeted intraoperative radiotherapy (TARGIT) yields very low recurrence rates when given as a boost (abstract SABCS-2005). Br Cancer Res Treat 94 [Suppl 1]:S180

57. Vaidya JS, Tobias JS, Baum M, Wenz F, Kraus-Tiefenbacher U, D'Souza D, Keshtgar M, Massarut S, Hilaris B, Saunders C, Joseph D (2005b) TARGeted Intraoperative radiotherapy (TARGIT): an innovative approach to partial-breast irradiation. Semin Radiat Oncol 15:84–91

58. Veronesi U, Luini A, Del Vecchio M, Greco M, Galimberti V, Merson M, Rilke F, Sacchini V, Saccozzi R, Savio T (1993) Radiotherapy after breast-preserving surgery in women with localized cancer of the breast [see comments]. N Engl J Med 328:1587–1591

59. Veronesi U, Orecchia R, Luini A, Gatti G, Intra M, Zurrida S, Ivaldi G, Tosi G, Ciocca M, Tosoni A, De Lucia F (2001) A preliminary report of intraoperative radiotherapy (IORT) in limited-stage breast cancers that are conservatively treated. Eur J Cancer 37:2178–2183

60. Veronesi U, Orecchia R, Luini A, Galimberti V, Gatti G, Intra M, Veronesi P, Leonardi MC, Ciocca M, Lazzari R, Caldarella P, Simsek S, Silva LS, Sances D (2005) Full-dose intraoperative radiotherapy with electrons during breast-conserving surgery: experience with 590 cases. Ann Surg 242:101–106

61. Wenz F, Steinvorth S, Wildermuth S, Lohr F, Fuss M, Debus J, Essig M, Hacke W, Wannenmacher M (1998) Assessment of neuropsychological changes in patients with arteriovenous malformation (AVM) after radiosurgery. Int J Radiat Oncol Biol Phys 42:995–999

62. Wyatt RM, Beddoe AH, Dale RG (2003) The effects of delays in radiotherapy treatment on tumour control. Phys Med Biol 48:139–155

Quality Assurance for Breast Brachytherapy

13

Bruce Thomadsen and Rupak Das

Contents

13.1 Quality Assurance During the Implantation Process

13.1.1 Interstitial Implants

13.1.1.1 Checking of the Implantation Equipment

Quality management begins before the implantation procedure with the check of the equipment. Preferably, the reusable equipment should be checked during cleaning after the previous case. Of particular importance for template-based implants is verification that all parts of the template system work correctly and are not broken. The templates themselves are relatively thin plastic; even the "thick" portions of many templates have had much of the template material removed to make the plate lighter. As a result, the plate may suffer breakage, particularly near the edges where the holes weaken the plastic. The rails on which the templates travel also may crack, although frank breakage is rare for most of the materials. A cracked rail could break during the subsequent implant, interrupting the procedure. Screws should be checked for operation and stripping. The condition of each of these things should be carefully inspected. The process of packaging should include verification that all parts are included.

Unfortunately (or fortunately), much of the implantation equipment comes sterilized so physical inspection before the procedure becomes difficult. The main items that could affect the quality of the implant (template or otherwise) are the needles, the catheters and buttons. Should these materials be purchased in bulk and prepared at the facility, one of the references (Thomadsen 2000) gives detailed guidance on quality management for such supplies.

At the time of replacement of the needles with catheters, each catheter should be checked visually for integrity. If the buttons that fix the catheter have numbers, the numbers should be checked for duplication. The most likely error would come from mistaking a "6" for a "9", and there have been packs of buttons where two of the same number were packaged instead of one of each. If the numbers do not differentiate between the "6" and "9" other than by orientation, some marking, such as a decimal point after each, should be added to avoid confusion later.

13.1.1.2 Verification of the Target

Each of the implant techniques provides image-based guidance, and each also carries particular challenges. For template-based implants, aligning the template often forms the most time-consuming part of the procedure. Once aligned, the rest of the implantation proceeds fairly quickly. However, a poor alignment will make covering the target very difficult.

Localizing the target for a template-based implant is discussed elsewhere in this book. However, one important control measure is assuring that the template and the images used for localization are not reversed. Most templates come with different markers on the right and left. Figure 13.1 shows a mammogram with the template in place. The right side shows two small markers while the left side shows only one (as seen as the needles enter the template). This allows a check for parity of the images. The markers also indicate a given row and hole position, for example, on this template, the right marker indicates position 5 in row C.

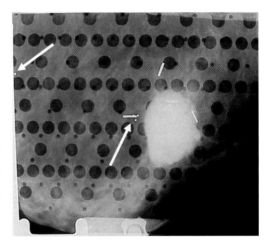

Fig. 13.1 A mammogram with the template in place. Small ball bearings orient the image, with one on the left side (indicated with an arrow), two on the right (just off the image) and three in the center (again with an arrow), looking as the needles enter the template. The ball bearings also indicate a particular row and hole

Implants performed under ultrasound (US), computer tomographic (CT) or magnetic resonance (MR) guidance make wrong-side errors in needle placement much less likely, but increase the difficulty in assuring placement of the needles in even, parallel rows. For US guidance, the target is drawn as projected on the skin directly anterior. That means that the implant needles run in planes quite a distance away from the transducer, adding to the difficulty of following the desired path. The images serve as the quality assurance (QA) on the placement.

13.1.1.3 Alignment of the Needles
Alignment of the needles during the implantation proper, while a certain part of quality control, is not discussed in this chapter. That is part of the implantation technique discussed previously. Assurance of proper needle placement is the function of the guiding template, or the guiding imagery.

13.1.1.4 Verification after Needle Placement
For all implants, regardless of the guidance approach, an image following insertion is always useful for verification. Such images can prevent treatment if a reversal of the guiding images was not detected previously, or without an adequate margin. Figure 13.2

shows such an image for a template-based implant. Any question that the implant coverage is not as expected or may not give an adequate margin should be carefully investigated and resolved before breaking the sterile field.

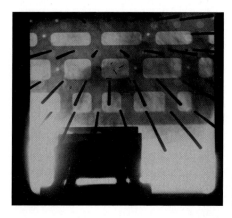

Fig. 13.2 A post-implantation image of a template-guided implant used to assure correct coverage of the target

A rule of thumb to follow for adequate coverage is to add needles to a margin if there is any question about coverage. Extra needles placed during the procedure add no discomfort for the patient. Later, unused catheters easily can be removed, but adding needles after localization indicates uncovered regions becomes a much more difficult procedure and uncomfortable for the patient.

13.1.2 Intracavitary Insertions

13.1.2.1 Checking the Intracavitary Equipment
The greatest concern about the equipment used for intracavitary breast insertions is loss of fluid in the balloon. Such a loss would lead to breast tissue coming closer to the source than calculated and potentially a large increase in dose. For a 4-cm diameter balloon, a 1-mm loss in radius produces a 10% increase in dose to the tissue at the balloon surface. Unfortunately, simply expanding the balloon before insertion is not the solution. Leaks may be slow, due to either poor seals at the syringe-end of the balloon or through small holes (or possibly diffusion), neither of which would be observed during a short inflation before insertion. However, major balloon failures would be evident, and the manufacturer recommends inflation of the balloons with about half the normal volume (about 60 to 90 cm³) as a check for integrity (and patency of the tube) before insertion.[1] For insertions performed after the tylectomy, rather than during, inflation before insertion can disrupt the smooth surface of the catheter making insertion more difficult. Much of the quality management before treatment focuses on assuring that the balloon diameter remains constant through the treatment.

---

1   Appreciation is extended to Gregory Edmundson for discussion on this topic.

13.1.2.2 Verification of Conformance with the Target

Intracavitary insertions eliminate many of the concerns with placing the sources in the target that accompany interstitial implants. In the intracavitary applications, the balloon catheter is often placed into the cavity at the time of the tylectomy. Questions of conformance of the applicator to the cavity then must wait for the localization phase of the procedure. In those cases where the catheter is placed later, the cavity still needs to be visible under imaging. Due to healing that may have taken place, positioning the balloon in the center of the cavity may be compromised, and such mispositioning could not be detected on the planning CT images. In addition, if the use of the balloon catheter was not planned at the time of the surgery, the cavity may not have been formed in a shape compatible to the use of the balloon. US imaging sometimes could serve to verify the correct positioning of the catheter during the insertion in such cases, but only where the cavity is still visible.

13.2 Quality Assurance during Localization and Reconstruction

The discussion of localization and treatment planning in this chapter assumes the use of CT or MR imaging. Two-dimensional radiographic imaging fails to delineate either the target or normal structures such as skin or lungs. Larger volumes of the patient must be treated to give reasonable assurance of covering the target, and yet such coverage is not assured. This becomes especially true for intracavitary treatments, where radiographic images fail to identify situations that can cause injury to the patient.

13.2.1 Interstitial Implants

Regardless of the position of the patient during implantation, treatment is almost always delivered with the patient supine. Localization requires the patient assume the same position as during treatment. Alternatively, if the bore of the imaging device (CT or MR) restricts the patient's position, treatment should be in the same position as localization. The position of the catheters will differ from the nice controlled array that existed during the implantation procedure, but through optimization during the treatment planning, the differences in catheter position seldom make any difference in the quality of the dose distribution.

13.2.1.1 Preparing the Catheters for Imaging

Before making the images, the catheters should have markers placed in them. The catheters do show on the images as dark spots, although it is sometimes difficult to visualize the actual end of the catheter. The uncertainty in the end position is aggravated by the interslice resolution. Special markers that indicate the end position of the source assist in obtaining the correct source positions for treatment planning. The limiting resolution of the slice thickness and interslice separation affects the accuracy of the calculation in all cases. If the catheters run perpendicular to the cuts, the position of the catheter are well defined but the position of the dwells along the catheter becomes uncertain by the slice thickness (assuming contiguous slices). If the catheters fall in a slice, the dwell positions in the catheter can be well located but the catheter position becomes uncertain, and if

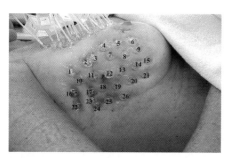

Fig. 13.3 A photograph of the exit side of an implant showing the catheter numbering as found from the entrance side

the catheters are perpendicular to the slice direction the dwell position becomes less certain.

The thickness of the breast changes over the duration of the treatment. Initially, when a template is used, it takes some time after the removal of the template for the breast to relax and assume a normal shape. The breast swells during, and for a time following, implantation. Because of these changes, the buttons fixing the catheters in place should not be placed too tightly immediately after the implant. By the next day, a common time for localization imaging, the breast will have reduced towards its normal size. However, during the course of treatment, the breast usually swells again in response to the radiation. Thus, at the time of localization, the buttons should not be fastened too tightly. Buttons that can slide along the catheter can be made snug at the time of localization and the pressure released as the breast swells. Buttons that fix solidly to the catheters must leave room for swelling. The changing contour of the breast during the course of treatment poses problems for correct localization of dwell positions. As the catheter shifts in the breast, the distances to the center of the target from the entry and the exit buttons do not remain constant – be they fixed or adjustable. Complicating the situation further, the target is seldom centered in the breast. Since there is no easy method to adjust for the change in the relative positions of the catheters with respect to the target, the margin in the direction of the catheter direction must include this uncertainty in expanding the clinical target volume to the planning target volume (PTV). The overall uncertainty can be approximately 1 cm. For consistency, it is probably best to keep the fixed end of the catheters (most distal with respect to the source travel) always against the skin, both during the localization and during treatments.

13.2.1.2 Catheter Numbering

Catheter identification, of course, becomes important both for input into the treatment planning and during catheter connection. Labeling catheters is discussed above. During input into the treatment planning system, it is useful to have photographs both from the tip end and the connector end. Figure 13.3 shows a photograph of the tip end. One of the easiest and surest ways to establish which exit button corresponds to which entrance catheter number is at the time of insertion of the imaging markers to watch for the marker to show at the bottom of the catheter (in most catheters the shadow of the marker can be seen in the center of the button) or to feel the marker hit the bottom of the button on insertion. These photographs serve for verification.

13.2.1.3 Checking the Length of Catheters or Catheter Inserts

The length to the first dwell position sets all subsequent positions, and must be correct for correct positioning of the dose distribution. On systems where the transfer tubes connect directly to the catheters and the catheters may be cut to arbitrary lengths, the distance to the end of the catheter must be measured. This can be done by inserting a wire down the transfer tube with the catheter connected and measuring the length on the wire. However, in doing so one must know the offset from the end of the transfer tube to the zero point of the afterloader, as well as the distance from the tip of the source cable to the center of the activity and any required margin from the end that the source cable must remain (to accommodate extra travel on the part of the check cable on some units). A better alternative is to use a tool sold by the manufacturers for performing just this measurement. Figure 13.4a shows the tool marketed by Nucletron (Veenendaal, The Netherlands) that connects to a transfer tube and catheter, consisting of a wire connected to a scale that directly reads the length of source travel. Units with "end-seek" functions, where the check cable goes to the end of the catheter and records the distance, could be confused by kinks or unexpected resistance in the catheter.

A different class of catheter systems uses special inserts attached to the transfer tube that slide into the catheters. The inserts have a constant length so the length of the catheters becomes irrelevant. However, that moves the task of verification of the length from checking the catheters to checking the inserts. Performing this check, though, is easier than checking the length of the catheters. For the most part, checking the length of the inserts can simply involve comparing the inserts to a standard insert that has been verified previously. Figure 13.4b shows a simple comparison. Of course, the comparison only has meaning following verification of the length of the standard insert.

13.2.2 Intracavitary Insertions

13.2.2.1 Verification of Length

The length becomes a much more critical parameter for intracavitary treatments than for interstitial treatments. With interstitial treatments, one catheter with an erroneous length alters the dose distribution locally around that catheter but usually does not make a large difference in the overall dose distribution. With an intracavitary treatment, however, any shift in the position of the source causes an equal shift in the dose distribution. A 1-mm misplacement in the length produces a 10% variation in dose at the surface of a 4-cm diameter balloon. Thus, verification of the length to send the source becomes of paramount importance, and the use of a special localization marker that indicates the location of the first dwell position becomes essential. At the time of treatment, coincidence between the dwell position and the center of the balloon again requires verification as discussed below.

13.2.2.2 Verification of Filled Diameter

Determining the correct diameter of the balloon requires as much care as determining the length because similar errors produce the same untoward results. During the localization procedure, there is no check of the diameter of the balloon other than comparison of that measured on the CT or MR to that expected given the filling. Before

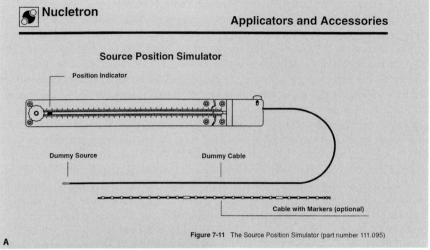

Figure 7-11 The Source Position Simulator (part number 111.095)

A

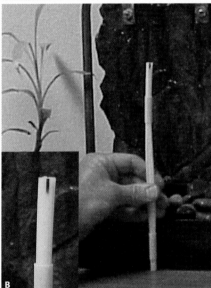

Fig. 13.4 A A tool for determining the length to the first dwell position (courtesy of Nucletron, Veenendaal, Netherlands). **B** Comparison of the lengths of catheter inserts to a standard, verified insert (marked with a *black line*). The *inset* shows a closer view of the tops of the inserts

treatment the balloon is checked to assure that the diameter is the same as that measured for the dosimetry. The balloons should never be used with smaller diameters than their specified range, for example treating a balloon of 4–5 cm filled only to a diameter of 3.5 cm. Doing so likely leaves the balloon in less than spherical shape.

13.2.2.3 Appropriateness of Application
Many aspects of an application would result in inappropriate, or even dangerous, dose distributions, and must be screened during localization.

Shape
Because the dose distribution is essentially spherical, the surface of the balloon should also be so. Significant variations from roundness constitute grounds to abort the procedure. The anisotropy of the source's dose distribution does allow for some constriction along the axis compared with the transverse direction, but such differences should remain within 3 mm.

Voids
One of the most common problems is voids at the surface of the balloon. During insertion of the applicator, air pockets can be trapped, holding target tissue away from the balloon and out of the range of the prescribed isodose surface. A void of 0.8 mm radial height reduces the dose to some target tissue to 95% for a 4-cm diameter balloon, and 1.6 mm reduces the dose to 90%. Volumetric assessment, looking at the volume of the void as a fraction of the target volume does not show much sensitivity to their effect. The same 4-cm diameter balloon produces a treatment volume of 80 cm^3 in the 1-cm wide rim (not counting the volume of the balloon). To use a volumetric-based criterion for evaluating the effect of a void, to have 10% of the volume pushed out of the treatment rind would require an 8 cm^3 void, which if hemispherical would have a radius of 1.6 cm. Obviously, the minimum dose criterion is more stringent.

Voids often seem to resolve over time. However, that resolution may be either the tissue filling back to contact the balloon, or as often is the case, simply fluid filling the void and leaving the target tissue at a distance from the balloon. CT images cannot distinguish between these cases, so the patient should be imaged using MR before deciding to initiate treatment. Placement of a vented catheter along the surface of the balloon to allow escape of any air in part defeats the intention because the venting catheter also pushes the target tissue out of the treatment volume. One mitigating aspect of the treatment modality is that the dose does not fall off very quickly. Even though not receiving the treatment dose, tissues moved 1.5 mm from the surface still receive about 90% of the prescribed dose. This slow gradient does provide some latitude.

Distance to Skin, Pectoralis, Lung and Heart
As discussed in a previous chapter, intracavitary treatment of the breast will deliver higher doses to the skin than will interstitial treatment. The skin dose should remain below 150% of the treatment dose. For this to hold the margin between the surface of the balloon and the skin, δ, must remain:

$$\delta \geq 8.2\,\text{mm} - 0.18 r_{ballon} \quad (1)$$

where $r_{balloon}$ indicates the radius of the balloon. For a 4-cm diameter balloon, the margin must be at least 4.6 mm. The general rule to allow for a safety margin is to have at least a 5-mm margin. While the concern for the pectoralis muscle is less than for the skin, it is usually considered prudent to allow this same margin to the muscle. The dose to the lung, and more so to the heart, seldom can become high enough or in a large enough volume to raise concern.

13.3 Quality Assurance of the Treatment Plan

Today, almost all treatment planning systems have the capability of importing CT/MRI/US images through a local area network (LAN). Delineation of critical structures such as the heart and lung along with defining the PTV by adding margins to the lumpectomy cavity has helped tremendously for conformal treatment plans. A dose volume histogram (DVH) for the region of interest to co-relate clinical outcome and toxicities (Kestin et al. 2000) and homogeneous dose distribution by optimization tools to reduce telangiectasia and fat necrosis (Clarke et al. 1983; Roston and El-Sayed 1987) has provided the radiation oncologist much needed, powerful tools to make clinical decisions during a patient's treatment plan. Finally, Quality Assurance (QA) for a complex HDR treatment plan with a single stepping source has always been a challenge to the physics community. A good and efficient QA program for treatment plan and delivery is extremely important and necessary for patient safety.

13.3.1 Interstitial Implants

13.3.1.1 Target Coverage
Ideally, both the lumpectomy cavity and the target volume should be covered by the prescription isodose line. Figure 13.5 shows a 3D view of one such plan. As can be seen, the 100% isodose cloud (blue) covers the lumpectomy cavity (deep pink) and also the PTV (light pink). In order to analyze the total coverage in 3D, the generation of a DVH is essential. Figure 13.6 shows the integral DVH with 100% of the lumpectomy cavity with a volume of 19.9 cm³ totally covered by the 100% isodose line. For the PTV, 95.4% of the target with a volume of 230.5 cm³ (i.e. 220 cm³) is covered by the prescription dose of 3.4 Gy per fraction. Critical structures such as heart, lung, skin and contralateral breast can also be delineated and their DVH can be generated to aid the physician in treatment planning.

13.3.1.2 High-Dose Volume
In any interstitial brachytherapy implant, the tissue around the radioactive source will be "hot". But the extent of this hot spot can be minimized by implanting catheters equidistant (1 to 1.5 cm) from one another. While optimizing the dose distribution, great care should be taken to distribute the "hot spot" (150% isodose line) among as many dwell positions as possible rather than among a few. A rule of thumb is not to let two adjacent 150% isodose surfaces coalesce or touch each other. A "good" or "optimal" implant with adequate catheters should be able to maintain this rule.

13.3.1.3 Uniformity Indices
One measure of the uniformity of dose distribution in a brachytherapy implant is termed the dose homogeneity index (DHI), defined by:

$$DHI = \frac{V_{100} - V_{150}}{V_{100}} \quad (2)$$

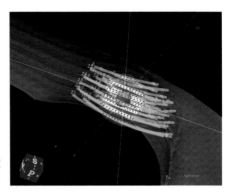

Fig. 13.5 A 3D view of the dose distribution with the lumpectomy cavity (*dark pink*) and the PTV (*light pink*)

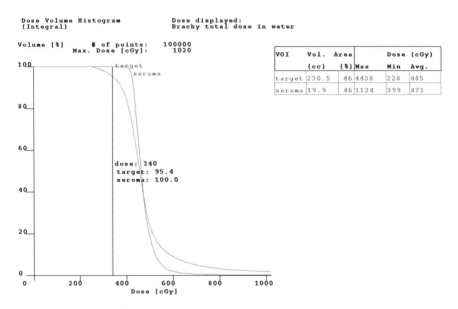

Fig. 13.6 Integral DVH of an interstitial breast implant

where V_{100} and V_{150} are the volume covered by the 100% and 150% isodose surface, respectively, and can be used to determine the level of dose homogeneity for the implant, which should be as high as possible (Wu et al. 1988). A DVH for the implant is generated to record V_{100} and V_{150} to calculate DHI. The ideal value for DHI is 1.0, which is realistically impossible since there will be some hot spots around the source.

13.3.1.4 Conformality Index

Target volume and the volume covered by the 100% isodose surface, V_{100}, should be as conformal as possible. Mathematically, a conformality index (CI) can be defined as (Das and Patel 2005; ICRU 1993):

$$CI = \frac{TargetVolume \cap V_{100}}{Target\ Volume \cup V_{100}} \quad (3)$$

The CI can be calculated as:

$$CI = \frac{Volume\ of\ PTV\ covered\ by\ 100\%\ isodoseline}{V_{100} + Volume\ of\ PTV\ not\ covered\ by\ 100\%\ isodoseline} \quad (4)$$

In an ideal implant, CI equals 1.0, indicating perfect conformance between the 100% isodose surface and the target volume. As explained above, a DVH of the brachytherapy implant and an integral DVH of the 3D treatment plan is necessary to generate the V_{100} and the volume of PTV covered/not covered by the 100% isodose line.

13.3.1.5 Skin Dose

For breast interstitial implants, a high dose to the skin can be detrimental to the cosmetic outcome and, in certain cases where the skin dose is very high, could lead to long-term complications. A quality assurance program to restrict the skin dose to a certain percentage of the prescription or the PTV to be at a certain depth below the skin (often taken as 5 mm) is essential. Figure 13.7 shows how a PTV generated by adding a 2-cm margin along the lumpectomy cavity is then modified to be 5 mm below the skin, which generally restricts the dose to the skin to about 80% of the prescription dose (Das et al. 2004).

13.3.1.6 Dwell Time vs. Volume

All remote afterloaders utilize the stepping source technology that enables the planner to maximize the dose uniformity while minimizing the implant volume needed to cover the target volume adequately. Such flexibility creates a challenge for the verification of the optimized calculations with practical manual calculation techniques taking only a few minutes and at the same time detecting significant errors. The Nuclear Regulatory Commission considers a difference of 20% between the administered dose and calculated dose a medical event (NRC 2005). Commonly, variations of greater than 5% in external-beam treatments are felt to potentially compromise outcomes. While the accuracy of brachytherapy treatments is less well defined, clearly there is a need for a quick method to verify the accuracy of an optimized plan. Using the Manchester volume implant table, calculated irradiation time can be used as a quality assurance for the HDR computed time very easily.

Table 13.1 shows the Manchester volume implant table with column 3 corrected for modern units and factors, conversion from mgRaEq-h/1000R to Ci-s/Gy and move the prescription to approximately 90% of the mean central dose (Williamson et al. 1994), while Table 13.2 gives the elongation factor as originally published (Paterson and Parker 1938).

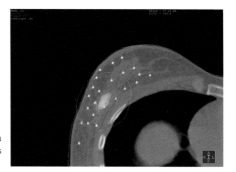

Fig. 13.7 Limiting the expansion of the seroma (*blue*) to the target (*red*) by the skin and pectoralis muscle

For a given treatment volume (V_{100}), the irradiation time in seconds needed to deliver a prescription dose in grays with a source activity in curies is given by:

$$\text{Time (s)} = \frac{R_v(\text{Ci} \cdot \text{s} / \text{Gy}) \cdot \text{Prescribed Dose (Gy)}}{\text{Activity (Ci)}} \qquad (5)$$

The time calculated from Eq. 5 can then be compared with the treatment planning time. A recent study of 50 breast interstitial plans showed that the two times agree within ±7% of each other (Das et al. 2004).

13.3.1.7 Lengths

As noted above, in an interstitial implant with many catheters of different lengths, great care should be taken in the measurement of the length of these catheters along with the transfer tubes. Accurate transfer of this measured length for each catheter to the treatment planning system is crucial and requires a quality assurance check. Moreover maintaining a record of these lengths and verifying the recorded length with the programmed length before each treatment is essential, since any discrepancies result in a totally different dose distribution to the PTV. One vendor (Nucletron Corporation) has come up with a fixed length catheter system (Comfort Catheter) as shown in Fig. 13.8. Even though the catheter button-to-button distance can vary, the length of the plastic tube that is inserted into the catheter is fixed. Instead of measuring the length of each catheter, a premeasured length applicable to all catheters can be used, reducing the simulation time. As noted in the section 13.2.1.3, the length of the inserts must be verified instead.

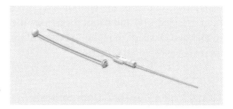

Fig. 13.8 Comfort catheter (courtesy of Nucletron, Veenendaal, Netherlands)

Table 13.1 Values of integrated decays to deliver a dose, R_V (Williamson et al. 1994)

Volume (cm³)	mRaEq-hr/1000R	R_V (Ci-s/Gy)
0	463	314
80	633	429
100	735	498
140	920	624
180	1087	737
220	1243	843
300	1529	1037
340	1662	1127
380	1788	1212

Ratio of length/diameter	Correction factor
1.5	1.03
2.0	1.06
2.5	1.10
3.0	1.15

Table 13.2 Elongation factors (Paterson and Parker 1938)

13.3.2 Intracavitary Insertions

13.3.2.1 Target Coverage

As in interstitial implants, integral DVH analysis for breast intracavitary implants should be performed to evaluate the PTV (surface of the balloon + 1 cm) covered by the prescribed dose. The assumption that the lumpectomy cavity and the balloon are isocentric and congruent does not hold for all patients. In those situations the V_{100} and the PTV do not overlap and an integral DVH is the ideal tool for clinical decision making.

13.3.2.2 Uniformity Indices

For intracavitary implants, Eq. 2 can be modified to:

$$DHI_{int\,racavitary} = \frac{V_{100} - V_{150}}{V_{100} - V_{ballon}} \quad (6)$$

where the volume of the balloon ($V_{balloon}$) needs to be assessed either by the amount of fluid injected into the balloon or from the integral DVH after delineating the balloon in all the CT slices. For the MammoSite balloon (Cytyc, Marlborough, MA) the DHI increases as $V_{balloon}$ increases.

13.3.2.3 Skin Dose and Dose to Other Structures

Unlike interstitial implants with multiple catheters, each with several active dwell positions, intracavitary applicators such as the MammoSite have limited dwells along the axis of the balloon. Conforming the V_{100} to the PTV or reducing the dose to critical structures such as the skin, heart, and lung is not an option. Great care should be taken in analyzing the DVH of the skin and other critical structures before making a clinical decision.

13.3.2.4 Dwell Time vs. Distance

Since the prescription point is determined from the center of the balloon to the equatorial surface of the balloon + 1 cm, a hand calculation of the time given by a point source Eq. 7 can be performed to compare the predicted time to the treatment planning time:

$$\text{Time (s)} = \frac{\text{Prescription Dose} \cdot r^2}{\Lambda \cdot S_k \cdot g(r)} \quad (7)$$

where, with values for the ^{192}Ir source in parentheses:
Λ is the dose rate constant (1.12 cGy/μGy m^2)
S_k is the air-kerma strength (μGy m^2 h^{-1})
g(r) is the radial dose function (1.02)
r is the radius of the balloon + 1 cm
Usually the timing agrees to within ±5%.

13.3.2.5 Length

For a MammoSite balloon, the center of the balloon needs to be located preferably by a source simulator and an imaging device. Diluted radioopaque material, strong enough to visualize the surface of the balloon, yet weak enough to see the dummy source of the source simulator, helps in locating the center of the balloon on the image as well as establishing the length for the source to be at the center.

13.4 Quality Assurance at the Time of Treatment

For both interstitial and intracavitary treatments, the first step is to assure that the patient assumes the same position on the treatment table as during localization. Variations in position can produce variations in geometry of the catheters and then in the dose distribution.

13.4.1 Interstitial Implants

13.4.1.1 Program Verification

Movement of the data from the treatment planning system to the treatment console station is either by LAN or by electronic memory devices. After the data have been transported, before the first treatment, the values in the program for patient name, total treatment time, step sizes or dwell locations, catheter lengths, and dwell times should be checked. For the most part, this check verifies that the correct plan has been imported into the treatment unit, since file corruption usually renders a file unusable rather than changing data. However, checking the program is not unwise. For subsequent fractions, each dwell time need not be checked – only as many as necessary to assure that the correct program is loaded.

13.4.1.2 Connection of the Catheters

Correct connection of the catheters, of course, is essential for a correct treatment. Errors in catheter connection can occur either while connecting the transfer tubes to the treatment unit or connecting the catheters to the transfer tubes. If more than one set of transfer tubes is available for catheter connection (e.g., for different lengths to the first dwell position), selection of the correct set of tubes should be part of the verification procedures. Many errors in connecting the transfer tubes to the treatment unit tend to be protected by design, for example, skipping a hole when inserting the tubes into the indexer. Such a mistake would cause the unit to pause during treatment until the tubes were moved to fill the empty location. Mixing the tubes is not protected: any tube may go in any hole. However, any error in the order must actually be *two* errors, for example, inserting tube no. 12 into hole no. 2 would leave hole no. 12 without a corresponding tube unless tube no. 2 were placed there, making the error less likely.

Mistakes in connecting the transfer tubes to the catheters are more likely, particularly when more catheters are treated than there are transfer tubes (i.e., holes in the indexer). In such cases, the catheters up to and including the highest number on the indexer are treated in a first set. Then, after disconnecting these catheters, the next numbers in line are connected. This process repeats until all the catheters are treated. With cases requiring multiple sets of connections, mistakes connecting catheters from different sets becomes a hazard. For example, while connecting the first set, catheter no. 32 could mistakenly be connected to hole no. 2 (or no. 3, depending on what the person connecting sees).

After connecting the catheters to the transfer tubes but before initiating treatment, the catheters must be moved so that the buttons on the exit side of the patient abut the skin, as they were for the localization imaging. Section 13.2.1.1 discusses this issue more completely.

Early in a breast brachytherapy program, it may be considered advisable to perform a patency check on all the catheters before starting the treatment to assure that the treatment does not get stuck because of a catheter with a kink. However, as experience grows, confidence in the procedure probably will lead to skipping this step. In our experience there has never been a catheter that the check cable detected as being kinked or blocked. Even without checking all the catheters before initiating treatment, the unit still checks each catheter immediately before sending the source. Such checks do find poor connections, but those are easily corrected.

13.4.2 Intracavitary Insertions

For intracavitary treatment all the above-mentioned checks for interstitial treatment should be performed along with a volume check and a check to ensure that the source goes to the correct location.

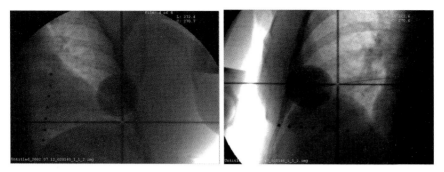

Fig. 13.9 Fluoroscopic images taken before treatment to verify the size of the balloon and the centering of the source position.

13.4.2.1 Volume Check

Before each treatment, an image of the balloon should be acquired to make sure that the volume of the balloon is the same and that the balloon has not collapsed or that fluid from the balloon has not leaked. Figure 13.9 shows fluoroscopic images of a MammoSite balloon in two patients. A ruler with small opaque spheres (1 cm apart) is placed at the same level as the center of the balloon to help determine the diameter of the balloon.

13.4.2.2 Source Going to Correct Location

A check of the source traveling at the center of the balloon should also be confirmed before each treatment. Figure 13.9 also shows the programmed check cable run at the center of the balloon before the radioactive source run.

13.5 Post-Treatment Verification

Immediately after the end of treatment, the operator must check the patient with a radiation detector to verify complete retraction of the source. A source, or part of a source, remaining in the patient after treatment would deliver enough dose locally in 1 minute to cause injury to the tissues. After the end of each treatment, the report of the treatment should be verified which includes the length of each channel, the total irradiation time, and the individual dwell time.

References

1. Clarke D, Curtis JL, Martinez A, et al (1983) Fat necrosis of the breast simulating recurrent carcinoma after primary radiotherapy in the management of early stage breast carcinoma. Cancer 52:442–445

2. Das RK, Patel R (2005) Breast interstitial implant and treatment planning. In: Thomadsen BR, Rivard MJ, Butler WM (eds) Brachytherapy physics, 2nd edn. Medical Physics Publishing, Madison

3. Das RK, Patel P, Shah H, et al (2004) 3D CT-based high dose-rate breast brachytherapy implants: treatment planning and quality assurance. Int J Radiat Oncol Biol Phys 59:1224–1228

4. ICRU (1993) Report 50, prescribing, recording, and reporting photon beam therapy. International Commission on Radiation Units and Measurements, Bethesda, MD

5. Kestin LL, Jaffray DA, Edmundson GK, et al (2000) Improving the dosimetric coverage of interstitial high-dose rate breast implants. Int J Radiat Oncol Biol Phys 46:35–43

6. NRC (2005) Code of Federal Regulations, part 35.3045. Nuclear Regulatory Commission, Washington DC

7. Paterson R, Parker HM (1938) A dosage system for interstitial Radium Therapy. Br J Radiol 11:313–339

8. Roston AY, El-Sayed ME (1987) Fat necrosis of the breast: an unusual complication of lumpectomy and radiotherapy in breast cancer. Clin Radiol 38:31

9. Thomadsen B (2000) Quality management for brachytherapy appliances. In: Thomadsen BR (ed) Achieving quality in brachytherapy. IOP Press, Bristol

10. Williamson JF, Ezzell GA, Olch A, et al (1994) Quality assurance for high dose rate brachytherapy. In: Nag S (ed) High dose rate brachytherapy: a textbook. Futura Publishing, Armonk, NY

11. Wu A, Ulin K, Sternick ES (1988) A dose homogeneity index for evaluating ^{192}Ir interstitial breast implants. Med Phys 15:104–107

New and Novel Treatment Delivery Techniques for Accelerated Partial Breast Irradiation

14

Mark J. Rivard, Alphonse G. Taghian and David E. Wazer

Contents

14.1 APBI: Established, New, and Novel Approaches

Many of the other chapters in this text discuss in detail the established techniques for APBI delivery with significant attention given to techniques specific to certain institutions. Furthermore, some chapters stress the cohesion of established techniques through multi-institutional clinical trials and implementation of uniform quality assurance practices. However, this chapter focuses on the possible directions for the future of APBI by looking at new and novel approaches to APBI delivery.

There are recent publications (see for example Hui and Das 2005, Formenti et al. 2004, or Butler and Butler 2005) in which patient positioning (prone or decubitus vs. conventional supine) are important improvements to established approaches. While quite useful in some cases, alteration of patient set-up alone does not satisfy the definition for a new or novel APBI treatment modality. Creative efforts should focus on developments of the treatment delivery system. Small but required steps forward from low dose-rate (LDR) ^{60}Co or ^{192}Ir temporary implants (Fourquet et al. 1995; Póti et al. 2004) would be the use of alternative brachytherapy radionuclides (e.g., high dose-rate, HDR, ^{169}Yb, ^{170}Tm, or ^{171}Tm) or the use of permanent LDR seed implants such as ^{103}Pd or ^{125}I. Application of other esoteric brachytherapy delivery systems to APBI would follow. In a similar context, utilization of teletherapy systems for APBI such as 3D conformal radiation therapy (3D-CRT) protons or intensity-modulated radiation therapy (IMRT) protons would offer increasing levels of complexity, yet potential for improved treatment delivery.

While one could consider using almost any new treatment modality for APBI, it is necessary to delineate what desirable features these modalities should have, and how they should improve upon the established techniques:

- Capability for the current team of care providers (surgeons, oncologists, radiation oncologists) to use the modality in a cost-effective and time-sensitive manner with ease-of-use
- Ability to deliver therapy in a controlled manner which may be quantitatively confirmed through measurements and calculations
- Provide therapy with improved homogeneity, conformity (non-target tissue sparing), and patient-specific compatibility

The majority of the new and/or novel approaches listed in the following sections have some or all of these desirable features. As these approaches to APBI may be categorized as to whether or not the therapy source emanates external to or within the patient, the following two sections are divided into teletherapy and brachytherapy, respectively.

14.2 Teletherapy

Conventional 3D-CRT for APBI is performed, but offers limited prospects due to the need to minimize irradiation of healthy breast tissues which limits forward treatment planning. IMRT with teletherapy photons has been used for the treatment of breast cancer since the mid-1990s. With this treatment modality, smaller planning target volumes (PTVs) may be obtained as compared to those available from CRT. While IMRT for APBI has been used now for over a decade, therapy delivery using the fraction schema common to current APBI approaches (e.g., 3.4 Gy/fraction, twice daily, total 34 Gy) has only recently been examined (Coles et al. 2005).

Intraoperative radiation therapy (IORT) has been used in general for radiotherapy since the 1960s. However, application to breast treatment has been limited. Further focusing of IORT to APBI, with its smaller clinical target volume (CTV) and decreased fractionation treatment schedule is discussed in Chapter 12. Herskind et al. (2005) have proposed using a spherical 50 kV x-ray source for single-dose or hypofractionated partial-breast IORT. The well-established LQ model was modified to determine the relative biological effectiveness as a function of dose, distance, and irradiation time for late-reacting normal tissues and tumor cells. The calculated relative biological efficiency (RBE) for late reactions was near unity at the applicator surface, but increased with increasing distance (lower dose rates). Furthermore, the RBE for tumor cells was favorably calculated to be larger than for late-reacting normal tissues. These factors provide the theoretical basis for IORT for APBI.

In contrast to photons, particles with mass such as electrons, neutrons, or exotic particles have not been utilized for APBI. Electrons have been used for recurrent disease (McKenzie et al. 1993; Nicolato and Franchini 1990), but not specifically for APBI. Murray et al. (2005) and Halpern et al. (1990) have used neutrons for irradiation of locally advanced breast cancer, but not for partial breast treatment or in an accelerated fashion. However, protons have been used recently and exhibit promise for APBI.

14.2.1 Proton Teletherapy for APBI

Protons have physical and radiobiological characteristics which differ from those of conventional radiotherapy (photons), and offer a number of theoretical advantages. Dose localization in the Bragg peak provides an ideal characteristic for dose conformation to the target volume, and at the same time reduced dose to non-target tissues (Koehler et al. 1972). This unique dosimetric feature of proton teletherapy makes it an attractive non-invasive modality. The main critical indications are proximity of the target area to critical structures where maximum selectivity of dose distribution is of paramount importance. A general review of proton teletherapy is provided by Orecchia et al. (1998), who have demonstrated success in the treatment of diseases such as uveal melanoma, base of skull chordoma and chondrosarcoma, central nervous system, soft-tissue sarcoma, and prostate cancer. However, the use of proton teletherapy for breast cancer has been very limited.

At Massachusetts General Hospital in Boston, Taghian and colleagues initiated an IRB-approved phase I/II clinical trial to evaluate the safety and feasibility of using a simple 3D-CRT APBI technique where the patient lies supine and treatment is delivered using either proton teletherapy or a three-field photon beam arrangement including an *en face* electron field. Use of protons was based on preliminary study suggesting superiority of proton dose distribution when compared with IMRT or 3D-CRT using photons and electrons (El-Ghamry et al. 2002). Figure 14.1 shows dose distribution comparisons between 3D-CRT photons, IMRT photons, and protons with the dose–volume histograms (DVHs) illustrating a 50% decrease in the dose received by the non-target breast tissue in favor of protons.

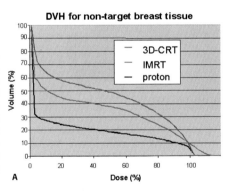

Fig. 14.1 Comparison of three treatment plans. **A** Non-target breast tissue DVHs for 3D-CRT, IMRT, and proton treatment plans. At the 50% isodose, there is improvement of approximately a factor of two going from 3D-CRT to protons, with IMRT falling somewhere in the middle. **B** Isodose lines for the same three treatment plans. It is clear that the proton teletherapy treatment plan, in comparison to 3D-CRT or IMRT, offers much more conformal targeting and minimizes the dosage to healthy tissue (from Taghian et al. 2005)

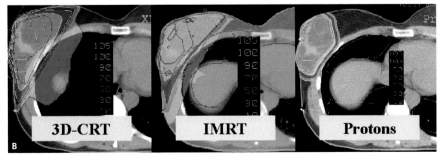

A summary of the clinical experience has been provided by Taghian et al. (2006). From May 2004 to June 2005, 25 patients were treated with proton-based APBI. Eligibility criteria included: invasive carcinoma of <2 cm; negative sentinel node; margin width >2 mm; and no lymphovascular invasion. The excision cavity represented the CTV, which was expanded by 1.5–2.0 cm to create the PTV, and then edited so the PTV came no closer than 5 mm to the skin surface and no deeper than the anterior chest wall or pectoralis muscles. The prescribed dose was 32 Gy in eight fractions, delivered twice daily over 4 days. One to three fields were used as necessary to keep dose inhomogeneity across the PTV less than 10%. Skin sparing with protons was less than that with photons, but was improved by the use of multiple fields. All 25 patients were treated with proton therapy. For 24 of them, a 3D plan using photon minitangents and an *en face* electron field was also generated. Dosimetric comparisons were made between photon/electron plans and proton plans using paired *t*-tests (Kozak et al. 2006). Figure 14.2 illustrates a plan using standardized 3D-CRT photons and electrons versus two proton fields (Taghian et al. 2006). Notice the difference in the dose received by the non-target breast tissue.

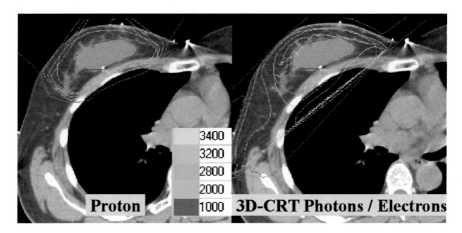

Fig. 14.2 Treatment plans for proton teletherapy (*left*) and 3D-CRT using photons and electrons (*right*). The dose to the chest wall, non-target breast, and lung are greatly minimized with proton teletherapy

Results for the first 25 patients showed that the median tumor size was 0.8 cm (range 0.2–1.8 cm). Fourteen patients had left-sided and eleven patients right-sided breast cancers. The median CTV was 19 cm³ (range 5–60 cm³) and the median PTV was 147 cm³ (range 46–307 cm³). The median percentage of the whole breast designated as PTV was 19% (range 7–37%). The mean doses delivered to the ipsilateral lung, heart, and non-target breast (whole breast minus PTV), for both proton and photon/electron plans are listed in Table 14.1. The use of protons resulted in lower doses to each of these normal structures. PTV coverage for both modalities was equivalent. The volume of non-target breast tissue receiving 50% of the dose (16 Gy) was 41% and 26% for photons/electrons and proton treatment, respectively (*P*=0.0001).

Table 14.1 Doses to lung, heart, and non-target breast illustrating significant improvements using 3D-CRT protons in favor of photons and electrons

	3D CRT photons/ electrons	3D-CRT protons	P-value
Ipsilateral lung			
Maximum dose (Gy)	28	19	0.001
Mean dose (Gy)	1.0	0.5	0.0001
D20 (Gy)	1.2	0.0	0.0001
D10 (Gy)	2.4	0.6	0.0001
D5 (Gy)	4.2	2.8	0.005
Heart			
Maximum dose (Gy)	3.2	0.8	0.0001
Mean dose (Gy)	0.4	0.1	0.002
D20 (Gy)	0.5	0.0	0.002
D10 (Gy)	0.7	0.0	0.002
D5 (Gy)	1.0	0.0	0.002
Non-target breast			
V16 Gy (%)	41	26	0.0001

D20, D10, D5 dose (Gy) received by 20%, 10% and 5% of the tissue
V16 Gy (%) percent of volume receiving 50% of the prescribed dose (i.e. 16 Gy)

Proton-based APBI treatments are technically feasible, and intensity modulation using protons may be even more promising. When compared to conventional 3D-CRT APBI treatments, doses delivered to normal structures such as the ipsilateral and contralateral lungs, heart, and non-target breast tissue were significantly lower without compromising PTV coverage. Proton therapy will soon become more readily available as two new facilities are under construction in Houston and Florida (Particle Therapy Co-Operative Group 2005), and may become an attractive tool for APBI. Furthermore, the cost estimate suggest that proton used in APBI may actually be less expensive than invasive techniques (Mammosite and interstitial HDR implants) (Taghian et al 2006). However, studies are needed on its long-term effect on cosmetic outcome and late normal-tissue complications.

14.3 Brachytherapy

While brachytherapy for APBI is well-established using temporary implants with conventional radionuclides such as ^{60}Co and ^{192}Ir, novel brachytherapy systems for APBI are being researched. The following summarizes three areas in which interstitial treatments for APBI are being investigated.

14.3.1 Seeds Containing Radionuclides

Unlike the conventional approach to use temporary implants, there is interest in permanently implanting brachytherapy sources at the time of lumpectomy. Due to their long half-lives of 5.27 years and 74 days, ^{60}Co and ^{192}Ir are not suitable candidates for this procedure. While ^{137}Cs has also been used for breast irradiation, it too has an unacceptably long half-life for permanent implantation. The remaining two radionuclides now regularly used for brachytherapy are ^{125}I and ^{103}Pd. While clinical results using LDR ^{125}I seeds have been reported for temporary implants in APBI (Vicini et al. 1997), clinical results have not been reported for permanent implants of ^{125}I or ^{103}Pd for APBI.

Recently, Keller et al. (2005) have reported on a feasibility study using both radionuclides for APBI. CT data from ten patients with early-stage breast cancer were used to simulate ^{125}I and ^{103}Pd implants. Calculations of radiobiological equivalence were used to estimate a teletherapy dose of 50 Gy delivered over 25 fractions to the appropriate source strengths and total activities in the simulations. Doses of 90 Gy and 124 Gy were needed for ^{103}Pd and ^{125}I, respectively. Based on the photon energies and resultant dose fall-off, ^{103}Pd was considered to be a suitable candidate for APBI permanent implants, while ^{125}I was not recommended for APBI permanent implants due to radiation safety concerns. The results of Keller et al. were not strongly dependent on breast size or tumor bed volume across the ten patients simulated. Consequently, a phase I/II investigator-initiated clinical trial was started at the Sunnybrook and Women's College Health Sciences Centre in 2004 using stranded ^{103}Pd, with promising clinical results so far (Pignol et al. 2005). With a ^{103}Pd implant, the dose rate would drop to one-fourth the initial dose rate after 1 month, and it is unclear if the ^{103}Pd half-life is appropriately suited to the growth rate of breast carcinoma. Also, it is not clear if the stranded implant would unduly obscure follow-up mammograms. More clinical investigation of this novel approach to APBI brachytherapy is required to fully access its potential role.

14.3.2 Microbrachytherapy

The new field of microbrachytherapy (μBx) takes the concept of brachytherapy to the domain of extremely small distances. While not classified as nuclear medicine, μBx employs tiny sealed sources of radionuclides, typically using ^{90}Y, and is both calibrated and administered in a manner similar to nuclear medicine. ^{90}Y μBx is currently used to treat non-resectable hepatic malignancies (Herba et al. 1988; Sarfaraz et al. 2003), and an in depth review of μBx is provided by Thomadsen et al. (2005). While animal studies have been performed to determine the effects of a ^{90}Y nuclear medicine agent on human breast cancer tumors (HBT 3477) implanted in athymic mice (DeNardo et al. 1998), there is no available literature at this time presenting the use of μBx in humans or subsequent clinical results for breast cancer let alone APBI. Since the principles currently exploited for μBx primarily rely on microvascular electrostatics for radionuclide localization primarily in the liver, new targeting systems will be needed to customize this therapy modality for APBI.

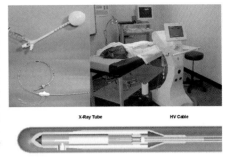

Fig. 14.3 X-ray generation system for the Axxent electronic brachytherapy source by Xoft. *Top-left* The balloon catheter for APBI applications is positioned above the flexible source component. *Top-right* The portable controller is positioned in front of a test phantom with a flexible shield over the implanted region. Beneath the table is the calibration system (electrometer and reentrant well ionization chamber). *Bottom* The internal geometry of the source component is shown inside the cooling catheter

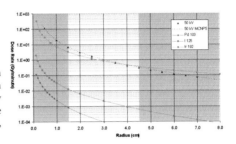

Fig. 14.4 Dose rates from the Axxent APBI system set to an operating voltage of 50 kV in comparison to conventional radionuclide-based brachytherapy sources. While the Axxent system has similar dose rates to HDR ^{192}Ir at clinically relevant distances, the dose fall-off is similar to that of ^{125}I

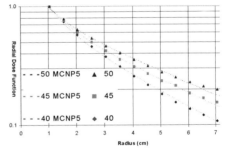

Fig. 14.5 The effect of running the Axxent electronic brachytherapy source at various operating voltages, as well as the level of agreement between ionization chamber measurements and Monte Carlo calculations at each operating voltage over a large range of distances

14.3.3 Electronic Brachytherapy

Since the discovery of ^{226}Ra, radionuclide-based brachytherapy sources have been in clinical use for over 100 years. Currently, the large majority of brachytherapy implants use the following radionuclides: ^{103}Pd, ^{125}I, ^{137}Cs, and ^{192}Ir. While well-established, radionuclides are limited due to:

1. Fixed dosimetric properties such as their radiation emission spectrum and tissue penetration.

2. Their source strength decays logarithmically requiring concerns for radiological waste storage and new source replacement.
3. National security and safety concerns by the U.S. Department of Homeland Security and U.S. Nuclear Regulatory Commission since 11 September 2001.

Thus, an alternative to radionuclide-based brachytherapy sources would be of interest.

With advances over the past few decades in the field of electrical miniaturization, it is now possible to create and use electronic brachytherapy (eBx) sources. Significant research over the past two decades has been performed to develop x-ray-emitting eBx sources. The interested reader is referred to a more detailed review article by Rivard et al. (2005) describing the current status of this field. While the Intrabeam IORT system from Carl Zeiss is the first and only eBx system currently having FDA approval, we will focus on the Axxent system by Xoft since this product is designed specifically to address the needs of APBI.

The company Xoft, initially incorporated to provide eBx sources for intravascular brachytherapy and treating coronary artery disease, focused in 2001 on developing eBx sources for APBI (Rusch and Rivard 2004). Similar to the Intrabeam system, a miniature x-ray tube operating at 50 kVp and 300 μA is available (Fig. 14.3) with a source strength similar to HDR ^{192}Ir, yet with dosimetric properties and shielding requirements similar to LDR ^{125}I. Xoft will sponsor a multicenter phase IV trial to assess safety and utility of their Axxent APBI system manner similar to that previously initiated by Proxima Therapeutics for the MammoSite system. Having their own assortment of balloon applicators, ten treatment fractions are to be delivered twice daily over 5 days with an radiation dose of 3.4 Gy at a distance of 10 mm from the balloon transverse plane, identical to the MammoSite approach. Figure 14.4 illustrates the potential dose rates of the Axxent APBI system at clinically relevant depths in comparison to HDR ^{192}Ir and LDR ^{125}I and ^{103}Pd brachytherapy sources. Compared to HDR ^{192}Ir, there is a slight increase in dose rate at radii closer than 3.0 cm with lower dose rates at larger distances. Figure 14.5 shows the effect of running the Axxent eBx source at various operating voltages, as well as the level of agreement between ionization chamber measurements and Monte Carlo calculations at each operating voltage over a large range of distances. At distances of 3 cm and 7 cm, going from 40 to 50 kV increases relative penetration by 20% and a factor of two, respectively. As the time of writing, FDA clearance for the Axxent is approved.

14.4 Summary

A variety of potential and novel modalities have been presented as treatment delivery techniques for APBI. Some of these approaches have already been used clinically, while others are still being developed at the benchtop. Just as conventional APBI techniques have advanced over the past decade to include interstitial HDR ^{192}Ir needles and the MammoSite system, it is anticipated that some of these new and novel treatment delivery techniques may eventually have a role for administering APBI.

References

1. Butler WM, Butler EG (2005) Partial breast irradiation using the MammoSite radiation therapy system. In: Thomadsen BR, Rivard MJ, Butler WM (eds) Brachytherapy physics: Joint AAPM/ABS Summer School, 2nd edn. Medical Physics Publishing, Madison, Wisconsin, pp 769–782

2. Coles CE, Moody AM, Wilson CB, et al (2005) Reduction of radiotherapy-induced late complications in early breast cancer: the role of intensity-modulated radiation therapy and partial breast irradiation. Part II–Radiotherapy strategies to reduce radiation-induced late effects. Clin Oncol 17:98–110

3. DeNardo SJ, Kukis DL, Miers LA, et al (1998) Yttrium-90-DOTA-peptide-chimeric L6 radioimmunoconjugate: efficacy and toxicity in mice bearing p53 mutant human breast cancer xenografts. J Nucl Med 39:842–849

4. El-Ghamry MN, Doppke K, Gierga D, Aboubaker F, Admas J, Taghian A, Powell S (2002) Partial breast irradiation using external beams: a comparison of 3-d conformal, IMRT, and proton therapy treatment planning using dose-volume histogram analysis (abstract). Int J Radiat Oncol Biol Phys 54:163

5. Formenti SC, Truong MT, Goldberg JD, et al (2004) Prone accelerated partial breast irradiation after breast-conserving surgery: preliminary clinical results and dose-volume histogram analysis. Int J Radiat Oncol Biol Phys 60:493–504

6. Fourquet A, Campana F, Mosseri V, et al (1995) Iridium-192 versus cobalt-60 boost in 3–7 cm breast cancer treated by irradiation alone: final results of a randomized trial. Radiother Oncol 34:114–120

7. Halpern J, Maor MH, Hussey DH, et al (1990) Locally advanced breast cancer treated with neutron beams: long-term follow-up in 28 patients. Int J Radiat Oncol Biol Phys 18:825–831

8. Herba MJ, Illescas FF, Thirlwell MP, et al (1988) Hepatic malignancies: improved treatment with intraarterial Y-90. Radiology 169:311–314

9. Herskind C, Steil V, Kraus-Tiefenbacher U, et al (2005) Radiobiological aspects of intraoperative radiotherapy (IORT) with isotropic low-energy X rays for early-stage breast cancer. Radiat Res 163:208–215

10. Hui SK, Das RK (2005) Optimization of conformal avoidance: a comparative study of prone vs. supine interstitial high-dose-rate breast brachytherapy. Brachytherapy 4:137–140

11. Keller B, Sankreacha R, Rakovitch E, et al (2005) A permanent breast seed implant as partial breast radiation therapy for early-stage patients: a comparison of palladium-103 and iodine-125 isotopes based on radiation safety considerations. Int J Radiat Oncol Biol Phys 62:358–365

12. Koehler A, Preston AB, Preston WM (1972) Protons in radiation therapy. Radiology 104:191–195

13. Kozak KR, Doppke K, Katz A, Taghian AG (2006). Dosimetric Comparision of Two Different Three-Dimensional Conformal External Beam Accelerated Partial Breast Irradiation Techniques. Int J Radiat Oncol Biol Phys (In press).

14. McKenzie MR, Freeman CR, Pla M, et al (1993) Clinical experience with electron pseudoarc therapy. Br J Radiol 66:234–240

15. Murray EM, Werner ID, Schmitt G, et al (2005) Neutron versus photon radiotherapy for local control in inoperable breast cancer. Strahlenther Onkol 181:77–81

16. Nicolato A, Franchini P (1990) Electron beam radiotherapy for loco-regional recurrence of breast cancer. Radiol Med 80S1:139–142

17. Orecchia R, Zurlo A, Loasses A, Krengli M, Tosi G, Zurrida A, Zucali P, Veronesi U (1998) Particle beam therapy (hadrontherapy): basis for interest and clinical experience. Eur J Cancer 34:459–468

18. Particle Therapy Co-Operative Group (2005) Particles: a newsletter for those interested in proton, light ion and heavy charged particle radiotherapy. Particle Therapy Co-Operative Group, January 2005

19. Pignol J-P, Keller B, Rakovitch E, Sankreacha R, Easton H, Que W (2005) First report of permanent breast (103)Pd seed implant as adjuvant radiation treatment for early-stage breast cancer. Int J Radiat Oncol Biol Phys 64:176–181

20. Póti Z, Nemeskéri C, Fekésházy A, et al (2004) Partial breast irradiation with interstitial ^{60}Co brachytherapy results in frequent grade 3 or 4 toxicity. Evidence based on a 12-year follow-up of 70 patients. Int J Radiat Oncol Biol Phys 58:1022–1033 (see also Int J Radiat Oncol Biol Phys 59:345–346)

21. Rivard MJ, DeWerd LA, Zinkin HD (2005) Brachytherapy with miniature electronic x-ray sources. In: Thomadsen BR, Rivard MJ, Butler WM (eds) Brachytherapy physics: Joint AAPM/ABS Summer School, 2nd edn. Medical Physics Publishing, Madison, Wisconsin, pp 889–900

22. Rusch TW, Rivard MJ (2004) Application of the TG-43 dosimetry protocol to electronic brachytherapy sources. Radiother Oncol 71(S2):S84

23. Sarfaraz M, Kennedy A, Cao Z, et al (2003) Physical aspects of yttrium-90 microsphere therapy for nonresectable hepatic tumors. Med Phys 30:199–203

24. Taghian A, Kozak KR, Adams J, et al (2005) Accelerated partial-breast irradiation (APBI) using protons for patients with early-stage breast cancer: a comparison with 3D conformal photon/electron based treatment. Int J Radiat Oncol Biol Phys 63S1:S8

25. Taghian A, Kozak KR, Doppke KP, et al (2006) Initial dosimetric experience using simple three-dimensional-conformal external-beam accelerated partial breast irradiation. Int J Radiat Oncol Biol Phys 64:1092–1099

26. Taghian A, Kozak, Katz A, et al (2006). Accelerated Partial Breast Irradiation using proton beams: Initial Dosimetric Experience. Int J Radiat Oncol Biol Phy (In press).

27. Thomadsen BR, Welsh JS, Hammes RJ (2005) Microspheres as microbrachytherapy. In: Thomadsen BR, Rivard MJ, Butler WM (eds) Brachytherapy physics: Joint AAPM/ABS Summer School, 2nd edn. Medical Physics Publishing, Madison, Wisconsin, pp 955–965

28. Vicini FA, Chen PY, Fraile M, et al (1997) Low-dose-rate brachytherapy as the sole radiation modality in the management of patients with early-stage breast cancer treated with breast-conserving therapy: preliminary results of a pilot trial. Int J Radiat Oncol Biol Phys 38:301–310

Overview of North American Trials

Rakesh R. Patel

15

Contents

15.1 Introduction

A major paradigm shift in locoregional management of breast cancer in the last two to three decades has been the acceptance of lumpectomy and whole-breast irradiation as a viable alternative to mastectomy. Similarly, axillary nodal evaluation has shifted in many centers from more extensive level I/II dissections to more limited sentinel node mapping procedures. The notion is to minimize morbidity, optimize cosmesis, and maintain treatment outcomes. Pathologic and clinical data suggest that the vast majority of ipsilateral breast recurrences occur in the vicinity of the index lesion and remote recurrences are uncommon whether whole-breast radiation is delivered or not, thereby lending credence to the concept of partial breast irradiation. The more limited treatment volume allows safe delivery of an accelerated hypofractionated regimen over a truncated course of 1 week. This effort represents yet another paradigm shift from standard whole-breast tangential external beam radiation therapy to investigation of accelerated partial breast irradiation (APBI).

Several studies utilizing APBI have shown promising early outcomes with few local recurrences, minimal toxicity, and excellent cosmetic outcome. There are several methods of APBI being investigated: brachytherapy involving multiple interstitial catheters or a single intracavitary balloon, external beam radiation either in the supine or prone position, and intraoperative irradiation. All of these share the common aim of treating a more limited volume allowing a higher dose per fraction resulting in a shortened overall treatment course; however, each of these modalities is logistically quite different for the patient. Each has distinct technical advantages and challenges in radiation delivery, and perhaps more importantly with each modality a different volume of breast tissue is irradiated. There is very little published information on treatment planning techniques and the quality assurance measures utilized to assure that the target volume was adequately covered.

Differences in target volume definition (variable margin around the surgical cavity), variable target delineation methods, as well as inconsistent methods of treatment planning have not allowed a standard method of dosimetry to be defined. Without this information, it is difficult to know if the results obtained in each study are dependent on the implant technique, dosimetry, differences in follow-up, or the selection criteria. The more frequent use of 3D-CT planning has allowed more rigorous comparisons between the techniques both within and between institutions. Dose optimization of implants by interactive graphics has allowed excellent target volume coverage and assessment of dosimetric quality concurrently, thereby allowing confidence that the dose is delivered to the desired partial breast region. Results of studies with modern planning systems, systematic quality assurance and stringent patient selection criteria thus far have been promising.

There are excellent and mature experiences of APBI from multiple European centers in addition to ongoing multicenter trials that are further outlined in another chapter. The ongoing NSABP B39/RTOG 0413 phase III randomized trial comparing conventional whole-breast irradiation with APBI allows patients to be treated with 3D external beam, multicatheter interstitial brachytherapy or balloon brachytherapy on the APBI arm. The initiation of this pivotal trial was based on a compilation of many experiences around the globe with significant technical advancements as well as improvements in treatment planning systems. In this chapter, key aspects of these published APBI trials from North America with each of these three treatment methods are highlighted.

15.2 Patient Selection

In order to be able to compare published trials between centers and between modalities, the selection criteria should be well-defined. The American Brachytherapy Society (ABS) and the American Society of Breast Surgeons (ASBS) have each recommended patient selection criteria and treatment guidelines. Both sets of selection criteria are more conservative than those in the published literature and applied in ongoing randomized trials. Both sets of criteria require negative margins, no axillary nodal involvement, and only non-lobular invasive breast cancer. There are differences in minimum age (45 years vs. 50 years), maximum tumor size (3 cm vs. 2 cm), and allowance of ductal carcinoma in situ (DCIS) (no vs. yes), respectively, between the ABS and ASBS criteria.

Several other selection criteria have been more controversial and have been debated vigorously; outcome analysis from the various experiences should prove useful in elucidating this issue. These factors include positive nodes, as the treatment of the axilla with external beam irradiation in patients with one to three positive nodes remains controversial. A randomized RTOG trial set to answer this question closed early due to poor accrual. Clearly, APBI can only be warranted when the draining lymphatic regions are confidently deemed to be at sufficiently low risk to not include them in the radiation portal. Many would not routinely encompass the axilla in this subset of patients and thus would allow more limited volumes if there is no compelling risk of residual microscopic disease such as extracapsular spread. Others would treat comprehensively in high-risk node-negative patients as well. Another group of patients with limited data include those with intraductal disease (DCIS). There is some pathologic evidence that patients with DCIS have a higher risk of multicentric disease, especially in the context of an extensive intraductal component (EIC). More recent pathologic data suggest that lumpectomy alone may be sufficient in select patients with widely negative margins, thereby refuting the notion that DCIS patients require wider volume treatment. Additionally, there are limited data revealing a multicentric recurrence pattern in DCIS patients after lumpectomy irrespective of whether whole-breast irradiation is administered. Similarly, patients with lobular carcinoma have been excluded in some series due to the heightened suspicion of multicentricity. Although clinical and pathologic data support smaller lesions with negative margin status, the specific maximal tumor size and minimal negative margin extent required are also not uniformly agreed upon and will require longer-term data from clinical trials.

The completed RTOG 95-17 and the ongoing NSABP B-39/RTOG-0413 randomized trials allow a more diverse population of women to be treated with APBI. The eligibility criteria include those with unicentric, small lesions ($\leq$3 cm), all carcinoma histologies including lobular and DCIS, positive nodes (up to three positive with no extracapsular spread), and negative margins ("no tumor on inked margin"). Distinct selection criteria used in each of the studies are mentioned in the relevant sections below (Table 15.1).

15.3 Interstitial Technique

The first APBI technique that was developed and is associated with the most mature results is the multicatheter interstitial brachytherapy approach. The initial implementation of this method dates back several decades when it was performed at the time of lumpectomy and used as a boost in conjunction with whole-breast irradiation. The technique and indications have evolved significantly to its current use as a sole modality following lumpectomy as described in the several studies below (Table 15.2). The premise is to place multiple needles/catheters through the breast tissue surrounding the lumpectomy cavity seroma correlating with the region at highest risk of harboring re-

Table 15.1 APBI trials: patient selection and dosimetric criteria (*NR* not reported)

Institution	Tumor size (cm)	Nodes	EIC	Margin definition (mm)	Technique	Radiotherapy details	Target definition	Median no. of needles
Interstitial series								
Ochsner	<4	Yes	Yes	Negative	HDR/LDR	32–34 Gy/8–10 fractions or 45 Gy/4 days	2–3 cm	15
William Beaumont Hospital	<3	Yes	No	≥2	HDR/LDR	32–34 Gy/8–10 fractions or 50 Gy/4 days	1–2 cm	14
Tufts/Brown	<5	Yes	Yes	≥2	HDR	34 Gy/10 fractions	2 cm	16
University of Kansas	<2	No	No	Negative	LDR	20–25 Gy/24–48 h	1 cm	NR
RTOG 95-17	<3	Yes	No	Negative	HDR/LDR	34 Gy/10 fractions or 45 Gy/4 days	2 cm	16
Virginia Commonwealth University	<3	Yes	No	Negative	HDR/LDR	34 Gy/10 fractions or 45 Gy/4 days	1–2 cm	15
University of Wisconsin	<3	Yes	No	Negative	HDR	32–34 Gy/8–10 fractions	1.5–2 cm	22
Massachusetts General Hospital	<2	No	No	Negative	LDR	50–60 Gy/4–5 days	3 cm	14
External beam								
William Beaumont Hospital pilot	<3	No	No	≥2	Three- to five-field, supine	34 Gy/10 fractions	1.5 + 1 cm	–
William Beaumont Hospital	<3	No	No	≥2	Three- to five-field, supine	38.5 Gy/10 fractions	1.5 + 1 cm	–
New York University	<2	No	No	≥2	Two-field, prone	30 Gy/6 fractions/10 days	1.5–2 cm + 7 mm	–
MammoSite								
FDA trial	<2	No	No	≥2	HDR	34 Gy/10 fractions	1 cm	–
Breast Care Center of the Southwest	<3	No	No	Negative	HDR	34 Gy/10 fractions	1 cm	–
Tufts/Virginia Commonwealth University/New England Medical Center	10	No	No	≥2	HDR	34 Gy/10 fractions	1 cm	–
St. Vincent's	<5	No	No	≥2	HDR	34 Gy/10 fractions	1 cm	–
Rush	<5	No	No	≥2	HDR	34 Gy/10 fractions	1 cm	–

sidual microscopic disease. The total number of catheters used is based on the size of the seroma cavity which involutes over the several weeks following surgery. Generally, basic brachytherapy principles are followed during implantation, and needles are spaced uniformly to optimally cover the planned target volume (PTV) while minimizing hot spots and proximity to normal tissues. This can require anywhere from 15 to 25 catheters in a given patient. The flexible catheters remain in the breast for the duration of the treatment course and are generally well-tolerated with minimal discomfort (Fig. 15.1). Following the outpatient procedure, treatment planning is performed to confirm proper coverage.

Recent advances in catheter placement techniques as well as an increased number of brachytherapy schools have led to more reproducible implantations. Specifically, advances in image-guidance measures such as CT, ultrasound, and stereotactic digital mammography have led to improvements in this APBI method. The complement of advanced 3D CT-based dosimetry with geometric volume optimization has further improved target volume delineation, coverage, and dose homogeneity (Fig. 15.2). As with all complex brachytherapy, including prostate and gynecologic, quality implantation does require a learning curve for radiation oncologists including additional time, skill and often specialized training, and this in turn has led to this method being deemed "technically challenging". However, it appears that in comparison to other APBI modalities, it affords the greatest control and tailoring of radiation dose delivery to accommodate the variations in lumpectomy cavity size, shape, or location within the breast, while potentially minimizing doses to normal tissues.

When reviewing studies regarding interstitial implants, it is important to realize that there has been significant disparity in the methods of performing these implants between physicians and institutions. One important difference is in target definition which comprises two critical components: target delineation and implant volume. The method of target delineation is important as there remains no consensus on which technique is preferred, thereby rendering comparison between reports in the literature less accurate. Some have advocated using surgical clips to define the seroma cavity, others have used contrast injection into the seroma to guide needle placement with digital mammography, and yet others have used the unenhanced seroma cavity visualized via CT or ultrasound (Fig. 15.3). The implant volume can also be different with some reports suggesting a 1-cm expansion while others favor a wider 2-cm expansion. Considerable differences also remain with the treatment planning process. Several reports have confirmed that CT-based treatment planning allows excellent visualization of the lumpectomy cavity and normal structures, thereby improving target volume delineation and optimal coverage, relative to conventional orthogonal film dosimetry (Fig. 15.4). However, CT-based planning with geometric optimization tools only became more commonly used recently and early studies used plain film 2D dosimetry (Fig. 15.5).

15.3.1 The Ochsner Clinic

The earliest experience of APBI utilizing interstitial brachytherapy was begun at the Ochsner Clinic by Kuske and colleagues. The method at the time was coined the "wide-volume" interstitial brachytherapy technique due to the larger number of catheters used (often more than 20) and volume of breast tissue irradiated compared to the earlier European studies (King et al. 2000). Between 1992 and 1993, 50 women with 51 breast can-

Table 15.2 APBI results: interstitial brachytherapy series with >2 years median follow-up (*NR* not reported)

Institution	No. of patients	Median follow-up (months)	5-year IBTR		Cosmesis (good/ excellent)	Grade 3/4 toxicity
			Total	Else-where		
Ochsner	160	84	2.5	1.2	75	8%
William Beaumont Hospital	199	65	1.2	0.6	92	0
Tufts/Brown	33	58	6	6	88	33
University of Kansas	25	47	0	0	100	NR
RTOG 95-17	99	44	3	0	NR	4
Virginia Common-wealth University	44	42	0	0	80	14
University of Wisconsin	240	30	1.4	1.4	96.5	8.9
Massachusetts General Hospital	48	23	0	0	92	12.5

cers were treated. Selection criteria included early-stage breast cancer following lumpectomy with unicentric Tis, T1, and T2 (T ≤4 cm) lesions and negative surgical margins by NSABP definition, and up to three involved lymph nodes were allowed. Although the eligibility was broad, 45% of lesions were occult and the mean size was only 1.4 cm. Brachytherapy catheters were placed intraoperatively at the time of lumpectomy using a freehand technique (45% of patients) or by closed technique via ultrasound guidance (55% of patients). The target volume was defined as at least a 2 cm expansion beyond the lumpectomy cavity which often encompassed a substantial proportion of the breast tissue. The mean number of catheters was 15. Patients were treated with either low dose-rate (LDR) to 45 Gy over 4 days or with high dose-rate (HDR) to 32 Gy in eight twice-daily outpatient fractions over 4 days. In a matched-pair analysis with similar patients treated with whole-breast external beam irradiation, the results were quite favorable at a median follow-up of 75 months. There were one and five local failures in the brachytherapy and external beam arms, corresponding to a crude ipsilateral breast tumor recurrence (IBTR) rate of 2% and 5%, respectively (*P*=0.24). There were also three nodal recurrences in the APBI group, which at 6% is slightly higher than would be expected for isolated recurrence after external beam radiation after a negative level I/II lymph node dissection (Harris et al. 2003). Most physicians would not routinely treat the axillary nodes to higher doses in this subset of patients, and thus it is possible that these recurrences may not have been avoided by standard whole-breast tangent beams. In an updated report, 160 patients with a median follow-up of 84 months were presented. The 5-year ipsilateral breast tumor recurrence rate was 2.5% with an overall 1.2% being elsewhere failures outside the partial breast volume. At 20 months median follow-up, 75% of women receiving brachytherapy had good to excellent cosmetic results; however, 8% of patients developed grade 3 or 4 toxicity and ultimately required surgical intervention for complications related to radiotherapy.

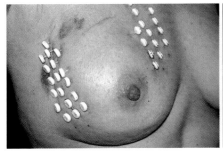 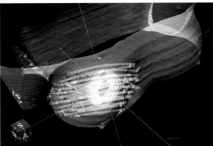

Fig. 15.1 Interstitial catheters intact. Tail-less Comfort catheter system that lies flush to the skin in a multiplane implant allowing improved patient tolerance and mobility

Fig. 15.2 3D reconstruction. 3D rendering of brachytherapy catheters demonstrating the PTV (*pink*) and 100% prescription dose cloud (*blue*)

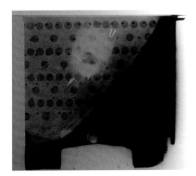 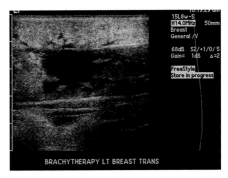

Fig. 15.3 Interstitial and ultrasound targets. *Left*: Digital mammogram demonstrating a contrast-enhanced seroma cavity and surgical clips after template application. *Right*: Ultrasound image depicting catheters placed above and below seroma cavity

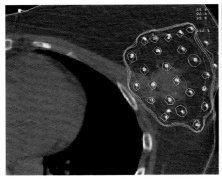 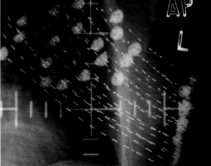

Fig. 15.4 Interstitial planning CT. Treatment planning CT scan with the 100% isodose line conforming to the PTV (*red*) and seroma (*purple*) after geometric volume optimization performed

Fig. 15.5 2D orthogonal films. Anteroposterior postimplant orthogonal film with dummy catheters with variable step sizes. Individual dwell times were delineated on the hard-copy film and digitized into the treatment planning system

15.3.2 William Beaumont Hospital

Vicini and colleagues at William Beaumont Hospital have played a pivotal role providing rigorous APBI data using several different methods. Their most mature results have been with interstitial brachytherapy and included a cohort of 199 women with stricter selection and treatment criteria than the Ochsner group (Vicini et al. 2003a). Inclusion criteria were age ≥40 years, tumor size ≤3 cm, and no EIC or lobular histology. Following lumpectomy and axillary node dissection in all patients, margins had to be clear microscopically by ≥2 mm. While women with up to three involved nodes were initially allowed (12% of patients enrolled), this was later restricted to no positive nodes once evidence emerged of potential survival benefits with chest wall radiotherapy in premenopausal women with one to three involved nodes in the randomized post-mastectomy trials (Overgaard et al. 1997; Ragaz et al. 1997). The average tumor size was small at 1.2 cm. Most patients had widely negative margins with 88% of patients having margins ≥2 mm and 55% margins ≥10 mm. Patients were treated with either LDR brachytherapy to a total dose 50 Gy continuously over 5 days (120 women, 1993–1995) or with HDR brachytherapy to a total dose of 32 Gy in eight fractions twice daily over 4 days or 34 Gy in ten fractions twice daily over 5 days (71 and 8 women, respectively, 1995–1999) (Baglan et al. 2001). The PTV was defined as a margin of 1–2 cm around the lumpectomy cavity, with catheters placed either at the time of the initial lumpectomy, or postoperatively. Uniquely, a rigid template system was used and kept in place during the treatment course in most women, which is unlike in other centers where a template system may be used during the implant procedure, but is replaced by flexible catheters for the duration of treatment. The majority of the patients were treated using 2D plain film dosimetry available at the time with 33% having received double plane implants and 66% triple plane implants. The average number of catheters was 14 (range 8–18).

Combined results from both phases of the trial were excellent at a median follow-up of 5.7 years. A total of 199 patients were treated and compared in a matched-pair analysis with patients receiving conventional whole-breast radiation. There were only five IBTR for a 5-year local recurrence rate of 1.2% with an elsewhere recurrence rate of 0.6%. Cosmetic outcome was also quite favorable with good to excellent cosmetic results obtained in 92% of patients, with no statistically significant difference between the LDR and HDR groups. In addition, the patients tolerated the treatment well with minimal complications and no acute grade 3 or 4 toxicity. However, the incidence of fat necrosis has increased over time (11% at 5 years) (Benitez et al. 2004).

15.3.3 University of Wisconsin

One of the largest experiences in the country has been reported by Patel and colleagues from the University of Wisconsin. Between 2000 and 2005, 268 patients were treated with HDR-APBI (240 multicatheter interstitial, 28 MammoSite balloon). Selection criteria were broad and included patients with unicentric, Tis-T2, N1 (<3 cm tumor size, up to three nodes positive with no extracapsular extension), negative surgical margins, and a negative post-lumpectomy mammogram. There were no age criteria, or exclusion based on histology (lobular and DCIS were allowed). The median tumor size was 1.1 cm. Two techniques, prone template with digital mammographic and template-guidance on the stereotactic biopsy table and supine free-hand with real-time ultrasound guidance, were used for catheter placement. The target volume was defined as the surgical cavity delineated by Omnipaque contrast and/or surgical clips with a margin of 1–2 cm modified to at least 5 mm deep to the skin surface or at the pectoral fascia. The group implemented CT-based 3D treatment planning in early 2002 thereby allowing more accurate target delineation, improved geometric coverage of the target volume with optimization, and dosimetric verification (Das et al. 2004).

The first 88 patients had orthogonal film dosimetry and were excluded from the dosimetric analysis. All patients were treated with fractionated HDR brachytherapy delivered in the supine position to a dose of 32–34 Gy in eight to ten twice-daily fractions over 4–5 days. The median follow-up for all patients was 30 months. The crude rate of total ipsilateral breast failure was 1.4% (four patients). All of these were elsewhere failures outside the treated volume. At 12 months, 96.5% of patients had good/excellent cosmesis (22.7% and 73.8% with good and excellent scores, respectively). The procedure was well-tolerated with minimal acute toxicity. The rate of symptomatic fat necrosis was 8.9% (24 patients). The target volume coverage with CT-planning was excellent. Importantly, the overall implant volume was larger than in other series with the median number of catheters being 22 (range 10–37) (Patel et al. 2005).

15.3.4 Virginia Commonwealth University

Arthur et al. at Virginia Commonwealth University from 1995 to 2000 treated 44 women with interstitial multicatheter brachytherapy (Arthur et al. 2003). Their selection criteria were similar to those of RTOG 95-17, allowing tumors <4 cm (median size 1.2 cm), no age restriction (median age 62 years), allowing limited positive nodes (18%), and negative surgical margins (72% of women had margins >2 mm). DCIS and lobular histologies were initially included; however, pure DCIS and node-positive patients were ultimately excluded. Most patients had catheters placed postoperatively. PTV was defined as the lumpectomy cavity plus a 2-cm margin, except where limited by skin or the chest wall. An average of 14.7 catheters were placed primarily using a free-hand technique with CT and fluoroscopic guidance. Patients received either LDR brachytherapy to a total dose of 45 Gy at 50 cGy/h or HDR for a total dose of 34 Gy in ten twice-daily fractions.

At a median follow-up of 42 months, there were no local or regional recurrences. Good to excellent cosmetic results were achieved in 79.6% and 90% with LDR and HDR, respectively. Toxicity was minimal, although six patients (14%) had cosmesis-altering fibrosis in the high-dose treatment region. Additionally, 43% of women receiving Adriamycin-based chemotherapy after brachytherapy developed a recall reaction which led to a detriment in cosmesis.

15.3.5 Tufts/Brown/Rhode Island

In a multiple institution series by Tufts-NEMC, Rhode Island Hospital and Brown University led by Wazer and colleagues, 32 women with 33 breast cancers were enrolled in an interstitial brachytherapy trial between 1997 and 1999 (Wazer et al. 2001). They allowed both T1 and T2 tumors (mean size 1.3 cm) with a requirement for tumor-free margins ≥ 1 mm (55% had margins of ≥ 2 mm). Age was not restricted although most women were postmenopausal with a mean age of 63 years. DCIS and invasive lobular cancer (ILC) were excluded, yet a high proportion of patients had EIC (55%) as well as up to three positive lymph nodes (27%). Catheter placement was either via a freehand technique at the time of lumpectomy or was postoperative. The PTV was the lumpectomy cavity plus a 2-cm margin. An average of 16 catheters were placed (range 8–25) kept 5–7 mm from the skin. All patients received HDR brachytherapy to 34 Gy in ten twice-daily fractions over 5 days. In an excellent analysis of dosimetric correlation with toxicity, fat necrosis was proportionally associated with larger tissue volumes receiving fractional doses of 340 cGy, 510 cGy, and 680 cGy.

In a separate report with 58 months of median follow-up, the 5-year crude local recurrence rate was 3% (Wazer et al. 2002). Cosmetic results were judged good to excellent in 91% of patients. RTOG/EORTC-defined grade 3 or 4 subcutaneous toxicity was seen in 33% of patients (3 patients grade 3, and 11 patients grade 4). Both the number of total dwell positions and the fractional volume of irradiated tissue at each isodose level were significantly associated with grade 3 or 4 toxicity. There was a trend toward a higher risk of clinically evident fat necrosis and among women who received Adriamycin-based chemotherapy. Further outcome analysis from experiences such as these should allow more accurate dose–volume constraints to be employed while treatment planning to minimize higher grade and symptomatic toxicities.

15.3.6 University of Kansas

Krishnan et al. treated 25 women at the University of Kansas from 1993 to 1998 (Krishnan et al. 2001). The selection criteria included patients with age ≥ 60 years, tumors ≤ 2 cm, and negative surgical margins. The mean tumor size was 1 cm. DCIS, EIC, and women with positive lymph nodes were excluded. The total dose was significantly lower than in the other APBI series at 20–25 Gy over 24–48 hours with LDR brachytherapy. Similarly, the minimum PTV margin was also smaller than in other interstitial series at 1 cm around the tumor bed. All patients had their catheters placed intraoperatively at the time of lumpectomy. At a median follow-up of 47 months, there were no local, regional, or distant recurrences. Patient tolerance was excellent with no reported RTOG grade 3 or 4 toxicity noted, and good to excellent cosmetic results in all patients.

15.3.7 Massachusetts General Hospital

Significant information about the impact of implant volume and dose on potential risk of toxicity and cosmetic outcome was first reported by Lawenda and colleagues at Massachusetts General Hospital. In their published series, 48 patients were enrolled between 1997 and 2001 (Lawenda et al. 2003). The eligibility criteria for the trial were more stringent than those mentioned previously and included patients with tumors ≤ 2 cm in size, with no DCIS, EIC, lymphovascular invasion or positive nodes. An average of 14 (range 10–16) brachytherapy catheters were placed. The PTV was formed by a 3-cm margin around the lumpectomy cavity usually in two or three planes. Patients were treated at three separate dose levels of 50, 55, and 60 Gy, respectively, with LDR brachytherapy. At a follow-up of 23 months, there were no local, regional, or distant recurrences. Cosmesis was good to excellent in 91.8% of patients. RTOG grade 2 or 3 complications were most common in the group with the largest treatment volume, >203 cm³ (27%). Significant fibrosis was noted in four patients (8.3%), and 17.4% had biopsy-proven fat necrosis.

15.3.8 RTOG 95-17

This phase II multicenter cooperative group study evaluating interstitial brachytherapy enrolled 99 patients between 1997 and 2000 (King et al. 2000). The selection criteria were broad and had no age limitations, allowed unifocal tumor sizes to up to 3 cm, required clear margins ("on tumor on ink"), and allowed women with up to three involved lymph nodes with no extracapsular extension. Patients with DCIS and ILC were excluded. APBI was delivered using either LDR with 45 Gy delivered over 3.5–5 days (33%) or HDR at a dose of 34 Gy in ten fractions over 5 days (66%). The PTV was intended to be a 2-cm margin around the lumpectomy cavity with a 5-mm minimum separation from the skin and chest wall. Most implants were multiplane (two or three planes). The median number of catheters was 16. At 3.7 years of median follow-up, the ipsilateral breast tumor recurrence rate was 3%, with a regional lymph node failure rate of 3%. The procedure was well-tolerated in both cohorts with 2% and 9% grade 2 toxicity in the HDR and LDR patients, respectively. There was minimal grade 3 or 4 toxicity (4%). Further outcome analysis awaits a longer patient follow-up.

15.4 MammoSite Balloon

Due to the invasiveness, implant technique variability and the perceived technical challenge of multicatheter interstitial implants, an alternative method for APBI was developed using an intracavitary balloon catheter treatment device, the MammoSite radiation therapy system (RTS; Proxima Therapeutics, Alpharetta, GA). This was originally designed to simplify the brachytherapy procedure thus lessening the learning curve while improving the reproducibility of dosimetric coverage of the target volume. The system is comprised of a single catheter located centrally within a balloon that is placed and inflated within the lumpectomy cavity (Fig. 15.6). The balloon can be inflated to a sphere of either 4–5 cm or 5–6 cm in diameter, although additional sizes and elliptical shapes have been developed. The device can be placed either at the time of lumpectomy in the operating room or postoperatively with the cavity closed; however, initial experience suggesting higher infection rates and the lack of known final pathologic margin status with the intraoperative approach has led to a recommendation of postoperative balloon placement. Early experiences have revealed several additional quality assurance measures necessary to improve optimal delivery. After inflation, balloon catheter placement is evaluated to assure balloon symmetry, an overlying skin distance of ≥7 mm, and tissue conformance with the balloon surface (Fig. 15.7). An important distinguishing factor from multicatheter brachytherapy is the target volume encompassed by the prescription isodose line. The treatment is typically delivered from a single, centralized, HDR source to a circumferential 1-cm distance from the surface of the balloon, while most of the published interstitial studies have used more extensive margins on the seroma cavity

(1–3 cm). Some have advocated the use of multiple dwell positions to enhance the conformality of the isodose distribution; however, most data presented have employed the single central dwell position method (Streeter et al. 2003). Thus far, patient tolerance has been excellent with minimal complications aside from high catheter pull-rate and initial infection rates. These should further decline as experience mounts and clinical and dosimetric factors are determined. Although efficacy and early institutional outcome data are still limited, a large registry database of 1500 patients has been collected and should provide key clinical, pathologic, and dosimetric data with the use of this technique. In the following section, initial experiences with this device are reviewed (Table 15.3).

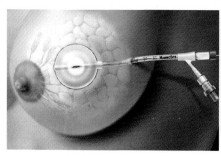 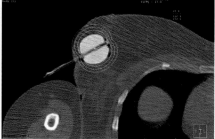

Fig. 15.6 MammoSite schematic. Single catheter located centrally within a balloon that is placed and inflated within the lumpectomy cavity

Fig. 15.7 MammoSite planning CT. Treatment planning CT scan demonstrating ideal balloon placement, tissue conformance, and skin thickness

Table 15.3 APBI results: MammoSite brachytherapy series (*NR* not reported)

Institution	No. of patients	Median follow-up (months)	IBTR (total)	Cosmesis, good/ excellent (%)	Infection (%)
FDA trial	43	48	0	80	4.7
Breast Care Center of the Southwest	21	NR	0	NR	NR
Tufts/Virginia Commonwealth University/New England Medical Center	28	19	0	93	NR
St. Vincent's	32	11	0	86	16
Rush	112	6	0	80	6

15.4.1 FDA Study

The MammoSite RTS was cleared by the US Food and Drug Administration (US FDA) in May 2002 based on results from an initial phase I/II trial designed to test the safety and performance of the device. The initial experience was reported by Keisch and colleagues and consisted of patients treated at a total of nine institutions. Selection criteria were more conservative than the interstitial APBI counterparts and included women with an age >45 years, tumor size ≤2 cm, negative lymph nodes, negative surgical margins (Keisch et al. 2003). Women with pure DCIS, EIC, and ILC were excluded. Of 54 patients who had the device inserted, 43 were eventually treated. The majority of catheters that were pulled were secondary to issues of poor tissue conformance (seven patients) and inadequate skin thickness (two patients) and resulted in no treatment. The catheter was placed with an open technique in 34 patients and with a postoperative closed technique in the other 20 patients. The prescription dose was 34 Gy in ten fractions delivered twice daily over 5 days prescribed to 1 cm from the balloon surface. A minimum skin-to-balloon surface distance of 5 mm was required for treatment. Device performance, complications, and cosmesis were assessed. At a median follow-up of 21 months, 88% of all treated patients had good to excellent cosmetic results. However, further experience indicated that cosmesis could be improved by increasing the skin-to-balloon thickness: with a thickness of ≥7 mm 97% of patients showed good to excellent cosmetic results versus 78% of those with a thickness of 5–7 mm. Local control and survival analysis have not been reported due to the shortness of the follow-up. Toxicity data have been reported at 48 months, and demonstrate excellent tolerability with no significant toxicity.

15.4.2 Tufts/New England Medical Center

There are limited data from the same institution comparing outcomes between different APBI techniques. One such report from the investigators from Tufts-New England Medical Center led by Wazer compared toxicity in 75 women receiving HDR interstitial brachytherapy and that seen in 20 women receiving intracavitary brachytherapy (Shah et al. 2004). Seven patients (20%) had the procedure aborted prior to treatment due to balloon rupture, hemorrhage, or inadequate skin thickness. In their series, grade 2–4 subcutaneous fibrosis was significantly less with the intracavitary than with the interstitial brachytherapy method (10% versus 32%). An important distinguishing point is that a much smaller volume of breast tissue was irradiated with the balloon technique (101 cm^3 versus 176 cm^3). The authors compared the volumes receiving 100% (34 Gy), 150% (51 Gy), and 200% (68 Gy) and concluded that the reduced fibrosis in the intracavitary patients was due to the smaller treatment volumes. However, when only multicatheter brachytherapy patients who did not have anthracycline-based chemotherapy were compared with those receiving intracavitary therapy, the toxicity difference was insignificant. The MammoSite-treated patients had a consistently greater skin dose which resulted in significantly higher mild erythema (42.9% and 17.3% with interstitial, respectively). Whether this will lead to higher rates of telangiectasias, fibrosis, or dermatitis remains to be seen. The dose homogeneity index (DHI), which is a reflection of the hot spots in the high dose region, was less with balloon brachytherapy than with HDR interstitial brachytherapy (0.73 versus 0.83, $P<0.001$). Longer follow-up will be needed to discern factors correlating with specific outcomes allowing rigorous dosimetric constraints that can be used during treatment planning to minimize late toxicity while optimizing local control rates.

15.4.3 Arizona

Zannis et al. from Breast Care Center of the Southwest reported 23 patients who underwent balloon placement of which 2 (9%) were explanted due to poor tissue conformance and poor balloon symmetry. Patients were selected with an age greater than 45 years, tumor ≤3 cm, negative margins with no EIC, ILC, or positive nodes. All patients had the balloon placed with the cavity closed under ultrasound guidance. The remainder underwent successful placement and tolerated the procedure well without serious complications (Zannis et al. 2003).

15.4.4 St. Vincent's

Richards and colleagues from St. Vincent's Cancer Center recently reported on their initial experience with the MammoSite balloon (Richards et al. 2004). This included 32 patients with a median follow-up of 11 months. Selection criteria included stage 1–2 patients with negative surgical margins. No acute toxicities occurred during the 5 days of treatment. Although all skin reactions were confined to the region overlying the balloon, 25% developed bright erythema and patchy moist desquamation. They also reported a high infection rate of 16% which may have been attributable to the minimal recommended catheter care when the device was initially implemented. Cosmesis was good to excellent in 86% of patients.

15.4.5 Rush University

The largest published experience is from Dowlatshahi and colleagues from Rush University and included 129 patients who had a balloon placed, of whom 112 underwent treatment (Dowlatshahi et al. 2004). Inclusion criteria were broad allowing women >40 years of age, stage T1-T2, node-negative or node-positive, negative surgical margins, plus DCIS, EIC and ILC. The primary reason for not treating was poor balloon/cavity conformance and inadequate balloon/skin spacing. Overall, the balloon was very well tolerated after the initial 24 hours. Six patients developed wound infections. At 6 months follow-up, 80% of patients had good to excellent cosmesis.

15.5 External Beam APBI

Given the technical challenges and skill-dependence of an invasive brachytherapy procedure, external beam APBI approaches have been investigated. The advent of 3D-CT-based treatment planning with highly conformal dose distributions and visualization and monitoring of the target volume has allowed several studies of clinical feasibility to be reported (Baglan et al. 2003; Formenti et al. 2004). The non-invasive and more accessible external beam treatment renders the similar APBI course significantly more convenient for both patients and treating physicians (Fig. 15.8). There remain, however, several important distinct challenges with this approach compared to brachytherapy that are being investigated. An important factor is that the integral dose can be significantly increased to normal tissue, especially the ipsilateral breast tissue (Fig. 15.9). This is due to concerns of target delineation, target motion due to respiration, and daily set-up variability. Alternate immobilization techniques have been utilized including prone positioning, alpha cradle bras, and respiratory-gating. Whether the higher integral dose will lead to increased long-term side effects remains to be seen. Rigorous dose–volume constraints have been proposed and will be evaluated in ongoing trials to assess the feasibility and safety of this approach, thereby making it more readily applied in the clinical setting.

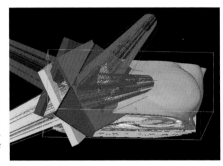

Fig. 15.8 3D-CRT field design. Four-field beam arrangement for external beam APBI on Pinnacle treatment planning system

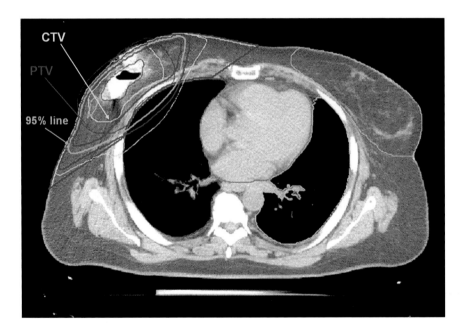

Fig. 15.9 3D-CRT isodose. 3D dose distribution with coverage of CTV (*yellow*) and PTV (*red*) by the 95% isodose line on the Pinnacle treatment planning system

There are limited data from North America yet reported with this technique, and further follow-up is needed to generate comparisons with the more established APBI methods. However, experience thus far has revealed high feasibility with minimal acute toxicity (Table 15.4). In addition to few single-institution series using variable techniques, a RTOG multi-institutional study has been completed and is outlined in the following section.

Table 15.4 APBI results: external beam radiation (*NR* not reported)

Institution	No. of patients	Median follow-up	IBTR (total)	Cosmesis, good/ excellent (%)	Grade 3/4 toxicity
William Beaumont Hospital pilot	9	8	0	100	NR
William Beaumont Hospital	31	10	0	100	0
New York University	47	18	0	100	NR

15.5.1 William Beaumont Hospital

Investigators at William Beaumont Hospital led by Vicini and colleagues were instrumental in complementing a long-term APBI experience with breast brachytherapy with 3D conformal APBI. In a small pilot study, nine patients were enrolled with similar criteria to those of their brachytherapy protocol: age >40 years, tumor size <3 cm, invasive ductal histology, negative margins >2 mm, and negative axillary nodes (Baglan et al. 2003). Details of the complex treatment planning process includes either a four-field (right breast) or five-field (left breast) non-coplanar beam arrangement with 6-MV photons. The CTV definition was similar to that for brachytherapy at 15 mm beyond the surgical cavity; however, an additional 10 mm was added to form the PTV (5 mm to account for normal respiration and 5 mm added for daily set-up variation). The surgical cavity was defined by the presence of surgical clips placed at the time of lumpectomy. A similar dose fractionation scheme was initially used at 34 Gy in ten fractions over 5 days, but was later escalated to a total dose of 38.5 Gy to account for the inherent homogeneity of the dose distribution in comparison to the brachytherapy plans. A follow-up report of a total of 31 patients demonstrated excellent tolerability of the procedure. At a median follow-up of 10 months, no grade 3 toxicity was observed and early cosmetic results were good to excellent in all patients. The authors concluded that there was less normal tissue irradiated compared to standard breast tangential beams including ipsilateral breast tissue, as well as underlying lung and heart tissue (Vicini et al. 2003b).

15.5.2 New York University

Formenti and colleagues from New York University have also explored external beam APBI. However, their focus has been on treating selected women in the prone position to minimize respiratory motion while displacing normal structures. A dedicated prone table was constructed to facilitate such positioning. Selection criteria in their pilot trial included women with clinically occult lesions of <2 cm, negative margins of >2 mm, negative axillary nodes, and estrogen receptor-positive tumors (Formenti et al. 2002, 2004). The PTV definition was variable and included the surgical cavity plus a margin of 1–2 cm. Initially 18 patients were treated at different dose levels ranging from 25 to 30 Gy delivered over five fractions over 10 days. Fraction sizes were 5 Gy, 5.5 Gy, and 6 Gy to the 95% isodose line. At a minimum follow-up of 36 months, all patients had tolerated the treatment well with minimal toxicity and had good to excellent cosmesis.

A second series of 47 patients was subsequently reported with all patients treated with the highest dose per fraction from their pilot series of 6 Gy for five fractions over 10 days with a total dose of 30 Gy (Formenti et al. 2004). Similar selection criteria were used in this cohort, although the median age of patients enrolled was older at 76.5 years. The predominant field design used was a pair of opposed minitangent beams. A larger proportional volume of breast was irradiated compared to the William Beaumont group with up to 45% of the breast encompassed by the prescription isodose line of 95%. However, prone positioning allowed a smaller region of underlying heart and lung in the high-dose region. At a median follow-up of 18 months, the treatment was well-tolerated with only mild erythema in 30% of patients. There were no ipsilateral breast tumor recurrences. The overall treatment time in this series was twice that with the other APBI regimens at 10 days versus typically 4–5 days. The initial results of this approach have nevertheless been favorable.

15.5.3 RTOG 0319

Building on the initial William Beaumont experience of Vicini and colleagues, a multi-institution phase I/II study, RTOG 0319, examined the feasibility of 3D conformal external beam partial breast irradiation. Selection criteria were similar to those for the previous RTOG 95-17 APBI trial of interstitial brachytherapy and included patients with unifocal, invasive non-lobular histology, size ≤3 cm, negative margins ≥2 mm, up to three positive nodes with no extracapsular spread. Patients were treated to a dose of 38.5 Gy in ten fractions (3.85 Gy per fraction) over 5 days. The trial enrolled 99 patients rapidly and is now closed to accrual. Although formal outcome analysis evaluating toxicity, cosmesis, and local control will require a longer follow-up, the successful completion and credentialing process of this trial formed the template of and was the impetus for the ongoing phase III NSABP B39/RTOG 0413 trial.

15.6 Conclusion

The rapid evolution of APBI has taken place significantly on both sides of the Atlantic in the past decade. Clearly, the concept of an accelerated, more limited irradiated volume approach represents one of the most important potential paradigm shifts in breast cancer treatment and will likely allow many more women access to breast-conservation therapy in a cost- and time-effective manner. However, rigorous analysis of evidence gained from single-institution and cooperative group trials will be required before this can be considered the new standard of care. Paramount to its success is appropriate patient selection criteria as studies with poor selection have shown higher than acceptable local control rates. Although slightly different amongst institutional series presented in this chapter, there is consistency in that the best results are seen in patients with small tumor size, negative margins, and minimally involved nodes. Clearly, if a patient is not a candidate for breast-conservation therapy with tangential whole breast radiation alone excluding the draining lymphatics then they should be excluded from regimens further reducing the volume of breast tissue irradiated.

There remains a significant difference between the three primary methods of APBI outlined in this chapter, multicatheter brachytherapy, balloon brachytherapy and external beam therapy. The highlighted differences include the amount of tissue irradiated, the technical challenge in radiation delivery and planning, and the logistics for the patient such as level of invasiveness. Additionally, there is a variable level of data supporting each modality as only the multicatheter approach has produced outcome data extending beyond 5 years and has been compared to matched or historical controls treated with whole-breast irradiation. The others have shown excellent feasibility and tolerability with minimal acute toxicity, but there are limited efficacy data available at this juncture. Clearly, the ongoing phase III NSABP B39/RTOG 0413 trial which allows treatment with any of these three methods on the APBI arm will allow controlled analysis between them, but more importantly will allow comparison with the current standard of care of whole-breast radiotherapy.

The advent of CT-based treatment planning has allowed significant advances in target delineation, dosimetric coverage, and quality assurance measures. Further outcome analysis linking toxicity with dosimetric parameters is needed to allow development of tighter dose–volume constraints that can be employed during treatment planning. It is not likely that just one method of APBI will remain superior and suitable for all patients, as the optimal technique will clearly need to be tailored to the individual patient. From the evidence presented in this review chapter, it appears that APBI has a high likelihood of being incorporated as a viable alternative treatment option for selected women with early-stage breast cancer.

References

1. Arthur DW, Koo D, Zwicker RD, et al (2003) Partial breast brachytherapy after lumpectomy: low-dose-rate and high-dose-rate experience. Int J Radiat Oncol Biol Phys 56(3):681–689

2. Baglan KL, Martinez AA, Frazier RC, et al (2001) The use of high-dose-rate brachytherapy alone after lumpectomy in patients with early-stage breast cancer treated with breast-conserving therapy. Int J Radiat Oncol Biol Phys 50(4):1003–1011

3. Baglan KL, Sharpe MB, Jaffray D, et al (2003) Accelerated partial breast irradiation using 3D conformal radiation therapy (3D-CRT) Int J Radiat Oncol Biol Phys 55(2):302–311

4. Benitez PR, Chen PY, Vicini FA, et al (2004) Partial breast irradiation in breast conserving therapy by way of interstitial brachytherapy. Am J Surg 188(4):355–364

5. Das RK, Patel R, Shah H, et al (2004) 3D CT-based high-dose-rate breast brachytherapy implants: treatment planning and quality assurance. Int J Radiat Oncol Biol Phys 59(4):1224–1228

6. Dowlatshahi K, Snider HC, Gittleman MA, et al (2004) Early experience with balloon brachytherapy for breast cancer. Arch Surg 139(6):603–607; discussion 607–608

7. Formenti SC, Rosenstein B, Skinner KA, et al (2002) T1 stage breast cancer: adjuvant hypo-fractionated conformal radiation therapy to tumor bed in selected postmenopausal breast cancer patients–pilot feasibility study. Radiology 222(1):171–178

8. Formenti SC, Truong MT, Goldberg JD, et al (2004) Prone accelerated partial breast irradiation after breast-conserving surgery: preliminary clinical results and dose-volume histogram analysis. Int J Radiat Oncol Biol Phys 60(2):493–504

9. Harris EE, Hwang WT, Seyednejad F, et al (2003) Prognosis after regional lymph node recurrence in patients with stage I-II breast carcinoma treated with breast conservation. Cancer 98:2144–2151

10. Keisch M, Vicini F, Kuske RR, et al (2003) Initial clinical experience with the MammoSite breast brachytherapy applicator in women with early-stage breast cancer treated with breast-conserving therapy. Int J Radiat Oncol Biol Phys 55(2):289–293

11. King TA, Bolton JS, Kuske RR, et al (2000) Long-term results of wide-field brachytherapy as the sole method of radiation therapy after segmental mastectomy for T(is,1,2) breast cancer. Am J Surg 180(4):299–304

12. Krishnan L, Jewell WR, Tawfik OW, et al (2001) Breast conservation therapy with tumor bed irradiation alone in a selected group of patients with stage I breast cancer. Breast J 7(2):91–96

13. Lawenda BD, Taghian AG, Kachnic LA, et al (2003) Dose-volume analysis of radiotherapy for T1N0 invasive breast cancer treated by local excision and partial breast irradiation by low-dose-rate interstitial implant. Int J Radiat Oncol Biol Phys 56(3):671–680

14. Overgaard M, Hansen PS, Overgaard J, et al (1997) Postoperative radiotherapy in high-risk premenopausal women with breast cancer who receive adjuvant chemotherapy. Danish Breast Cancer Cooperative Group 82b Trial. N Engl J Med 337(14):949–955

15. Patel R, Ringwala S, Shah H, Das R (2005) Multi-catheter breast brachytherapy following lumpectomy in select early stage breast cancer patients: the University of Wisconsin Experience (abstract). Int J Radiat Oncol Biol Phys 63 [Suppl 1]:S7–S8

16. Ragaz J, Jackson SM, Le N, et al (1997) Adjuvant radiotherapy and chemotherapy in node-positive premenopausal women with breast cancer. N Engl J Med 337(14):956–962

17. Richards GM, Berson AM, Rescigno J, et al (2004) Acute toxicity of high-dose-rate intracavitary brachytherapy with the MammoSite applicator in patients with early-stage breast cancer. Ann Surg Oncol 11(8):739–746

18. Shah NM, Tenenholz T, Arthur D, et al (2004) MammoSite and interstitial brachytherapy for accelerated partial breast irradiation: factors that affect toxicity and cosmesis. Cancer 101(4):727–734

19. Streeter OE Jr, Vicini FA, Keisch M, et al (2003) MammoSite radiation therapy system. Breast 12(6):491–496

20. Vicini FA, Kestin L, Chen P, et al (2003a) Limited-field radiation therapy in the management of early-stage breast cancer. J Natl Cancer Inst 95(16):1205–1210

21. Vicini FA, Remouchamps V, Wallace M, et al (2003b) Ongoing clinical experience utilizing 3D conformal external beam radiotherapy to deliver partial-breast irradiation in patients with early-stage breast cancer treated with breast-conserving therapy. Int J Radiat Oncol Biol Phys 57(5):1247–1253

22. Wazer DE, Lowther D, Boyle T, et al (2001) Clinically evident fat necrosis in women treated with high-dose-rate brachytherapy alone for early-stage breast cancer. Int J Radiat Oncol Biol Phys 50(1):107–111

23. Wazer DE, Berle L, Graham R, et al (2002) Preliminary results of a phase I/II study of HDR brachytherapy alone for T1/T2 breast cancer. Int J Radiat Oncol Biol Phys 53(4):889–897

24. Zannis VJ, Walker LC, Barclay-White B, et al (2003) Postoperative ultrasound-guided percutaneous placement of a new breast brachytherapy balloon catheter. Am J Surg 186(4):383–385

An Overview of European Clinical Trials of Accelerated Partial Breast Irradiation

16

Csaba Polgár, Tibor Major,
Vratislav Strnad, Peter Niehoff,
Oliver J. Ott and György Kovács

Contents

16.1 Introduction

In the last two decades there has been an increasing interest in Europe in treating selected patients with early-stage breast cancer with accelerated partial breast irradiation (APBI) using external beam irradiation (EBI) (Magee et al. 1996; Ribeiro et al. 1993), interstitial brachytherapy (BT) (Cionini et al. 1995; Clarke et al. 1994; Fentiman et al. 1991, 1996, 2004; Johansson et al. 2002; Mayer and Nemeskéri 1993; Ott et al. 2004, 2005a, 2005b; Polgár et al. 2000, 2002a, 2002b, 2004a, 2004b, 2005; Póti et al. 2004; Samuel et al.

Table 16.1 Results of early European APBI trials (NR not reported)

Institution	References	Technique	RT scheme (dose [Gy]× fraction no.)	Median follow-up period (years)	Total LR, % (n)	True recurrence/marginal miss, % (n)	Elsewhere failure (%)	Annual LR (%)	Cosmesis excellent/good
Christie Hospital	Magee et al. 1996; Ribeiro et al. 1993	Electron	5×8	8	20 (69 of 353)	NR	NR	2.5	NR
Uzsoki Hospital	Mayer and Nemeskéri 1993; Póti et al. 2004	Medium dose-rate	50×1	12	24 (17 of 70)	17 (12 of 70)	7 (5 of 70)	2	50
Guy's Hospital I	Fentiman et al. 1991, 1996	Low dose-rate	55×1	6	37 (10 of 27)	33 (9 of 27)	4 (1 of 27)	6.2	83
Guy's Hospital II	Fentiman et al. 2004	Medium dose-rate	11×4	6.3	18 (9 of 49)	14 (7 of 49)	4 (2 of 49)	2.9	81
Florence Hospital	Cionini et al. 1995	Low dose-rate	50–60×1	4.2	6 (7 of 115)	2 (2 of 115)	4 (5 of 115)	1.4	NR
Royal Devon/Exeter Hospital	Clarke et al. 1994	High dose-rate	10×2; 8×4; 6×6	1.5	16 (7 of 45)	9 (4 of 45)	7 (3 of 45)	10.7	95
All patients				1.5–12	18 (119 of 659)	11 (34 of 306)	5 (16 of 306)	1.4–10.7	50–95

Table 16.2 Results of early breast conservation trials using conventional whole-breast irradiation

Institution	Reference	Study period	Whole-breast irradiation dose (Gy)	Boost dose	Median follow-up period (years)	LR (%)	Annual LR
NCI	Jacobson et al. 1995	1979–87	45–50.4	15–20	10	18[a]	1.80
W. Beaumont Hospital	Pass et al. 2004	1980–85	45	15	12.3	21[b]	1.75
EORTC 10801	Van Dongen et al. 1992	1980–86	50	25	8	13c	1.63
Christie Hospital	Magee et al. 1996	1982–87	40	0	8	13c	1.63
Ontario	Clark et al. 1996	1984–89	40	12.5	7.6	11.3	1.48
Uzsoki Hospital	Lövey et al. 1994	1986–90	50	10–20	3.8	5.5	1.45
Uzsoki Hospital	Lövey et al. 1994	1986–90	50	0	3.8	10.7	2.82

[a] 10-year actuarial rate
[b] 12-year actuarial rate
[c] 8-year actuarial rate

1999; Strnad et al. 2004), or intracavitary (MammoSite) BT (Niehoff et al. 2005). In this chapter, we give an overview of these European clinical trials of APBI including their implications for optimal patient selection, target definition, treatment technique, and quality assurance (QA). Finally, we discuss the development and status of the new European multicentric phase III APBI trial conducted by the Breast Cancer Working Group of the Groupe Européen de Curiethérapie – European Society for Therapeutic Radiology and Oncology (GEC-ESTRO). European experience with intraoperative radiotherapy for APBI is discussed elsewhere (see Chapter 12).

16.2 Early European APBI Trials

Several European centers pioneered the use of different APBI regimens for unselected patients in the early 1980s (Cionini et al. 1995; Clarke et al. 1994; Fentiman et al. 1991, 1996, 2004; Mayer and Nemeskéri 1993; Póti et al. 2004). However, results in all but one of these early studies were poor, with high local recurrence (LR) rates (Table 16.1). The high rates of local failure seen in these early APBI studies reflect inadequate patient selection criteria and/or suboptimal treatment technique and lack of appropriate QA procedures (Polgár et al. 2004b, 2005). Of note, these results are quite similar to those of earlier breast conservation trials using conventional whole-breast radiotherapy (Table 16.2) (Clark et al. 1996; Jacobson et al. 1995; Lövey et al. 1994; Pass et al. 2004; Van Dongen et al. 1992), which suggests that this problem was not due to omitting irradiation of the whole breast.

16.2.1 Christie Hospital External Beam APBI Trial

The first APBI trial using EBI was conducted at the Christie Hospital in Manchester, UK, between 1982 and 1987 (Magee et al. 1996; Ribeiro et al. 1993). Patients were randomly assigned to receive either 40–42.5 Gy electron beam irradiation in eight fractions to the tumor bed only (limited field, LF, group), or 40 Gy whole breast plus regional photon irradiation (wide field, WF, group). The 8-year actuarial LR rate was significantly higher in the LF group than in the WF group (25% vs. 13%). However, there was no significant difference in disease-specific survival in the two groups (73% vs. 72%). The average field size used in the LF arm was 6×8 cm, and no attempt was made to localize the excision cavity by means of surgical clips or CT-based treatment planning. Of note, the majority of ipsilateral breast recurrences were in the treated quadrant. Patients with tumor size up to 4 cm (75% T2) were enrolled on the study, and axillary dissection was omitted. Specimen margins were not evaluated microscopically, and no adjuvant systemic therapy was administered. The authors concluded that with improved patient selection and refinement of technique, radiotherapy restricted to the tumor bed may be an adequate local treatment.

16.2.2 Uzsoki Hospital Cobalt-Needle Study

One of the first prospective APBI studies using interstitial implants was conducted in Hungary at the Uzsoki Hospital between 1987 and 1992 (Mayer and Nemeskéri 1993;

Polgár et al. 2005; Póti et al. 2004). Due to the limited availability of modern teletherapy equipment and the lack of iridium-192 wires in Hungary, special cobalt-60 sources were designed and manufactured to allow manual afterloading of interstitial BT catheters. (These cobalt-60 needles were used in the late 1980s to replace the conventional radium-226 needles previously used in Hungary, in order to increase radiation safety of the staff and allow more patients to have the option of breast conserving therapy.) During this period, 70 patients were treated with these needles following conservative surgery without the use of whole-breast irradiation (Póti et al. 2004). Any patient with a pathological T1 or T2 tumor that was clinically unifocal was eligible. A median of five (range two to eight) catheters with an active length of 4 cm were implanted into the tumor bed (which was not delineated by surgical clips or by the use of CT) in a single plane without template guidance. A dose of 50 Gy was prescribed at 5 mm from the surface of the sources, given in a single session of 10–22 hours with 2.3–5.0 Gy per hour (medium dose rate, MDR). The volume included within the reference isodose surface was quite small (median 36 cm³).

The first interim analysis of this series was published in 1993 (Mayer and Nemeskéri 1993). With a median follow-up time of 3.8 years, 8 of 44 patients (18%) had developed a LR. Because of poor cosmetic results (a high incidence of changes in skin pigmentation, development of telangiectasias, and fibrosis), the study was closed in 1992 (Mayer and Nemeskéri 1993; Póti et al. 2004). Updated 12-year results of this series showed that the crude LR rate was 24%, with 59% of patients having grade 3 or 4 complications (Póti et al. 2004).

The investigators noted that modern imaging methods (mammography and ultrasound) were not available during this particular study period in their hospital's healthcare area (Mayer and Nemeskéri 1993). Therefore, most patients did not have pre- or postoperative mammographic evaluation. The vast majority of pathology reports did not contain such important information as pathological tumor size or the presence of multifocality. Hence, it is likely that even their very limited predefined patient selection criteria were frequently violated. Other important pathological factors were also not assessed, such as pathological axillary node status (unknown for 80% of patients) and margin status (unknown for all patients). Hence, perhaps many or most of the patients treated in this study would not be considered eligible today for breast-conserving therapy. Therefore, it is likely that the high rate of LR in this study was due to having persistent (not recurrent) tumor due to inadequate patient selection criteria and radiological and pathological evaluation, as well as a very small, inadequate implant volume. The high rate of toxicity may have resulted from giving a high total dose (86 to 134 Gy low dose-rate, LDR, equivalent dose) delivered within a short overall treatment time without fractionation.

American, Japanese, and European experts have declared that the defects in the Uzsoki Hospital's study cannot be used to discredit the concept of APBI, if properly performed (Polgár et al. 2004b, 2005; Vicini et al. 2004a). Despite its obvious limitations, the reported annual LR rate of 2% in this study is quite similar to those observed in other early breast-conservation trials using whole-breast irradiation (Table 16.2). In addition, the pioneering experience of the Uzsoki Hospital subsequently served as a basis for the development of the later more successful APBI series at the National Institute of Oncology, Budapest (Polgár et al. 2002b, 2004a, 2005).

16.2.3 Guy's Hospital Studies

Fentiman et al. (1991, 1996, 2004) also explored the feasibility and limitations of partial breast BT in two consecutive pilot trials performed at Guy's Hospital, London, UK. In the first study, conducted from May 1987 to November 1988, 27 patients were treated with LDR implants using rigid needles (Fentiman et al. 1991, 1996). The target volume included a 2-cm margin around the tumor bed. Doses were prescribed using the Paris dosimetry system with a dose of 55 Gy given over 5–6 days using manually afterloaded ^{192}Ir wires. The authors stated that a systematic QA procedure was not used at that time. With a median follow-up of 6 years, 10 of 27 patients (37%) experienced recurrence in the treated breast (Fentiman et al. 1996). All relapses were within the irradiated volume, except in one patient. None of the patients developed breast fibrosis, and only one patient had telangiectasias. The cosmetic outcome was good or excellent in 83% of patients.

A second Guy's Hospital study enrolled 50 patients between 1990 and 1992 (Fentiman et al. 2004). Patient selection criteria, and surgical and implant techniques were similar to those in the first Guy's Hospital series except for three aspects. First, only patients aged 40 years or older were eligible. Second, to reduce radiation exposure to medical and nursing staff, a MDR remote-controlled afterloading system employing caesium-137 was used to give a total dose of 45 Gy in four fractions over 4 days. Third, 92% of patients received adjuvant systemic therapy. At a median follow-up of 6.3 years, 8 of 49 eligible patients (18%) developed a breast relapse, which was located in the index quadrant in seven (78%). Only one LR (4%) occurred among patients with lesions smaller than 2 cm, while the rate was 35% among patients with tumors of 2 cm or larger. Cosmetic outcome was considered excellent or good in 81% of patients.

With hindsight, it can be easily seen that there were many flaws in the design of these trials, particularly with regard to surgical technique and patient selection. No attempt was made to achieve a wide excision either grossly or microscopically. As a consequence, the surgical margins were involved in 56% of patients in the first study and in 43% of patients in the second. Although only patients with tumors measuring no more than 4 cm in diameter were eligible for the first study, there were three patients with larger tumors. Furthermore, in the first study, 11 patients (41%) had tumors containing an extensive intraductal component (EIC), and 12 patients (44%) had positive axillary lymph nodes; in the second study, 44% of patients had positive nodes.

16.2.4 Florence Series

Between 1989 and 1993, Cionini et al. (1995) in Florence, Italy, treated 115 patients with T1-2N0-1 tumors with quadrantectomy, axillary dissection and LDR BT of the entire quadrant and the nipple, giving a dose of 50–60 Gy using ^{192}Ir implants. Young patients (52% of the population were premenopausal), patients with positive or unknown margins (15%), and patients with infiltrating lobular carcinoma (20%) were included in the study. Patients with positive axillary nodes (38%) received chemotherapy or tamoxifen. At a median follow-up of 50 months, seven breast recurrences (6%) were observed (two in the tumor bed and five elsewhere in the breast). The 5-year actuarial LR, disease-free survival (DFS), and overall survival (OS) rates were 6%, 83%, and 96%, respectively. Cosmetic outcome and side effects were not reported.

16.2.5 Royal Devon and Exeter Hospital Series

In a pilot study performed at the Royal Devon and Exeter Hospital in the UK, fractionated high dose-rate (HDR) interstitial BT was used to treat the quadrant after tumor excision in 45 patients (Clarke et al. 1994). Patients selected for BT alone had tumors smaller than 4 cm, grade 1 or 2 tumors, and clear or close margins. Three different fractionation schedules were used: 20 Gy given in two fractions; 28 Gy given in four fractions; and 32 Gy given in six fractions. The crude LR rate was 15.6% at 18 months. A true recurrence/marginal miss within the treated volume was observed in four patients, and three patients had elsewhere failures. However, this study was also limited by the surgical techniques and pathological reports used, as axillary dissection was not performed routinely, and in many cases detailed histological findings were not available. Cosmetic outcome was excellent in 95% of patients.

16.3 Contemporary European APBI Trials

Based on the controversial results of earlier studies, a number of European groups created APBI trial protocols incorporating strict patient selection criteria and systematic QA procedures. As a result, the outcomes of these studies have been much improved (Table 16.3) (Johansson et al. 2002; Ott et al. 2004, 2005a; Polgár et al. 2002b, 2004a, 2005; Samuel et al. 1999; Strnad et al. 2004).

16.3.1 Ninewells Hospital Study

Samuel et al. (1999) reported their experience of a small pilot study (11 patients) performed in Dundee, Scotland, using perioperative double-plane LDR ^{192}Ir implants. The mean reference dose (prescribed according to the Paris system) was 51 Gy (range 46–55 Gy). Stringent patient selection criteria were used. Eligible patients had a single unilateral tumor with a diameter of 2 cm or less. Women with EIC-positive, multifocal cancers, or invasive lobular carcinomas were excluded. All patients were older than 40 years. Only one patient had positive surgical margins, and all but one patient were pathologically node-negative. At a median follow-up time of 67 months, there were no LR or breast cancer-related deaths. Cosmetic results were felt to be satisfactory as judged by the authors in all patients except in one patient who developed an abscess.

16.3.2 Örebro Series

The first APBI study using pulsed dose-rate (PDR) BT was begun in 1994 at the Örebro Medical Centre in Sweden (Johansson et al. 2002; Polgár et al. 2005). Inclusion criteria included age 40 years or older with a unifocal breast cancer measuring 5 cm or less (with 80% of patients having tumors ≤2 cm) without an EIC which was excised with clear inked margins, and up to three positive axillary lymph nodes (although 86% of patients were node-negative). Free-hand plastic tube implants were used to cover the planning

Table 16.3 Results of contemporary European APBI trials (*NR* not reported)

Institution	Reference	Technique	RT scheme (dose [Gy]× fraction no.)	Median follow-up period (years)	Total LR, % (n)	True recurrence/ marginal miss, % (n)	Elsewhere failure (%)	Annual LR (%)	Cosmesis excellent/ good (%)
Ninewells Hospital	Samuel et al. 1999	Low dose-rate	46–55×1	6	0 (0 of 11)	0 (0 of 11)	0 (0 of 11)	0	91
NIO, Budapest I	Polgár et al. 2004, 2005a	High dose-rate	4.33×7; 5.2×7	8.3	6.7 (3 of 45)	0 (0 of 45)	6.7 (3 of 45)	0.81	84
NIO, Budapest II	Polgár et al. 2002, 2005a	High dose-rate	5.2×7	4.2	4.6 (4 of 86)	2.3 (2 of 86)	2.3 (2 of 86)	1.09	86
NIO, Budapest II	Polgár et al. 2002, 2005a	Electrons	2×25	4.2	5.0 (2 of 40)	2.5 (1 of 40)	2.5 (1 of 40)	1.19	71
Örebro Medical Centre	Johansson et al. 2002; Polgár et al. 2005	Pulsed dose-rate	50/0.83b	4.6	4 (2 of 49)	2 (1 of 49)	2 (1 of 49)	0.87	NR
Germany–Austria	Ott et al. 2004, Strnad et al. 2004c	Pulsed dose-rate/high dose-rate	50/0.6b; 4×8	1.3	0.7 (2 of 274)	0.35 (1 of 274)	0.35 (1 of 274)	0.54	96
MammoSite Trials	Niehoff et al. 2005d	High dose-rate	3.4×10	1	0 (0 of 50)	0 (0 of 50) 0	(0 of 50)	0	NR
All patients				1–8.3	2.3 (13 of 555)	0.9 (5 of 555)	1.4 (8 of 555)	0–1.19	71–96

a Updated results by Polgár C
b Total dose/pulse dose
c Updated results by Strnad V
d Updated results by Kovács G

target volume (PTV) defined as the excision cavity plus 3-cm margins. In this study, 49 patients were treated with a total dose of 50 Gy using pulses of 0.83 Gy delivered over 5 days. At a median follow-up time of 55 months, only two patients (4%) had developed LR. Cosmetic results have not yet been analyzed.

16.3.3 National Institute of Oncology (Hungary) Studies

Between 1996 and 1998, 45 selected patients with early-stage invasive breast cancer were treated with APBI using interstitial HDR implants at the National Institute of Oncology (NIO), Budapest, Hungary (Polgár et al. 2002b, 2004a, 2005). Patients were eligible for sole BT if they met all of the following conditions: unifocal tumor; tumor size ≤20 mm (pT1); microscopically clear surgical margins; pathologically negative axillary nodes or only axillary micrometastases (pN1mi); histological grade 1 or 2; and technical suitability for breast implantation. Exclusion criteria were: pure ductal or lobular carcinoma in situ (pTis); invasive lobular carcinoma; or the presence of EIC. During surgery, the boundaries of the excision cavity were marked with titanium clips. Implantation was performed 4–6 weeks after surgery under local anesthesia. A preimplant radiographic simulation was performed using a template placed on the breast in order to determine the entrance and exit points of the implant strand from a "needle's-eye" view. The PTV was defined as the excision cavity (delineated by the surgical clips) plus a margin of 1–2 cm. Single-, double-, and triple-plane implants were performed on 3, 34, and 8 patients (7%, 75%, and 18%), respectively. After all the rigid guide needles were implanted, they were replaced with flexible plastic tubes. Dose planning was based on a three-dimensional reconstruction of the locations of catheters, surgical clips, and skin points. Two postimplant isocentric radiographs were taken on a simulator with variable angles and the radiographic films were used for digitizing the positions of catheters (Fig. 16.1). A total dose of 30.3 Gy ($n=8$) or 36.4 Gy ($n=37$) in seven fractions over 4 days was delivered to the PTV. The mean volume encompassed by the 100% isodose surface was 50 cm³. Only 7 patients (16%) received adjuvant tamoxifen therapy.

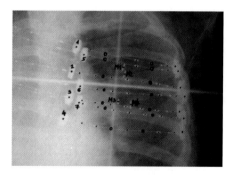

Fig. 16.1 Radiographic verification of a typical two-plane implant for the phase II Hungarian APBI study (*M1–M4* surgical clips, *small circles* first and last active source positions)

A 7-year update of this study was reported, including comparison with results of a control group treated during the same time period with conventional breast-conserving therapy (Polgár et al. 2004a). The control group comprised 80 consecutive patients who met the eligibility criteria for APBI, but who were treated with 50 Gy whole-breast radiotherapy with (n=36) or without (n=44) a 10 to 16 Gy tumor bed boost. The crude rates of total ipsilateral breast failure were 6.7% (3 of 45) and 10% (8 of 80) in patients treated with multicatheter BT and whole-breast RT, respectively. LR occurred as a first event in three (6.7%), and five patients (6.3%), respectively. The 7-year actuarial rate of ipsilateral breast recurrence was not significantly different between patients treated with APBI (9%) and whole-breast irradiation (12%). There were no significant differences in either the 7-year probability of DFS (80% and 75%, respectively), or cancer-specific survival (both 93%). The 7-year actuarial rate of failure elsewhere in the breast was similar for both groups (9% and 8.3%, respectively). All three patients with isolated breast recurrences in the APBI group underwent a second breast-conserving surgery followed by 46–50 Gy of whole-breast radiotherapy. So far, there have been no further LR in these three patients, yielding a 100% mastectomy-free survival rate for patients treated with APBI. In contrast, three (3.8%) patients in the control group underwent salvage mastectomy. The rate of excellent or good cosmetic results was 84.4% in the APBI group and 68.3% in the control group (P=0.04). The incidence of grade 2 or worse late radiation side effects was similar in both groups (26.7% and 28.6%, respectively). Only one patient (2.2%) in the APBI group developed symptomatic fat necrosis and underwent re-excision. Similar incidences of asymptomatic fat necrosis were identified in both the APBI group (20.0%) and control group (20.6%).

According to the last update of this study (unpublished results by Polgár C, August 2005), no further LR had occurred in the APBI group at a median follow-up of 8.3 years, yielding an annual LR rate of 0.81 (see Table 16.3).

Based on the encouraging results of the first NIO study, a randomized study was conducted between 1998 and 2004 at the same institution in Budapest (Polgár et al. 2002b, 2005). Initial eligibility criteria were similar to those for the previous study, although following the publication of the European Organization for Research and Treatment of Cancer (EORTC) boost trial in 2001, patients aged 40 years or younger were excluded. In addition, the trial allowed patients with a breast technically unsuitable for performing interstitial implantation to enroll and be treated with an external-beam approach. By May 2004, 255 eligible patients had been randomized to receive either 50 Gy whole-breast radiotherapy (n=129) or partial-breast irradiation (n=126). The latter consisted of either 36.4 Gy (given over 4 days using seven fractions of 5.2 Gy each) with HDR multicatheter BT (n=86) or limited-field electron irradiation (n=40) giving a dose of 50 Gy in 25 fractions (prescribed to the 80% isodose line) over 5 weeks. One-, two-, three-, or four-plane implants were performed in 1 (1%), 47 (55%), 37 (43%), and 1 patients (1%), respectively. The mean volume encompassed by the reference isodose surface was 62 cm^3. The majority of patients in both arms (70%) received adjuvant hormone therapy.

The most recent interim analysis (unpublished results by Polgár C, August 2005), at a median follow-up time of 4.2 years, has revealed no significant difference in local and regional tumor control, disease-free, cancer-specific or distant metastasis-free survival between the two treatment arms (Tables 16.3 and 16.4). Analysis of cosmetic results is pending. However, to date there have been significantly fewer grade 2/3 skin side effects in patients treated with sole HDR BT compared to those treated with whole-breast irradiation (3.7% vs. 14.3%, respectively; P=0.01), and similar rates of fat necrosis (35.3% vs. 29.6%, respectively; P=0.85) and grade 2/3 fibrosis (both 16%) have been observed.

Table 16.4 Four-year actuarial results of the Budapest phase III trial (unpublished results)

Treatment arm	Recurrence		Survival		
	Local, % (n)	Regional, % (n)	Cancer-specific (%)	Disease-free (%)	Distant metastasis-free (%)
Partial breast irradiation	5.0 (6 of 126)	1.1 (1 of 126)	97.7	90.7	96.7
Whole breast irradiation	6.2 (4 of 129)	1.9 (3 of 129)	98.2	91.5	97.6
P-value	0.61	0.25	0.67	0.55	0.71

16.3.4 German–Austrian Multicentric Trial

In the year 2000 four institutions decided to start the first European multi-institutional phase II trial to investigate the effectiveness and safety of APBI (Ott et al. 2004, 2005a, 2005b; Polgár et al. 2005; Strnad et al. 2004). Radiation oncology departments of the University Hospitals of Erlangen and Leipzig from Germany and University Hospital of Vienna and the Barmherzige Schwestern Hospital of Linz from Austria recruited 274 patients between November 2000 and April 2005.

Patients were eligible for APBI if they had histologically confirmed breast cancer, a tumor diameter ≤3 cm, complete resection with clear margins of 2 mm at least, pathologically negative axillary lymph nodes (pN0), or singular nodal micrometastasis (pN1mi) with at least nine lymph nodes removed and histologically examined, no evidence for distant metastasis or contralateral breast cancer, ECOG performance status ≤2, estrogen and/or progesterone receptor-positive tumors, and patient age ≥35 years. Patients were excluded from the protocol if they initially showed a multicentric invasive growth pattern, poorly differentiated or undifferentiated tumors, had postoperative residual microcalcifications, an EIC, lymph vessel invasion, or unknown, involved or close margins.

After breast-conserving surgery, an interval of 4–6 weeks was designated for wound healing and for proper histological analysis of the tumor specimen to guarantee the selection of the appropriate patients. Partial breast irradiation was solely performed as multicatheter BT according to the Paris system rules (Figs. 16.2 and 16.3). The median duration of the interval between surgery and BT was 59 days (range 4–159 days). The tumor bed was localized by the use of surgical clips, preoperative mammography and ultrasound examination and/or postoperative planning CT scans. In contrast to the USA and some other European countries, where the surgical cavity remains open, breast-conserving surgery is performed with a closed cavity in Germany and Austria. In case of closed-cavity surgery, CT-based planning often does not lead to a clear delineation of the target volume; therefore, it was not stipulated in the protocol. The PTV was confined to the tumor bed plus a safety margin of 2–3 cm in each direction, if possible. Two- or three-plane implants were used in 57.7% and 42.3%, respectively. The median number of afterloading tubes was 13 (range 6–18). Treatment planning was done with either CT scans or conventional radiographs taken with a simulator. Dose specification was performed according to the Paris system. The reference isodose was defined to 85% of the mean central dose (MCD). Implant volumes for all 274 patients were 75.0±34.3 cm³ (range 22.4–205.1 cm³) enclosed by the reference isodose (Vref), for the volume V150 (1.5 × reference isodose) 14.7±6.9 cm³ (range 5.3–54.0 cm³), and for the volume of $V_{1.5}$×MCD 8.6±3.6 cm³ (range 3.2–23.5 cm³). The median dose homogeneity index (DHI) was 0.81 (range 0.49–0.91). The prescribed reference dose in HDR BT was 32 Gy in eight fractions of 4 Gy twice daily with an intraday interval of at least 6 hours. The prescribed reference dose in PDR BT was 49.8 Gy in 83 fractions of 0.6 Gy every hour. Total treatment time was 4 days. PDR and HDR BT were performed in 63.6% and 36.4% of the patients, respectively.

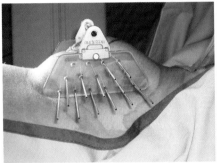
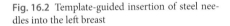
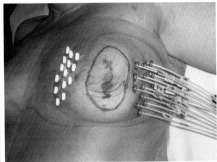

Fig. 16.2 Template-guided insertion of steel needles into the left breast

Fig. 16.3 Interstitial multicatheter breast implant in the same patient as in Fig. 16.2. The steel needles have been replaced by 14 flexible afterloading tubes

Preliminary results of the trial have already been published (Ott et al. 2004, 2005a, 2005b; Strnad et al. 2004). According to the last update of this study (unpublished results by Strnad V and Ott OJ, August 2005), two patients had developed ipsilateral breast recurrence. One of these had a true in-field recurrence 13 months after the primary therapy, and the other had a multicentric relapse in the treated breast 53 months after initial breast-conserving surgery. This gives a 2% LR rate relating to the first 100 patients with a median follow-up of 37 months, and a 0.7% LR rate for the whole group after a median follow-up of 16 months.

Data on perioperative complications and side effects were available in all of the 274 patients. Bacterial infection developed in six patients (2.2%). The incidence of hematoma was also 2.2%. Acute toxicity was low: 3.6% of the patients experienced mild and 1.1% moderate radiodermatitis. To date late toxicity was mild: 6.6% of the women experienced hypersensation/mild pain related to the tumor bed, and 2.6% intermittent but tolerable pain. Mild dyspigmentation of the skin above the BT implant was found in 8.8%, and moderate dyspigmentation in 1.8% of the patients. Grade 1 fibrosis was palpated in 6.6%, grade 2 fibrosis in 7.7%, and grade 3 fibrosis in 0.4% of the patients in the region of the surgical scar. Grade 1 telangiectasia of the involved skin was found in 3.3%, grade 2 telangiectasia in 1.5%, and grade 3 telangiectasia 0.4% of the women, respectively.

Ott et al. (2005b) recently investigated the incidence of fat necrosis in a subgroup of patients (n=33) treated in the German–Austrian study. At a median follow-up of

35 months the incidence of fat necrosis was 15.2%, and no patient underwent surgical intervention because of fat necrosis-related pain.

Data on cosmetic outcome were available for 94.5% of the patients. At a median follow-up of 16 months, physicians judged the cosmetic results as excellent or good in 96.1%, and as fair in 3.9% of the women. Patients subjectively judged the cosmetic outcome as excellent or good in 95.0%, fair in 4.6%, and poor in 0.4%. Immediately before the beginning of BT, physicians and patients declared cosmetic outcome as good to excellent in 93.4% and 91.5%, respectively. This indicates that the use of multicatheter BT did not impact cosmetic outcome after a median follow-up of 16 months.

Recruitment for the German–Austrian phase II trial was stopped in April 2005. The four participating institutions are concentrating their energy on the randomized GEC-ESTRO phase III APBI trial (Polgár et al. 2005).

16.4 European MammoSite Brachytherapy Trials

APBI with interstitial BT using multicatheter systems requires high experience in all members of the staff. For that reason a new and simple BT system was developed in the US (Edmundson et al. 2002). The MammoSite radiation treatment system (RTS) is a dual lumen spherical balloon catheter. One lumen allows inflation of the balloon to diameter of 4–5 cm; the other provides a pathway for the ^{192}Ir source. The advantage of this system is that only one applicator is implanted to perform fractionated radiotherapy of the tumor bed as compared to interstitial BT, which requires up to 20 needles. Since 2002 this system has been available for commercial use. In the US, the system is used by many institutions in the their daily practice. In Europe several feasibility studies have been initiated to investigate the practicability and safety of the system (Niehoff et al. 2005). Most of these trials were designed to test the device as the sole method for APBI and for delivery of a boost dose in combination with whole-breast EBI.

Up to June 2005 the MammoSite applicator had been implanted in 87 patients in different institutions in Europe (Table 16.5). Eligibility criteria for the sole modality (boost modality in parenthesis) were: age ≥60 years (boost: age ≥40 years); tumor ≤2 cm (boost: ≤2.5 cm); invasive ductal histology; grade 1/2 (boost: grade 2–3); margins ≥5 mm (boost: negative margins); applicator placement within 10 weeks of final lumpectomy procedure; and excision cavity with one dimension of at least 3.0 cm. In contrast to the American studies (Harper et al. 2005; Shah et al. 2004; Vicini et al. 2004b) a skin–balloon distance of at least 7 mm was demanded. Exclusion criteria were: presence of EIC, pure intraductal cancer (pTis), lobular histology, multifocal or multicentric lesions, or collagen vascular disease. The implantation, treatment planning and treatment performance was similar to the American trials described in Chapter 10. The applicators were preferably implanted during the final lumpectomy. In one institution a drain was inserted into the cavity to prevent air bubbles and hematoma, and to maintain optimal tissue conformance to the balloon surface. For sole MammoSite therapy a total dose of 34 Gy in ten fractions (prescribed at 1 cm from the balloon surface) was delivered over 5–7 days. In the boost group a total dose of 10–20 Gy was delivered with a fraction dose of 2.5 Gy over 2–4 days. In both groups, two daily fractions were delivered with a minimum of 6 hours between fractions. Patients were treated with various commercially available HDR remote afterloading machines.

Table 16.5 Implanted patients in European MammoSite studies listed by country

Country	Primary	Boost	Not treated	Total
France	22	–	11	33
Germany	10	2	7	19
Italy	13	–	2	15
Hungary	1	11	1	13
Switzerland	2	3	–	5
Austria	2	–	–	2
All countries	50	16	21	87

Overall 87 patients were enrolled in the European studies. Out of 87 implanted patients 21 (24.1%), had to be excluded from the clinical trial. The most common reason for exclusion was the final pathology. At the final decision, 50 patients were eligible for BT alone and 16 patients were treated with a boost BT followed by whole-breast EBI. No LRs have been reported after a mean follow-up of 12 months (range 1–31 months). One patient died of intercurrent disease 2 years after treatment, and another disease-free patient suffers from stomach carcinoma. In all patients the anatomic position of the device to the skin and to the chest wall was verified before and during the treatment. With the daily fluoroscopic simulations a balloon rupture was detected in two patients, one prior to and one in the course of treatment. One patient was excluded; the other patient finished the treatment after reimplantation of a new balloon. The devices were returned to the manufacturer for analysis and in each case the balloon damage was consistent with contact with a suturing needle or suture material. Because of this, we recommend cavity closure with a deflated balloon.

CT-based treatment planning is required to define the balloon–skin distance and to detect air pockets and hematoma. An insufficient skin distance of less than 7 mm leads to an overdosage at the small skin vessels. A subgroup analysis of the 32 German and Hungarian patients showed that the mean balloon-to-skin distance was 12 mm (range 3–36 mm), and it has a strong correlation with the breast cup-size. Calculated skin dose was between 65% and 132% of the reference dose. The DHI of 0.71 (range 0.61–0.83) was the same as the DHI (0.71) using multicatheter BT (Polgár et al. 2000).

Air pockets and hematoma of more than 3 mm lead to an underdosage of relevant breast tissue. The air gap volumes of 31 patients were analyzed in the German–Hungarian study. The measured mean air gap volume with or without a drain was 0.01% (range 0–2%) and 0.97% (range 0–4.8%) of the PTV, respectively ($P=0.01$).

The side effects in patients ($n=24$) treated in Germany and Hungary are listed in Table 16.6. The most common toxicity was mild or moderate erythema in the high skin dose area with or without desquamation. Other less-common events were: hyperpigmentation, mastitis, seroma, abscess, edema and fistula. Five serious adverse events were recorded, three of which were device related (two abscesses and one fistula). Patients who developed an abscess show only minor cosmetic deterioration at a follow-up of 1 year. No abscess was observed in patients receiving antibiotic prophylaxis.

For the Hungarian and German patients the D90 (minimum dose to 90% of the target volume) was 98% (range 84–112%), which is higher than that reported in the literature

Side effect	n (%)
Erythema	21 (88%)
Hyperpigmentation	13 (54%)
Seroma	10 (42%)
Abscess	2 (8%)
Mastitis	1 (4%)
Desquamation	2 (8%)
Fistula	1 (4%)
Fibrosis	3 (13%)
Edema	3 (13%)
Fat necrosis	1 (4%)
Telangiectasia	2 (8%)
Serosanguine-ous leakage	1 (4%)

Table 16.6 Side effects in 24 patients irradiated (subgroup analysis of the German–Hungarian MammoSite study)

(Edmundson et al. 2002). High dose volumes never exceeded the literature reported volumes for fat necrosis (Shah et al. 2004; Wazer et al. 2001).

Antibiotic prophylaxis and stringent wound care recommendations seem to be indispensable. The abscess rate (8%) in the German–Hungarian study was lower than that reported by others (Harper et al. 2005; Shah et al. 2004; Vicini et al. 2004b). No abscess was seen after introduction of antibiotic prophylaxis. Harper et al. (2005) reported a 16% abscess rate. An infection rate of 9.2% including breast infection, mastitis, cellulites and abscess was observed in the American Society of Breast Surgeons Registry study (Shah et al. 2004; Vicini et al. 2004b).

The balloon surface to skin distance is a critical point in terms of avoiding toxicity. In Europe a minimum skin distance of 7 mm was allowed. Van Limbergen et al. (1989) reported that the risk of telangiectasia is increased if doses for the subcutaneous skin vessels exceed 46 Gy. Van Limbergen et al. (1987, 1990) also emphasized that any overlapping of the high dose areas of the interstitial implants with the upper 5 mm of the subcutaneous tissue should be avoided. Turreson (1990) reported that there is an interval of 5 years before telangiectasia appears. We observed telangiectasia in 8% of our patients 1 year after irradiation with the MammoSite RTS. It has to be underlined that we need a longer follow-up to know the final risk of telangiectasia after using balloon BT.

Based on the early European experience, the MammoSite device is simple and safe to handle. The acceptance of the system by the patients is very high and we believe that the device will offer an alternative method for postoperative partial breast brachytherapy for a highly selected group of patients. Additional studies and long-term follow-up of existing studies are recommended in order to further define and potentially expand the patient selection criteria as well as to assess long-term local tumor control and late toxicities. Reimbursement in Europe is as yet unclear. In most European countries the immense costs of the applicator are not taken over from the health insurance companies, but an all-inclusive amount is paid for the treatment. Until the issue of reimbursement is clarified the MammoSite RTS will remain financially unattractive in Europe.

16.5 European (GEC-ESTRO) Multicentric Randomized APBI Trial

Based on the success of the Hungarian and German–Austrian studies of APBI, a phase III multicentric APBI protocol has been developed by the Breast Cancer Working Group of the GEC-ESTRO (Polgár et al. 2005). As long-term results beyond 5 years are available only with interstitial implants, proving that multicatheter BT can be used with adequate reproducibility, low toxicity, and appropriate local control, it has been decided that only interstitial HDR/PDR BT will be allowed for the APBI arm of this European multicentric phase III trial.

The first patient was randomized in May 2004 at the European Data Center in Erlangen, Germany. To date seven centers from four European countries—Austria (Vienna), Germany (Erlangen, Leipzig and Rostock), Hungary (Budapest), and Spain (Barcelona and Valencia)—have activated the protocol.

Patients in the control group are treated with 50 Gy whole-breast EBI plus 10 Gy electron boost (Fig. 16.4). Patients in the APBI arm are treated with HDR or PDR multicatheter BT. The primary end-point of the study is LR as a first event within 5 years. The scientific hypothesis to be assessed and statistically tested is "non-relevant non-inferiority" of the experimental treatment. Compared to the estimated 4% 5-year LR rate in the control arm, an absolute increase of up to 3% (e.g. 7%) in the APBI arm is regarded as non-relevant non-inferior. For adequate statistical power, 1170 patients will be enrolled, based on the desire to detect a difference of 3% in LR rates between the arms. Secondary end-points will address overall, disease-free and distant metastasis-free survival, contralateral breast cancer, early and late side effects, cosmesis, and quality of life. Eligibility criteria include unifocal ductal carcinoma in situ (DCIS) or invasive carcinoma of the breast, tumor size ≤3 cm, microscopic negative margins of at least 2 mm (5 mm for DCIS or invasive lobular carcinoma), no EIC, no lymphovascular invasion, no more than one micrometastasis in axillary lymph nodes (pN1mi), and patient age ≥40 years. Patients are stratified before randomization according to the treatment center, having DCIS or invasive carcinoma, and menopausal status. The QA program for partial breast BT includes preimplant PTV definition by surgical clips and/or preimplant CT image-based preplanning of the implant geometry (Fig. 16.5). The PTV is defined as the excision cavity plus 2 cm margin minus the minimum clear pathological margin (Fig. 16.6). Postimplant CT scans are mandatory for the documentation of target coverage and dose homogeneity (Fig. 16.7). Acceptable treatment parameters for CT image-based treatment planning include:

- DVH analysis of target coverage confirming that the prescribed dose covers ≥90% of the PTV (coverage index ≥0.9)
- DNR ≤0.35
- Maximum skin dose <70% of the prescribed dose

Fig. 16.4 Scheme of the GEC-ESTRO multicentric randomized APBI trial (*BCS* breast-conserving surgery, *EBI* external beam irradiation, *ELE* electron, *HDR-BT* high-dose-rate brachytherapy, *PDR-BT* pulse-dose-rate brachytherapy)

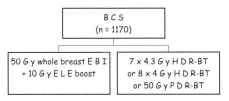

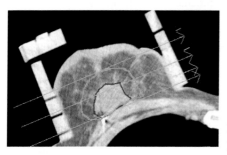

Fig. 16.5 CT-based preplanning of the implant geometry for multicatheter brachytherapy (*red line* excision cavity, *green line* PTV, *yellow arrows* pre-planned implant planes)

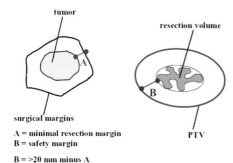

Fig. 16.6 PTV definition for the GEC-ESTRO multicentric randomized APBI trial

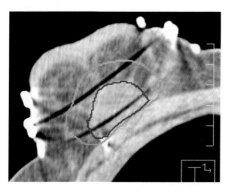

Fig. 16.7 PTV definition on postimplant CT scan for multicatheter brachytherapy (*red line* excision cavity, *green line* PTV)

The GEC-ESTRO APBI trial is financially supported by a grant from German Cancer Aid (Deutsche Krebshilfe) for a study period of 4 years from 2005 to 2009.

16.6 Summary and Future Directions

APBI is an attractive treatment approach with considerable advantages over standard whole-breast radiotherapy. Earlier European APBI studies with less than satisfactory results failed to identify the ideal subset of patients and/or applied suboptimal treatment techniques. Indeed, by modern pathological and surgical standards, the majority of patients treated in these earlier APBI studies were not acceptable candidates even for conventional breast-conserving therapy. Consequently, results of these so-called "negative" APBI trials only prove that radiotherapy confined to the surgical bed with localization uncertainties is not appropriate treatment for unselected patients and reinforce the necessity for meticulous QA. Contemporary European APBI trials have been based on this hard-won lesson. These series using multicatheter or MammoSite BT with strict patient selection criteria, and systematic QA procedures have shown an annual LR rate ranging between 0 and 1.19%. The 5- to 8-year results from single-institution phase I/II APBI studies certainly support the continuation of the current European multicentric phase III trial. Issues of patient selection, PTV definition, total dose, and fractionation will be addressed and refined in such randomized trials. As data from this and other trials mature, they will hopefully support the implementation of APBI into routine clinical practice.

References

1. Cionini L, Marzano S, Pacini P, et al (1995) Iridium implant of the surgical bed as the sole radiotherapeutic treatment after conservative surgery for breast cancer (Abstract). Radiother Oncol 35 [Suppl l]:S1

2. Clarke DH, Vicini F, Jacobs H, et al (1994) High dose rate brachytherapy for breast cancer. In: Nag S (ed) High dose rate brachytherapy: a textbook. Futura Publishing Company, New York, pp 321–329

3. Clark RM, Whelan T, Levine R (1996) Randomized clinical trial of breast irradiation following lumpectomy and axillary dissection for node-negative breast cancer: an update. J Natl Cancer Inst 88:1659–1654

4. Edmundson GK, Vicini F, Chen P, et al (2002) Dosimetric characteristics of the MammoSite® RTS, a new breast brachytherapy applicator. Int J Radiat Oncol Biol Phys 4:1132–1139

5. Fentiman IS, Poole C, Tong PJ, et al (1991) Iridium implant treatment without external radiotherapy for operable breast cancer: a pilot study. Eur J Cancer 27:447–450

6. Fentiman IS, Poole C, Tong D, et al (1996) Inadequacy of iridium implant as a sole radiation treatment for operable breast cancer. Eur J Cancer 32A:608–611

7. Fentiman IS, Deshmane V, Tong D, et al (2004) Caesium[137] implant as sole radiation therapy for operable breast cancer: a phase II trial. Radiother Oncol 71:281–285

8. Harper J, Jenerette JM, Vanek KN, et al (2005) Acute complications of MammoSite® brachytherapy: a single institution's initial clinical experience. Int J Radiat Oncol Biol Phys 61:169–174

9. Jacobson JA, Danforth DN, Cowan KH (1995) Ten-year results of a comparison of conservation with mastectomy in the treatment of stage I and II breast cancer. N Engl J Med 332:907–911

10. Johansson B, Karlsson L, Liljegren G, et al (2002) PDR brachytherapy as the sole adjuvant radiotherapy after breast conserving surgery of T1-2 breast cancer (abstract). Program and Abstracts, 10th Nucletron International Brachytherapy Conference, Madrid, p 127

11. Lövey K, Nemeskéri C, Mayer A (1994) Analysis of local recurrences developed after conservative surgery of breast cancer (in Hungarian). Magyar Onkológia 38:179–183

12. Magee B, Swindell R, Harris M, et al (1996) Prognostic factors for breast recurrence after conservative breast surgery and radiotherapy: results of a randomised trial. Radiother Oncol 39:223–227

13. Mayer A, Nemeskéri C (1993) Forms of radiotherapy complementing operations of reduced radicality for early cancer of the breast (prospective clinical study) (in Hungarian). Magyar Sebészet 46:65–68

14. Niehoff P, Kovacs G, Polgar C, et al (2003) Feasibility of a new applicator system for interstitial brachtherapy of breast cancer. Radiother Oncol 67 (Suppl. 1):S13

15. Ott OJ, Pötter R, Hammer J, et al (2004) Accelerated partial breast irradiation with iridium-192 multicatheter PDR/HDR brachytherapy. Preliminary results of the German-Austrian multicenter trial. Strahlenther Onkol 180:642–649

16. Ott OJ, Pötter R, Hildebrandt G, et al (2005a) Partial breast irradiation for early breast cancer: 3-year results of the German-Austrian phase II trial. Rofo 177:962–967

17. Ott OJ, Schulz-Wendtland R, Uter W, et al (2005b) Fat necrosis after breast conserving surgery and interstitial brachytherapy and/or external beam irradiation in women with breast cancer. Strahlenther Onkol 181:638–644

18. Pass H, Vicini FA, Kestin LL, et al (2004) Changes in management techniques and patterns of disease recurrence over time in patients with breast carcinoma treated with breast-conserving therapy at a single institution. Cancer 101:713–720

19. Polgár C, Major T, Somogyi A, et al (2000) CT-image-based conformal brachytherapy of breast cancer. The significance of semi-3-D and 3-D treatment planning. Strahlenther Onkol 176:118–124

20. Polgár C, Fodor J, Major T, et al (2002a) Radiotherapy confined to the tumor bed following breast conserving surgery: current status, controversies, and future prospects. Strahlenther Onkol 178:597–606

21. Polgár C, Sulyok Z, Fodor J, et al (2002b) Sole brachytherapy of the tumor bed after conservative surgery for T1 breast cancer: five-year results of a phase I-II study and initial findings of a randomized phase III trial. J Surg Oncol 80:121–128

22. Polgár C, Major T, Fodor J, et al (2004a) HDR brachytherapy alone versus whole breast radiotherapy with or without tumor bed boost after breast conserving surgery: seven-year results of a comparative study. Int J Radiat Oncol Biol Phys 60:1173–1181

23. Polgár C, Major T, Strnad V, et al (2004b) What can we conclude from the results of an out-of-date breast-brachytherapy study? Int J Radiat Oncol Biol Phys 60:342–343

24. Polgár C, Strnad V, Major T (2005) Brachytherapy for partial breast irradiation: the European experience. Semin Radiat Oncol 15:116–122

25. Póti Z, Nemeskéri C, Fekésházy A, et al (2004) Partial breast irradiation with interstitial ^{60}Co brachytherapy results in frequent grade 3 or 4 toxicity: evidence based on a 12-year follow-up of 70 patients. Int J Radiat Oncol Biol Phys 58:1022–1033

26. Ribeiro GG, Magee B, Swindell R, et al (1993) The Christie Hospital breast conservation trial: an update at 8 years from inception. Clin Oncol 5:278–283

27. Samuel LM, Dewar JA, Preece PE, et al (1999) A pilot study of radical radiotherapy using a perioperative implant following wide local excision for carcinoma of the breast. Breast 8:95–97

28. Shah NM, Tenenhoz T, Arthur D, et al (2004) MammoSite® and interstitial brachytherapy for accelerated partial breast irradiation: factors that affect toxicity and cosmesis. Cancer 101:727–734

29. Strnad V, Ott OJ, Pötter R, et al (2004) Interstitial brachytherapy alone after breast conserving surgery: interim results of a German-Austrian multicenter phase II trial. Brachytherapy 3:115–119

30. Turreson I (1990) Individual variation and dose dependency in the progression rate of skin telangiectasia. Int J Radiat Oncol Biol Phys 19:1569–1574

31. Van Dongen JA, Bartelink H, Fentiman IS (1992) Randomized clinical trial to assess the value of breast-conserving therapy in stage I and II breast cancer, EORTC 10801 Trial. J Natl Cancer Inst Monogr 11:15–18

32. Van Limbergen E, van den Bogaert W, van der Schueren E, et al (1987) Tumor excision and radiotherapy as primary treatment of breast cancer. Analysis of patient and treatment parameters and local control. Radiother Oncol 8:1–9

33. Van Limbergen E, Rijnders A, van der Schueren E, et al (1989) Cosmetic evaluation of breast conserving treatment for mammary cancer. II. A quantitative analysis of the influence of radiation dose, fractionation schedules and surgical treatment techniques on cosmetic results after tumor excision and radiotherapy. Radiother Oncol 16:253–267

34. Van Limbergen E, Briot E, Drijkoningen M (1990) The source-skin distance measuring bridge: a method to avoid radiation telangiectasia in the skin after interstitial therapy for breast cancer. Int J Radiat Oncol Biol Phys 18:1239–1244

35. Vicini F, Edmundson G, Arthur D (2004a) In regard to Poti et al.: partial breast irradiation with interstitial (60)co brachytherapy results in frequent grade 3 or 4 toxicity: evidence based on a 12-year follow-up of 70 patients (Int J Radiat Oncol Biol Phys 2004;58:1022-1033). Int J Radiat Oncol Biol Phys 60:345

36. Vicini FA, Beitsch P, Quiet C, et al (2004b) First analysis of patient demographics and technical reproducibility by the American Society of Breast Surgeons (ASBS) MammoSite® breast brachytherapy registry trial in 801 patients treated with accelerated partial breast irradiation (APBI). Proceedings of the San Antonio Breast Cancer Symposium. 2004, San Antonio, TX, USA

37. Wazer DE, Lowther D, Boyle T, et al (2001) Clinically evident fat necrosis in women treated with high-dose-rate brachytherapy alone for early-stage breast cancer. Int J Radiat Oncol Biol Phys 50:107–111

Normal Tissue Toxicity after Accelerated Partial Breast Irradiation

17

David E. Wazer

Contents

17.1 Introduction

A number of studies in recent years have detailed the rationale for and the various technical considerations involved in partial breast irradiation, which is defined as radiation of the site of excision and adjacent breast tissue only. Partial breast irradiation can be delivered with brachytherapy or external modalities. Accelerated partial breast irradiation (APBI) is defined as radiotherapy that employs fractions higher than 1.8–2.0 Gy per day over a period of less than 5–6 weeks and uses any of the following four techniques: (1) interstitial brachytherapy; (2) the MammoSite device (a registered trademark of Proxima Therapeutics, Alpharetta, GA); (3) highly conformal external beam; and (4) intraoperative radiation therapy with photons or electrons. Several clinical reports (reviewed by Kuerer et al. 2004) of predominantly nonrandomized treatment groups with a follow-up of 7–8 years have produced substantial interest in APBI amongst surgeons, radiation oncologists, and patients. With the approval by the United States Food and Drug

Administration in 2002 of the MammoSite catheter, APBI is now commonly practiced in both academic and non-academic settings. In 2005, the NSABP and RTOG began accruing patients to a phase III randomized trial to compare APBI with conventional whole-breast radiotherapy.

To date, the primary focus of many APBI studies has been on local control with limited information available on normal tissue toxicity. Further, the studies that have provided detailed data pertaining to normal tissue toxicity have been limited mostly to brachytherapy techniques: multiple catheter interstitial and MammoSite. Very little information has been presented thus far regarding the toxicity associated with APBI delivered by conformal external beam or intraoperative techniques.

A comprehensive systemic evaluation of early, intermediate, and late toxicity associated with APBI has not previously been performed particularly as related to the wide variety of clinical and treatment-related technical variables that are inherent in the different treatment modalities. In this chapter, a summary of the current information regarding toxicity after APBI is presented. Where possible, an attempt is made to distil the currently available data into specific clinical recommendations designed to minimize the risk of normal tissue toxicity.

17.2 Terminology, Techniques, and Radiation Biology

Any comparison of toxicity between the various methods of APBI is complicated by the distinctive dosimetry and radiation biology inherent in interstitial, intracavitary, or external beam techniques. Table 17.1 summarizes the four most commonly practiced APBI modalities in general terms of prescription points, fractionation schemes, total delivered dose, and a rough comparison of biological effective doses (BED) as calculated at the prescription point (which ignores critical dose gradients). The interpretation of toxicity data can be further complicated when one considers, for example, such operator-specific variables as the method of catheter placement for interstitial brachytherapy. Controlling for needle placement technique can be difficult as complex interstitial breast brachytherapy systems have tended to develop as institution-specific protocols that may entail the use of customized rigid templates (Das et al. 2004; Vicini et al. 1999), specialized devices to guide free-hand placement (Wazer et al. 1997), or CT-guided placement (Arthur et al. 2003). There are no clear data to suggest that there are differences in normal tissue toxicity related to specific interstitial brachytherapy techniques.

It is again important to emphasize that virtually all of the limited toxicity data currently available for APBI were derived from the use of brachytherapy with either interstitial or MammoSite techniques. Early data are becoming available for conformal external beam APBI but little exist for single fraction intraoperative applications of electrons or low-energy photons. As such, this chapter focuses primarily on studies of APBI by brachytherapy.

Prior to reviewing the results of clinical studies, it would be useful to briefly explain some terminology that has been employed to describe the dosimetric characteristics of both interstitial and MammoSite implants. The V100, V150, and V200 represent the volume of breast tissue encompassed by the 100%, 150%, and 200% isodose lines, respectively. The dose homogeneity index (DHI) has been defined as a method for evaluating the dosimetric quality of an implant (Wu et al. 1988). The higher the, the more uniform is the dose distribution within the treatment volume. Numerous methods have been

Table 17.1 A comparison of the common APBI modalities for prescription point, total dose, fractionation/dose-rate, and biological effective dose (BED)

APBI technique	Typical prescription point (PTV)	Total dose (Gy)	Fractionation or dose rate	BED (Gy) Normal tissue	Tumor
Interstitial brachytherapy					
HDR	Tumor bed plus 1.5 cm	34	Ten fractions twice daily	72.5	45.6
LDR	Tumor bed plus 2.0 cm	45	50 cGy/h	75	54
MammoSite	1 cm from balloon surface	34	Ten fractions twice daily	72.5	45.6
3D conformal external beam	Tumor bed plus 2.5 cm	38.5	Ten fractions daily or twice daily	164.9	53.3
Intraoperative electrons	"Operative bed"	21	Single fraction	168	65.1
Intraoperative 50-kV photons	1 cm from surface of applicator	5	Single fraction	13.3	7.5

Table 17.2 RTOG/EORTC normal tissue late toxicity scoring criteria

Grade	Description
Skin	
0	No change from baseline
1	Slight atrophy; pigmentation change; some hair loss
2	Patchy atrophy; moderate telangiectasia; total hair loss
3	Marked atrophy; macroscopic telangiectasia
4	Ulceration
Subcutaneous tissues	
0	No change from baseline
1	Slight induration (fibrosis) and loss of subcutaneous fat
2	Moderate fibrosis (asymptomatic); slight field contracture; <10% linear reduction
3	Severe induration and loss of subcutaneous tissue; field contracture; >10% linear measurement
4	Necrosis

proposed to calculate the DHI, but the formula commonly used in the assessment of APBI brachytherapy (Edmundson et al. 2002) is:

$$DHI = (V100 - V150)/V100$$

APBI brachytherapy has been delivered with both low dose-rate (LDR) and high dose-rate (HDR) techniques. Typically, LDR implants have been performed at a dose-rate of 40–60 cGy/h to a total dose of 45–60 Gy (Arthur et al. 2003; Kuerer et al. 2004; Kuske et al. 1998; Vicini et al. 1997). HDR implants have most commonly been prescribed to a total dose of 32–34 Gy at 3.4–4.0 Gy per fraction delivered twice daily.

The normal tissue toxicity end-points commonly evaluated after APBI are early and late changes to skin and subcutaneous tissues. These are scored using the established grading criteria of the RTOG/EORTC (Table 17.2). There is not a uniformly accepted scoring system for cosmetic outcome and, as such, there is considerable variability in the criteria applied across studies. In general, a four-tiered grading of excellent, good, fair, and poor has been applied in the majority of studies.

17.3 Interstitial Brachytherapy

17.3.1 Toxicity Reports from Selected Single- and Multi-Institutional Studies

One of the original efforts to explore the role of interstitial brachytherapy APBI was developed by Kuske while at the Ochsner Clinic. His group initially reported on 51 patients (25 LDR, 26 HDR) with a median follow-up of 75 months (King et al. 2000). The interpretation of the late normal tissue effects observed by these authors is limited by the fact that they employed their own three-tiered institution-specific grading scheme where grade I/II reflected primarily early events and grade III reflected late events. Nonetheless, they reported grade I/II and grade III toxicity in 22% and 8% of patients, respectively. The cosmetic outcome was rated as good/excellent in 75% of patients. Kuske pursued interstitial brachytherapy APBI after moving to the University of Wisconsin and in an updated oral presentation (personal communication) of 310 patients (a mix of LDR and HDR techniques), he stated that "The rate of fat necrosis reduced over time from 10% to 1%". Further, with evolution of his template-guided catheter placement technique and the application of three-dimensional treatment planning, "The DHI is never below 0.85".

Stimulated in part by these early results from the Ochsner Clinic, the RTOG launched in 1995 a phase II trial (protocol 95-17) to further investigate the potential role of interstitial brachytherapy APBI in a multi-institutional setting. Enrollment allowed for randomization to two different dose delivery schedules: LDR (45 Gy in 3.5–5 days) or HDR (34 Gy twice daily in ten fractions). This afforded the first opportunity to directly compare the effect of dose-rate technique on outcome. A toxicity analysis was reported on 99 patients (33 LDR, 66 HDR) after a median follow-up of 27 months (Kuske et al. 2002). The mean DHI for the entire study cohort was 0.82. Major acute toxicity was more commonly seen with LDR than with HDR techniques with grade 3/4 toxicity found in 9% and 3%, respectively. Similarly, late toxicity was found to be more severe with LDR technique with a 9% incidence of grade 3/4 skin thickening and a 12% incidence of grade 3/4 subcutaneous fibrosis. This was in contrast to patients treated with HDR where grade 3/4 skin thickening and subcutaneous fibrosis was seen in 1.5% and 3%, respectively.

A detailed analysis of normal tissue effects after interstitial brachytherapy has been performed by another group of APBI pioneers at the William Beaumont Hospital. Benitez et al. (2004) presented the results of an institutional protocol that enrolled 199 patients (120 LDR, 79 HDR) with a median follow-up of 5.7 years. This is a particularly noteworthy study as the authors clearly documented that normal-tissue changes after APBI will dramatically evolve over time. Further, this time-dependent evolution

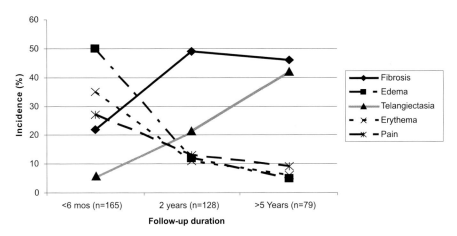

Fig. 17.1 The incidence of normal tissue toxicity as a function of time after interstitial brachytherapy APBI at the William Beaumont Hospital (data plotted from Benitez et al. 2004)

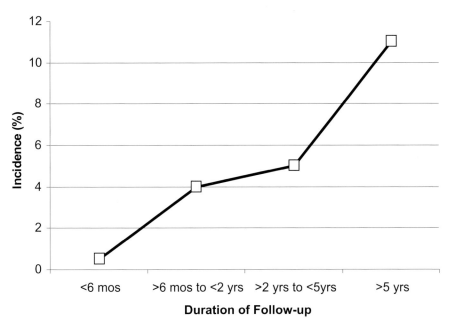

Fig. 17.2 The incidence of fat necrosis as a function of time after interstitial brachytherapy APBI at the William Beaumont Hospital (data plotted from Benitez et al. 2004)

can be for both the better and the worse. Some end-point measures significantly improved with time. For example, the cosmetic rating was scored as excellent/good in 95% at a median follow-up of ≤6 months but improved to 99% after 60 months. Breast pain, present in 27% at ≤6 months, decreased to 9% at ≥5 years. Similarly, edema and erythema progressively improved over the observation period (Fig. 17.1). In contrast, other measured end-points clearly worsened with prolonged follow-up. Over time, the incidence of fat necrosis, subcutaneous fibrosis, and telangiectasias all progressively increased (Figs. 17.1–17.4). Of particular note, the incidence of fat necrosis rose from 0.5% at <6 months to 11% at >5 years (Fig. 17.2). These findings underscore the complexity inherent in the assessment of late normal-tissue effects after APBI as the incidence of any given endpoint will be highly dependent upon when the measurement was obtained. As such, all short follow-up, "snap-shot" views of normal tissue effects, as is the norm in most studies of APBI reported to date, must be interpreted with caution.

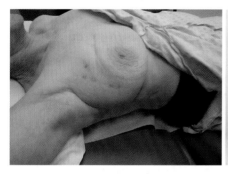
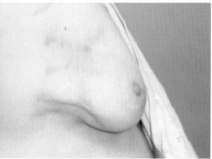

Fig. 17.3 Grade 1 late skin toxicity after interstitial brachytherapy APBI. Note the telangiectasias at the catheter entry sites in the lateral aspect of the breast

Fig. 17.4 Grade 3 late subcutaneous toxicity after interstitial brachytherapy APBI. Note the fibrotic contracture of tissues within the implant volume

17.3.2 LDR versus HDR

The APBI toxicity data reported from the Ochsner Clinic/University of Wisconsin, the RTOG, and the William Beaumont Hospital employed a mix of LDR and HDR techniques. The interpretation from these trials of specific variables that may influence complications is limited due to the markedly distinct normal tissue radiobiology of LDR versus HDR (described more fully in Chapter 5). In order to address this concern, more recent studies have focused exclusively on patients treated with either LDR or HDR applications.

As noted above, in the RTOG 95-17 trial, LDR implants prescribed to 45 Gy were found to be associated with a greater incidence of clinically significant normal tissue toxicity than HDR implants. However, Lawenda et al. (2003) reported on 48 patients enrolled on a phase I/II dose escalation study of LDR brachytherapy APBI and found a low rate of normal-tissue injury. The implants were delivered at 50 cGy/h to total doses of 50 Gy, 55 Gy, and 60 Gy. After a median follow-up of 23 months, cosmetic results were rated as very good to excellent in 91.8% of patients. As expected, total dose appeared to be a critical factor in that fibrosis was scored as "firm to moderate" in 9% of the entire patient cohort but with the highest dose level of 60 Gy, the incidence increased to 25%. Unfortunately, apart from total dose, limited dosimetric data are available from this study to correlate outcome with treatment-related variables.

In a subset analysis of the William Beaumont Hospital experience, Baglan et al. (2001) reported on 38 patients treated exclusively with HDR interstitial brachytherapy after a median follow-up of 31 months. APBI was delivered as 32 Gy in eight twice-daily fractions. The median DHI, V100, and V150 were 0.878, 216 cm³, and 26 cm³, respectively. The cosmetic outcome was rated as good or excellent in 100% and "mild residual fullness" was noted in 9%. No patients were found to have either persistent breast pain or symptomatic fat necrosis.

At the National Institute of Oncology in Budapest, Hungary, a series trials of APBI have been performed that have predominantly employed HDR interstitial brachytherapy (Polgar et al. 2002, 2004). The treatment scheme for APBI included HDR interstitial brachytherapy consisting of seven fractions to a total dose of either 30.3 Gy (17.8% of patients) or 36.4 Gy (82.2% of patients). In this cohort of patients, the mean V100 was 50 cm³ and the mean dose non-uniformity ratio was 0.45. After a median follow-up of 7 years, good/excellent cosmetic outcome was seen in 84.4% of cases. Late skin effects were generally mild with only 4.4% reported as grade 2/3. Grade 2/3 subcutaneous fibrosis was observed in 20% of patients and fat necrosis, asymptomatic and symptomatic, was seen in 20 % and 2.2%, respectively.

In order to more fully understand the clinical and treatment-related variables that could affect normal tissue toxicity, investigators from Tufts University, Brown University, and Virginia Commonwealth University pooled their data for patients treated with HDR interstitial APBI. Patients at all three institutions were treated in an identical manner with respect to selection criteria, implant technique, dosimetric evaluation, and follow-up assessment (Wazer et al. 2006). The entire cohort consisted of 75 patients with a median follow-up of 60 months and, similar to the RTOG 95-17 trial, the "worst toxic event" was recorded for analysis. Clinical variables including patient age, volume of ex-

Table 17.3 Summary of results from the Tufts/Brown/VCU analysis of variables associated with late normal tissue effects after interstitial brachytherapy APBI

End-point measure	Significantly associated variable	
Cosmetic outcome (excellent vs. good/fair/poor)	No. of dwell positions	211 vs. 250; P=0.04
	V150	43 cm³ vs. 59 cm³; P=0.03
	DHI	0.77 vs. 0.73; P=0.05
Late skin toxicity (grade 0 vs. grade 1/2)	V150	44 cm³ vs. 62 cm³; P=0.04
	DHI	0.77 vs. 0.71; P=0.009
Late subcutaneous toxicity (grade 0/1 vs. grade 2/3/4)	DHI	0.73 vs. 0.77; P=0.02
Clinically evident fat necrosis	V150	44 cm³ vs. 69 cm³; P=0.02

cised tissue, tumor diameter, and a history of diabetes or hypertension were not found to be significantly associated with either cosmetic score or normal tissue toxicity. In contrast, several implant-associated variables could be identified as having significant influence on the risk of an adverse cosmetic outcome or increased risk of late skin toxicity, late subcutaneous toxicity, and clinically evident fat necrosis (Table 17.3) (Wazer et al. 2006). In general, the volume of the implant, the volume of dose "hotspots" as defined by the V150 and V200, and the global dose homogeneity of the implant as described by the DHI were strongly correlated with adverse outcome. This study was the first to provide some specific dosimetric parameters to guide clinicians in defining, at least with respect to late tissue effects, what constitutes an optimal interstitial HDR implant.

17.3.3 Is there an Adverse Interaction between Interstitial Brachytherapy and Chemotherapy?

The answer is "possibly". The first evidence presented in this regard was reported by Kuske et al. (2002) from the RTOG 95-17 trial. In their study, grade 3 toxicity was significantly increased with the use of chemotherapy. This was true for both HDR and LDR techniques, but particularly so for LDR implants. Similarly, Arthur et al. (2003) found that APBI with an LDR interstitial technique was associated with a significant decrement in cosmetic outcome when patients also received Adriamycin-based chemotherapy. In the combined Tufts/Brown/VCU series (Wazer et al. 2006) of HDR interstitial brachytherapy, the use of Adriamycin-based chemotherapy was associated with an increased risk of clinically evident fat necrosis, grade 1/2 skin toxicity, and suboptimal cosmetic scores. In contrast, no adverse interactive effect has yet been found between the use of chemotherapy and the MammoSite catheter (Vicini et al. 2005).

17.3.4 Toxicity Avoidance Guidelines

As clinical data continue to accumulate, toxicity avoidance guidelines can, at best, be considered preliminary and subject to future revision. The guidelines that will be put forward are, by and large, limited to the use of HDR interstitial brachytherapy. To date, the amount and dosimetric specificity of data regarding LDR implants is simply too sparse to make even limited recommendations. With these caveats, current data do suggest the following:
- Volume probably matters; that is, keep it as low as practically achievable within the constraints imposed by adequate coverage of the PTV. Ideally, less than 60% of the normal whole breast reference volume should receive greater than or equal to 50% of the prescribed dose.
- Minimize hot spots. The dosimetric parameter that appears to be particularly sensitive in this regard is the V150. Most certainly, this value needs to be ≤70 cm3 though it appears preferable to strive for <45 cm3.
- Try to maintain a high level of global dose uniformity as defined by a DHI value of at least >0.75, even better >0.85. This is achievable with all of the common currently employed interstitial catheter placement techniques but does require attention to the detail of catheter position.

- The dose/volume limits to the skin and chest wall are as yet not defined. In general, the dose delivered to these structures should be less than the prescribed dose. Delineate the PTV such that it is at least 5 mm from the skin.
- Proceed with caution if chemotherapy is to be used after interstitial brachytherapy APBI.

17.4 MammoSite Brachytherapy

The first and perhaps most critical factor to consider in assessing risk of normal tissue effects with MammoSite brachytherapy is that, from the perspective of both dosimetry and radiobiology, it is a distinctly different implant from interstitial brachytherapy. As such, one must be cautious in transferring the lessons learned from interstitial brachytherapy APBI as they likely have limited relevance to this applicator system. As an example of these inherent differences, Shah et al. (2004) reported a series of interstitial and MammoSite implants and found significant differences in critical dosimetric parameters. MammoSite implants are associated with significantly less irradiated tissue and smaller volume "hotspots" as compared to interstitial brachytherapy (for example, V150 of 26 cm^3 with MammoSite vs. 40 cm^3 with interstitial technique, $P<0.0001$). In contrast, the global uniformity as reflected in the calculated DHI is superior with an interstitial implant (DHI of 0.83 with interstitial technique vs. 0.73 with MammoSite, $P<0.0001$). The relative importance of these variables in predicting normal tissue toxicity after MammoSite brachytherapy has yet to be fully elucidated.

In addition to the standard toxicity endpoints as described in the RTOG/EORTC rating scale, there are events that are, for the most part, specific to the MammoSite catheter that can result in implant failure. These include:

- Non-conformance of the applicator to the excision cavity (Fig. 17.5)
- Hemorrhage (Fig. 17.6)
- Balloon rupture (Fig. 17.7)
- Suboptimal balloon-to-skin spacing (Fig. 17.8)
- Inadequate tumor excision margin or nodal status (for intraoperative placement)

The initial safety and performance multi-institutional trial of the MammoSite catheter was performed by Keisch et al. (2003). This study of 43 patients investigated acute toxicity encountered up to 4 weeks after treatment. The most common side effects of the procedure included mild erythema (57.4%), drainage (51.9%), pain (42.6%), ecchymosis (31.5%), seroma (11.1%), and an infection rate of 3.7% (Figs. 17.9 and 17.10). Post-procedure infections have been the focus of some controversy in the early experience with the MammoSite catheter (Harper et al. 2005). However, it does appear that with meticulous wound care during the 1–2 weeks required to complete irradiation, the infection rate can be kept acceptably low even when assessed amongst a broad base of users. In a report of the American Society of Breast Surgeons (ASBS) Breast Brachytherapy Registry trial, the device-related infection rate among 793 patients was only 5.9% (Vicini et al. 2005). Prophylactic antibiotic use is advocated by some (Harper et al. 2005), but its role in modifying the rate of device-related infections remains unclear.

The incidence of seroma after MammoSite APBI is another area of on-going study (Fig. 17.11). The acute incidence of 11% reported by Keisch et al. (2003) likely underrepresents the frequency of persistent asymptomatic and symptomatic seroma seen

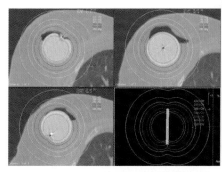

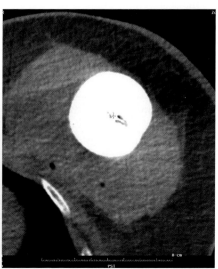

Fig. 17.5 An example of unacceptable non-conformance to target breast tissue of the fully inflated MammoSite catheter

Fig. 17.6 Intracavitary hemorrhage 24 hours after intraoperative placement of a MammoSite catheter

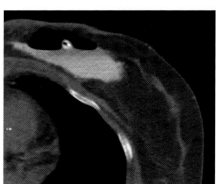

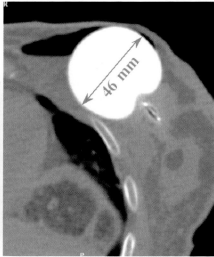

Fig. 17.7 Spontaneous rupture of a MammoSite catheter 48 hours after placement results in partial filling of the lumpectomy cavity with dilute contrast material

Fig. 17.8 Suboptimal balloon-to-skin spacing after intraoperative MammoSite placement necessitating catheter removal

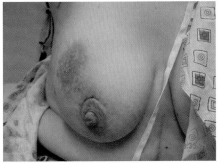

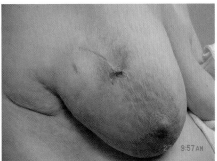

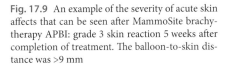

Fig. 17.9 An example of the severity of acute skin affects that can be seen after MammoSite brachytherapy APBI: grade 3 skin reaction 5 weeks after completion of treatment. The balloon-to-skin distance was >9 mm

Fig. 17.10 Infection in the operative bed 8 weeks after completion of MammoSite brachytherapy APBI

Fig. 17.11 Persistent and painful seroma (with associated mammogram) at the operative bed in the upper outer quadrant 9 months after completion of MammoSite brachytherapy APBI

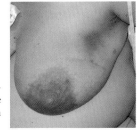

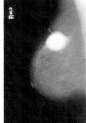

after several months of follow-up. The factors that contribute to the risk of persistent seroma as well as the most effective clinical management strategy have yet to be fully elucidated.

As the MammoSite catheter was approved for clinical use in May 2002 by the United States Food and Drug Administration, few data exist on the intermediate and late tissue effects. Keisch et al. (2004) have reported on a more extended evaluation of their original 43 patient cohort with a median follow-up of 29 months. These data show that cosmetic scores are clearly related to balloon-to-skin spacing such that suboptimal results are seen when the spacing is ≤6 mm. Further, these authors report asymptomatic fat necrosis in 4.9%, subcutaneous fibrosis in 29%, and telangiectasia in 27%. In light of the time-dependent evolution of late effects reported with interstitial brachytherapy APBI by the Beaumont Hospital group (Fig. 17.2), a reasonable expectation is that similar changes may be seen with further follow-up of the MammoSite experience.

Additional data regarding intermediate and late effects on normal tissue after MammoSite APBI are being actively collected through the ASBS Registry trial (Vicini et al. 2005). In a report of 702 patients, factors found to be significantly associated with favorable cosmetic outcome are balloon-to-skin spacing, both as a continuous variable and at a cut-off value of ≥7 mm, and larger bra size (C/D versus A/B) (Vicini et al. 2005). The use of chemotherapy or tamoxifen was not found to adversely affect cosmetic outcome.

How do MammoSite and interstitial brachytherapy compare with respect to normal tissue side effects? One might expect that, with the smaller volume of irradiated tissue seen with MammoSite, that MammoSite would be clearly superior in this regard. To address this question, Shah et al. (2004) used an expanded dataset from the Tufts/Brown/VCU collaboration to perform a comparison of normal tissue toxicity encountered with interstitial brachytherapy (75 cases) versus MammoSite (28 cases). When all patients were included, the use of the MammoSite catheter was associated with a higher rate of grade 1 acute skin toxicity (42.9% vs. 17.3%, $P = 0.01$) whereas subcutaneous fibrosis was more commonly seen with interstitial brachytherapy (32% vs. 10.7%). However, when interstitial brachytherapy patients who received chemotherapy were excluded from the analysis (as none of the MammoSite patients received chemotherapy), the only significant difference that remained between the groups was a higher rate of grade 1 skin toxicity with MammoSite.

17.4.1 Toxicity Avoidance Guidelines

As with interstitial brachytherapy, toxicity avoidance guidelines for use of the MammoSite catheter for APBI must be considered preliminary and subject to change with the emergence of longer term follow-up studies. Nonetheless, based upon currently available information, the following guidelines are offered:

- Meticulous attention to wound care is essential throughout the duration of a MammoSite catheter placement. Adherence to wound care instructions should result in a minimal rate (<5%) of device-related infections.
- Under all circumstances, strive to maintain a balloon-to-skin separation of >6 mm.
- Never allow the balloon-to-skin separation to be <5 mm.

17.5 3D Conformal External Beam APBI

The data available to assess normal tissue effects after 3D conformal external beam APBI are very limited and conclusions are, at best, preliminary. One of the largest experiences reported to date is that from the William Beaumont Hospital (Baglan et al. 2003; Vicini et al. 2003) where 31 patients were treated with 34 or 38.5 Gy in ten twice-daily fractions. After a median follow-up of 10 months, no significant immediate toxicity was seen beyond grade 1 skin erythema. At 4–8 weeks of follow-up, only grade 1 and 2 toxicity was seen in 61% and 10%, respectively. Cosmetic results were rated good or excellent in all patients with up to 2 years of follow-up. These promising preliminary data have lead to multi-institutional prospective phase II and phase III trials (RTOG 0319, RTOG 0413/NSABP B-39) to further test this approach.

Formenti et al. (2004) have used a conformal external beam partial breast irradiation technique with patients in the prone position. In contrast to the Beaumont Hospital group, an even more extreme hypofractionation scheme was employed with 30 Gy at 6 Gy per fraction delivered in five fractions over 10 days. In 47 patients with a median follow-up of 18 months, the normal tissue effects were found to be minor with nothing more than grade 1 acute or late toxicity.

17.5.1 Toxicity Avoidance Guidelines

As noted, the actual clinical toxicity data on 3D conformal external beam APBI is sparse and specific dose–volume relationships cannot yet be stated with confidence. Nonetheless, based upon the preliminary practice at William Beaumont Hospital (Baglan et al. 2003; Vicini et al. 2003), the following are suggested:

- Less than 60% of the whole breast normal reference volume should receive greater than or equal to 50% of the prescribed dose and less than 35% of the whole breast normal reference volume should receive the prescribed dose.
- The contralateral breast should receive less than 3% of the prescribed dose to any point.
- Less than 10% of either lung can receive 5% of the prescribed dose.
- For right-sided lesions, less than 5% of the heart should receive 5% of the prescribed dose. As for left-sided lesions, acceptable dose–volume limits are still uncertain and are subject to further analysis of data accumulated in the phase II trial of 3D conformal external beam APBI (RTOG 0319).
- A maximum point dose to the thyroid should be no more than 3% of the prescribed dose.

17.6 Intraoperative APBI

There are two intraoperative partial breast irradiation techniques currently under investigation. In Milan, Italy, Veronesi et al. (2005) are testing an approach that employs 3–9 MeV electrons to deliver 21 Gy as a single fraction to the excision bed. In a report of 590 patients with a median follow-up of 20 months, the authors claim a low rate of complications. They report mild to severe fibrosis in 3.2%, "that resolved in 24 months". Overt fat necrosis was seen in 2.5% of patients within 1–4 weeks after treatment.

Another approach pioneered by Vaidya et al. (2004) uses a device with a spherical tip that is inserted intraoperatively into the lumpectomy cavity. A 50-kV x-ray beam is generated to deliver a single fraction of 5 Gy prescribed at 1 cm from the surface of the applicator. A prospective randomized trial is underway in the United Kingdom and, to date, no normal tissue toxicity data are available.

17.7 Conclusion

Current techniques of APBI differ markedly in their dosimetric and radiobiological properties. As such, normal tissue toxicity data must be carefully collected in a prospective fashion for each treatment modality and fractionation scheme. Ongoing assessment of both clinical and treatment-related factors that may contribute to adverse normal tissue effects is required in order to minimize the risk of both early and late toxicity. To date, our most complete understanding of the incidence and variables associated with normal tissue injury after APBI is based upon the experience with interstitial brachytherapy and, to a lesser degree, the MammoSite catheter. The general applicability of the lessons learned with these catheter systems to other APBI modalities must be approached with caution.

References

1. Arthur DW, Koo D, Zwicker RD, et al (2003) Partial breast brachytherapy after lumpectomy: low-dose-rate and high-dose-rate experience. Int J Radiat Oncol Biol Phys 56:681–689

2. Baglan KL, Martinez AA, Frazier RC, et al (2001) The use of high dose-rate brachytherapy alone after lumpectomy in patients with early stage breast cancer treated with breast conserving therapy. Int J Radiat Oncol Biol Phys 50:1003–1011

3. Baglan KL, Sharpe MB, Jaffray D, et al (2003) Accelerated partial breast irradiation using 3D conformal radiation therapy (3D-CRT). Int J Radiat Oncol Biol Phys 55:302–311

4. Benitez PR, Chen PY, Vicini FA, et al (2004) Partial breast irradiation in breast-conserving therapy by way of interstitial brachytherapy. Am J Surg 188:355–364

5. Das RK, Patel R, Shah H, et al (2004) 3D CT-based high-dose-rate breast brachytherapy implants: treatment planning and quality assurance. Int J Radiat Oncol Biol Phys 59:1224–1228

6. Edmundson GK, Vicini FA, Chen PY, et al (2002) Dosimetric characteristics of the MammoSite RTS, a new breast brachytherapy applicator. Int J Radiat Oncol Biol Phys 52:1132–1139

7. Formenti SC, Minh TT, Goldberg JD, et al (2004) Prone accelerated partial breast irradiation after breast conserving surgery: preliminary clinical results and dose-volume histogram analysis. Int J Radiat Oncol Biol Phys 60:493–504

8. Harper JL, Jenrette JM, Vanek KN, et al (2005) Acute complications of MammoSite brachytherapy: a single institution's initial clinical experience. Int J Radiat Oncol Biol Phys 61:169–174

9. Keisch M, Vicini F, Kuske RR, et al (2003) Initial clinical experience with the MammoSite breast brachytherapy applicator in women with early stage breast cancer treated with breast conserving therapy. Int J Radiat Oncol Biol Phys 55:289–293

10. Keisch M, Vicini F, Scroggins T, et al (2004) Thirty month results with the MammoSite breast brachytherapy applicator: cosmesis, toxicity, and local control in partial breast irradiation. Int J Radiat Oncol Biol Phys 60 [Suppl]:272

11. King TA, Bolton JS, Kuske RR, et al (2000) Long-term results of wise-field brachytherapy as the sole method of radiation therapy after segmental mastectomy for T(is,1,2) breast cancer. Am J Surg 180:299–304

12. Kuerer HM, Julian TB, Strom EA, et al (2004) Accelerated partial breast irradiation after conservative surgery for breast cancer. Ann Surg 239:338–351

13. Kuske R, Bolton JS, McKinnon WP, et al (1998) Five-year results of a prospective phase II trial of wide-volume brachytherapy as the sole method of breast irradiation in Tis, T1, T2, N0-1 breast cancer (abstract). Int J Radiat Oncol Biol Phys 42 [Suppl]:181

14. Kuske RR, Winter K, Arthur D, et al (2002) A phase II trial of brachytherapy alone following lumpectomy for select breast cancer: toxicity analysis of Radiation Therapy Oncology Group 95-17. Int J Radiat Oncol Biol Phys 54 [Suppl]:87

15. Lawenda BD, Taghian AG, Kachnic LA, et al (2003) Dose-volume analysis of radiotherapy for T1N0 invasive breast cancer treated by local excision and partial breast irradiation by low-dose-rate-interstitial implant. Int J Radiat Oncol Biol Phys 56:671–680

16. Polgar C, Sulyok Z, Fodor J, et al (2002) Sole brachytherapy of the tumor bed after conservative surgery for T1 breast cancer: five year results of a phase I-II study and initial findings of a randomized phase III trial. J Surg Oncol 80:121–128

17. Polgar C, Major T, Fodor J, et al (2004) High dose rate brachytherapy alone versus whole breast radiotherapy with or without tumor bed boost after breast conserving surgery: seven year results of a comparative study. Int J Radiat Oncol Biol Phys 60:1173–1181

18. Shah NM, Tennenholz T, Arthur D, et al (2004) MammoSite and interstitial brachytherapy for accelerated partial breast irradiation: factors that affect toxicity and cosmesis. Cancer 101:727–734

19. Vaidya JS, Tobias JS, Baum M, et al (2004) Intraoperative radiotherapy for breast cancer. Lancet Oncol 5:165–173

20. Veronesi U, Orecchia R, Luini A, et al (2005) Full-dose intraoperative radiotherapy with electrons during breast-conserving surgery: experience with 590 cases. Ann Surg 242:101–106

21. Vicini FA, Chen PY, Fraile M, et al (1997) Low-dose-rate brachytherapy as the sole radiation modality in the management of patients with early stage breast cancer treated with breast-conserving therapy: preliminary results of a pilot trial. Int J Radiat Oncol Biol Phys 38:301–310

22. Vicini FA, Kestin LL, Edmundson GK, et al (1999) Dose-volume analysis for quality assurance of interstitial brachytherapy for breast cancer. Int J Radiat Oncol Biol Phys 45:803–810

23. Vicini FA, Remouchamps V, Wallace M, et al (2003) Ongoing clinical experience utilizing 3D conformal external beam radiotherapy to deliver partial breast irradiation in patients with early stage breast cancer treated with breast conserving therapy. Int J Radiat Oncol Biol Phys 57:1247–1253

24. Vicini F, Beitsch P, Quiet C, et al (2005) First analysis of patient demographics, technical reproducibility, cosmesis and early toxicity by the American Society of Breast Surgeons MammoSite Breast Brachytherapy Registry trial in 793 patients treated with accelerated partial breast irradiation (APBI). Cancer 104:1138–1148

25. Wazer DE, Kramer B, Schmid C, et al (1997) Factors determining outcome in patients treated with interstitial implantation as a radiation boost for breast conservation therapy. Int J Radiat Oncol Biol Phys 39:381–393

26. Wazer DE, Kaufman S, Cuttino L, et al (2006) Accelerated partial breast irradiation: An analysis of variables associated with late toxicity and long-term cosmetic outcome after high-dose-rate interstitial brachytherapy. Int J Radiat Oncol Biol Phys 64:489–495

27. Wu A, Ulin K, Sternick E (1988) A dose homogeneity index for evaluating Ir-192 interstitial breast implants. Med Phys 15:104–107

Future Directions: Phase III Cooperative Group Trials

18

Joseph R. Kelley and
Douglas W. Arthur

Contents

18.1 Introduction

Through the past 15 years, several single-institutional trials in Europe and the United States have been published with results that maintain that the use of accelerated partial breast irradiation (APBI) yields acceptable toxicity and comparable local control to standard breast-conservation therapy with whole-breast irradiation (WBI) (Arthur et al. 2003; King et al. 2000; Lawenda et al. 2003; Polgar et al. 2002; Vicini et al. 2003; Wazer et al. 2002). The follow-up periods in these trials range from 3 to >5 years and the numbers of patients included in these trials amount to a combined experience of several hundred patients. These trials have helped to provide the needed data to allow initial definition of patient selection criteria and the development of basic rules for treatment delivery and quality assurance for those physicians who choose to offer APBI in their clinical practice (American Society of Breast Surgeons 2005; Arthur 2003; Arthur et al. 2002). However, it must be recognized that the concept of APBI challenges the present standard treatment paradigm for early-stage breast cancer and introduces new treatment concepts that include target volume reduction to a partial breast target and the intensification of the treatment fractionation scheme to deliver the total dose in 5 days. To fully understand the impact of these new concepts and the role of APBI in the management of early-stage breast cancer, additional data are needed. This additional information can only be obtained through properly designed clinical trials and a joint effort by all physicians in supporting these trials.

Presently two large, multi-institutional phase III clinical trials are actively accruing, one in Europe and one in the United States. They are both designed to definitively compare APBI with WBI in a prospective randomized fashion and to further define the role of APBI in the management of early-stage breast cancer. The European Brachytherapy Breast Cancer GEC-ESTRO (Groupe Européen de Curietherapie–European Society for Therapeutic Radiology and Oncology) Working Group has opened a multicenter phase III trial, potentially including 12 institutions from seven European countries, with a goal of randomizing 1170 women between standard WBI and APBI utilizing multicatheter brachytherapy, see Fig. 18.1 (Strnad and Polgar 2004). This trial has been statistically designed as a noninferiority trial. With the patient accrual goal of 1170, the study is powered with a significance level set to 0.05 to detect greater than the set non-relevant 3% increase in local failure rate above the 5-year in-breast failure reference value of 4%. If the local failure rate in the APBI arm does not exceed 7%, then APBI will be judged to be "non-inferior" to adjuvant WBI.

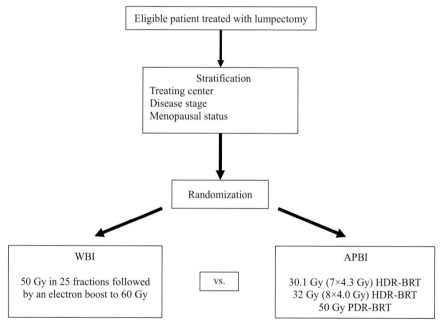

Fig. 18.1 GEC-ESTRO multicenter phase III trial (*HDR-BRT* high dose-rate brachytherapy, *PDR-BRT* pulsed dose-rate brachytherapy)

The National Surgical Adjuvant Breast and Bowl Project (NSABP) jointly with the Radiation Therapy Oncology Group (RTOG) subsequently opened a 3000-patient phase III trial in the United States. This trial will also compare standard whole-breast radiotherapy to APBI utilizing multicatheter brachytherapy, MammoSite balloon brachytherapy or the three-dimensional conformal external beam (3D-CRT) technique (Fig. 18.2)

(Vicini et al. 2004). This trial is statistically designed as a trial of equivalence. Based on previous NSABP trial data, the estimated 10-year cumulative incidence of in-breast recurrence is 6.1% for the population to be included in this trial and an acceptable variance from this result set as ±3%. If the risk of in-breast tumor recurrence following APBI relative to the risk of in-breast tumor recurrence following WBI is ≥1.5, then APBI will be defined as inferior to WBI. If the risk of in-breast tumor recurrence following APBI relative to the risk of in-breast tumor recurrence following WBI is ≤1/1.5 (0.667), then WBI will be defined as inferior to APBI. If neither APBI is inferior to WBI nor WBI inferior to APBI, then APBI will be defined as equivalent to WBI.

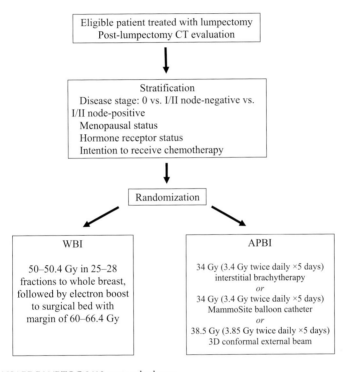

Fig. 18.2 NSABP B39/RTOG 0413 protocol schema

The primary objective in both trials is to determine if local control is equivalent between APBI and WBI. Secondary objectives are also similar in that acute and late toxicities will be reviewed, cosmetic outcome compared, quality of life differences evaluated and failure patterns including distant metastases-free survival, disease-free survival and overall survival assessed. The key components of successful partial breast irradiation are patient selection, target delineation, technique, dosimetry, and quality assurance. These components are clearly outlined in the European phase III trial (GEC-ESTRO multicenter phase III trial) and the American phase III trial (NSABP B-39/RTOG 0413). In review of these trials, many similarities are appreciated, subtle differences are seen and both trials are constructed to generate important additional and needed information regarding APBI. In this chapter the key aspects of these two trials are reviewed and their similarities and differences highlighted.

18.2 Patient Selection/Study Eligibility

Proper conservative patient selection appears to be crucial to the success of APBI, yet clear boundaries of inclusion and exclusion criteria have yet to be fully tested. The goal of patient selection is to identify those patients without a significant risk of harboring microscopic disease outside the immediate vicinity of the lumpectomy cavity. To provide guidance for those practitioners offering APBI, selection criteria have been endorsed and published by the American Brachytherapy Society (ABS) and the American Society of Breast Surgeons (ASBS) (American Society of Breast Surgeons 2005; Arthur et al. 2002). These selection criteria were based on the early APBI published experiences, are conservative in nature and indicate that patients should only be treated with APBI if they present with infiltrating ductal histology [the ASBS did include ductal carcinoma in situ (DCIS) as appropriate], lesions <3 cm, negative margins of resection and negative axillary lymph nodes, and are older than 45–50 years. Many factors (including non-infiltrating ductal histologies, younger age, extensive intraductal carcinoma or up to three positive lymph nodes without extracapsular extension) have been excluded based on speculation, rather than solid data, suggesting that patients with these features may have a higher risk of harboring disease elsewhere within the breast and therefore require whole-breast radiotherapy. Although the patient selection criteria published by the ABS and ASBS appear appropriate, this set of criteria is conservative and may exclude many appropriate patients. The American and European phase III trials are designed to explore the bounds of patient selection and both phase III trials have broadened the inclusion criteria (Table 18.1). Patients will be stratified at the time of randomization. There will be stratification for disease stage and menopausal status in both trials with the GEC-ESTRO multicenter phase III trial additionally stratifying for treatment center and the NSABP B39/RTOG 0314 additionally stratifying for hormonal receptor status and intent to receive chemotherapy (Figs. 18.1 and 18.2).

The GEC-ESTRO phase III multicenter trial will include only patients who are ≥40 years old, tumors which are unifocal/unicentric and histopathologically assured to be ≤3 cm, and will include all invasive histologies and DCIS alone. DCIS lesions are only eligible if they are classified as low or intermediate risk group as defined as a Van Nuys prognostic index of <8 (Silverstein 2003). Margins of resection must be clear by a confirmed 2 mm in any direction and if the histology is lobular or DCIS, then this margin must be at least 5 mm. Axillary lymph node evaluation in invasive histologies is to be by dissection, with a minimum of six axillary lymph nodes if positive, or by a negative sentinel node and the resected nodes must be negative or with no greater than microscopic involvement (pN1mi). Additional exclusion criteria include evidence of lymphatic invasion, vascular invasion and/or extensive intraductal component (EIC).

Eligibility criteria for NSABP B39/RTOG 0314 are similar but are less restrictive. This trial will include all ages, unifocal/unicentric tumors that are histopathologically assured to be ≤3 cm, and will include all invasive histologies and the entire spectrum of DCIS. Margins of resection must be clear; however, the NSABP definition of clear (no tumor

Table 18.1 Cooperative group phase III trials: core patient eligibility criteria

	NSABP B39/RTOG 0413	GEC-ESTRO multicenter phase III trial
Patient age	All ages	≥40 years
Tumor size (cm)	≤3	≤3
Histology	All invasive histologies; ductal carcinoma in situ	All invasive histologies; ductal carcinoma in situ; (Van Nuys Prognostic index[a] <8 only)
Margin status	Negative (no tumor extending to inked margin)	Non-lobular invasive histologies – >2 mm; invasive lobular carcinoma – >5 mm; ductal carcinoma in situ – >5 mm
Node status	pN0–pN1; up to three positive nodes; extracapsular extension negative	pN0–pN1mic; negative or microscopic involvement only

[a] Silverstein (2003)

extending to and involving the inked margin) is used for all histologies. Axillary lymph nodes require evaluation in invasive histologies and either a sentinel node negative or greater than six lymph nodes on dissection is required. Patients must be node-negative or no more than three positive lymph nodes involved without evidence of extracapsular extension. The presence of lymphatic invasion, vascular invasion or extensive intraductal component will not be used as exclusion criteria and will not be reported in this trial.

18.3 Target Delineation

As the post-lumpectomy radiation target decreases from the whole breast to partial breast, the precision of target delineation becomes increasingly important. A universally accepted target definition has not been established and the present definitions used vary depending on physician preferences and biases, specific pathologic findings and the treatment technique used. The partial breast target has most often been defined as a 1–2 cm margin of normal breast tissue beyond the lumpectomy cavity, bounded by breast tissue extent. Although the definitions are within a range of only 1 cm, this can represent a significant volume of breast tissue and it is the burden of further investigation to identify a universally accepted definition. Visualizing the cavity and clearly delineating the target are essential for APBI to be successful. Originally, target delineation was based on clinical parameters. This can often be misleading and is considered unacceptable by contemporary standards. Both phase III trials require clear radiographic visualization of the lumpectomy cavity. The GEC-ESTRO multicenter phase III trial recommends surgical clip placement at the time of lumpectomy to accurately define the cavity. If the clips are present, then any form of imaging to locate and visualize the target is acceptable. CT is recommended and preferred, but in cases where surgical clips have not been placed, CT evaluation is mandatory. In the NSABP B39/RTOG 0314 trial, surgical clips are optional and CT evaluation for cavity localization and target delineation is required in all cases. Any patient in whom the cavity is not clearly visualized is considered ineligible in both trials.

Once the location of the clinical target volume has been established, the planning target volume (PTV) must then be defined. In the European trial, an elegant approach is used. In this trial, the PTV is defined using a "safety margin" of 2 cm beyond the original tumor. This safety margin is the amount of normal breast tissue beyond the edge of the tumor in all directions that is to be treated. This is the expanded treatment target and is to be restricted to 5 mm below the skin surface and 5 mm above the ribs. This 2 cm treatment distance is covered through a combined surgical margin and designed radiation target (Fig. 18.3). For instance, a cavity with a medial surgical margin clear by 1 cm, a superior surgical margin clear by 5 mm, and all other surgical margins clear by 2 mm would result in an eccentric PTV covered by radiation dose that would extend from the cavity edge 1 cm medially, 1.5 cm superiorly and 1.8 cm in all others directions. This requires thorough pathologic evaluation, documentation and communication. The opportunity to customize the radiation target based on the extent of surgery provides the potential for treating smaller volumes of normal breast tissue.

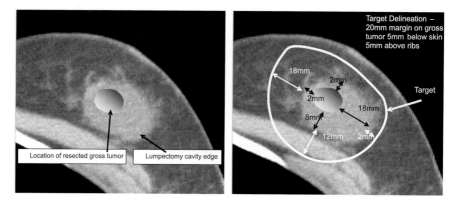

Fig. 18.3 GEC-ESTRO multicenter phase III target definition

The American trial works from a simplified approach but must deal with the challenge of equating target coverage goals between three different partial breast treatment techniques. The goal is to treat a 1.5 cm distance from the cavity edge and bounded to 5 mm below the skin surface anteriorly and the chest wall and pectoralis muscles posteriorly (Fig. 18.4). In the case of multicatheter brachytherapy, target coverage is achieved with proper catheter placement and radioactive source dwell positioning (Fig. 18.5A). Target coverage with MammoSite brachytherapy is not as adaptable as multicatheter brachytherapy and can only safely treat to a nominal 1 cm distance from the balloon surface (Fig. 18.5B). However, it is known that the actual treatment distance reaches beyond 1 cm due to the stretching, conforming and compacting effect that the inflation of the balloon has on the surrounding targeted breast tissue (Edmundson et al. 2002). This is dependent on the post-surgical size and shape of the lumpectomy cavity and cannot be controlled, but actually treatment distances beyond 1 cm that approach 1.5 cm are expected in the majority of cases. 3D-CRT presents a unique challenge that is not confronted with brachytherapy techniques: the need to account for breathing motion and set-up error. When treating with 3D-CRT, the protocol defines the clinical target volume as a 1.5 cm expansion beyond the cavity edge but adds an additional 1 cm to define the PTV to account for potential variations in target coverage due to breathing motion and set-up error (Fig. 18.5C). This results in a larger volume of breast tissue receiving radiation as compared to brachytherapy techniques.

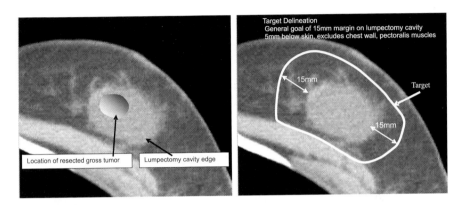

Fig. 18.4 NSABP B39/RTOG 0413 target definition—general goals

18.4 Technique and Dosimetry

The largest distinction between the NSABP B39/ RTOG 0413 and the GEC-ESTRO multicenter phase III trial is the technique of delivering partial breast irradiation and the dose delivery schemes used. Intraoperative dose delivery techniques are not included in either study, reflecting the investigators desire for complete pathologic evaluation to assure eligibility prior to protocol enrollment and the need for clear target delineation and confirmation of dose delivery to the target. Interstitial multicatheter implants have been the predominant method investigated to date in Europe and are the only method of partial breast irradiation that will be used on the GEC-ESTRO multicenter phase III trial. The dose delivery schemes allowed reflect the European experience with APBI. Low dose-rate brachytherapy is not allowed and investigators have a choice of high dose-rate (HDR) or pulsed dose-rate (PDR). If HDR, then they can treat with a total dose of 32 Gy in eight fractions treating twice daily over 4 days or a total dose of 30.3 Gy in seven fractions treating twice daily. The PDR dose scheme is 0.6–0.8 Gy per hour to 50 Gy (one pulse per hour, 24 hours per day). All brachytherapy plans require imaging on simulator or CT scanner. Dose parameters to assure dose homogeneity and the reporting of the dose distribution characterization are clearly outlined. Dose coverage goals include confirmation that 100% of the prescribed dose covers 90% of the target and that the maximum skin dose is <70% of the prescribed dose.

Multicatheter brachytherapy is also one of the techniques that can be used for APBI in the NSABP B39/RTOG 0314 trial. Despite the long history of multicatheter brachytherapy in the United States, it is recognized that this approach can be technically challenging and far less appealing to patients due to the appearance and potential pain. In

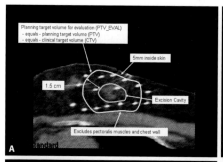

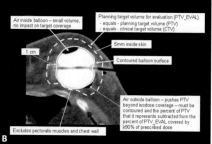

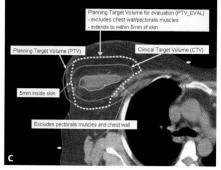

Fig. 18.5 Target definition specifics for NSABP B39/RTOG0413 treatment techniques: **A** multicatheter brachytherapy, **B** MammoSite brachytherapy, **C** 3D-conformal external beam radiotherapy

response, the MammoSite radiation treatment system was developed in an attempt to simplify breast brachytherapy for both the physician and patient. As a result of this innovation, the MammoSite radiation treatment system has become the dominant method of delivering APBI in the United States and will also be included as an APBI treatment method. Lastly, 3D-CRT will also be included in the American trial. Utilizing CT planning for design of multiple conformal external beam fields, this technique has been developed to provide a noninvasive method of APBI.

After eligibility determination and enrollment, patients will be randomized between standard whole-breast radiotherapy and APBI. If randomized to APBI, the treating physician will choose which APBI technique to be used: multicatheter brachytherapy, MammoSite brachytherapy, or 3D-CRT. The decision will be based on facility preference, patient preference and technical feasibility for that unique case. In each of the two brachytherapy approaches, the dose delivery scheme has been standardized to a total dose of 34 Gy delivered in ten fractions twice daily over 5 days. Brachytherapy dose delivery is inherently non-homogeneous and therefore to properly adjust the homogeneous dose delivery scheme of 3D-CRT to a dose delivery scheme that is radiobiologically equivalent, an increase in dose is required. The dose scheme calculated to provide equivalence and used in the phase I/II RTOG 0319 protocol is a total dose of 38.5 Gy delivered in ten fractions twice daily over 5 days. All APBI plans require CT-based planning. Dose parameters to assure dose homogeneity and the reporting of the dose distribution characterization are clearly outlined. Dose coverage goals include confirmation that 90% of the prescribed dose covers 90% of the target, that skin dose is controlled and, that when treating with 3D-CRT, the dose to surrounding normal tissues is restricted to defined dose volumes.

18.5 Quality Assurance

Standard breast-conservation therapy, where standard WBI follows lumpectomy, has proven to be successful and therefore it is our responsibility to assure that APBI maintains comparable in-breast control and toxicity rates. The ethical predicate to do no harm is thus very high and consequently, the quality assurance procedures in both trials are stringent. To prevent unacceptable toxicity and ensure a meaningful comparison between results, quality control dominates both trials. Dosimetric parameters governing target coverage and dose homogeneity are thorough with details provided within each protocol. In the GEC-ESTRO multicenter phase III trial, a traditional approach of submitting requested dosimetric information is used and site visits are planned. Measured and calculated parameters are provided for data collection and subsequent review and to compare with clinical outcome.

The quality assurance program of the NSABP B39/RTOG 0413 trial is based on an innovative electronic data submission system developed and managed by the Image-Guided Therapy Center (ITC). The CT data set for each APBI case will be submitted to the ITC for review and evaluation where normal tissue structures and target volumes are checked for accuracy and the dosimetric target coverage and dose homogeneity evaluated to assure guidelines are followed. These cases are reviewed by members of the ITC and the principle investigators of the study. The complexity of the guidelines is recognized, and therefore a system of monitoring was developed to help sites quickly understand all of the details involved. This all starts with a credentialing process that comprises two questionnaires and CT-based test cases. The questionnaires test the facility's capabilities and assess the physician's understanding of the protocol. A CT-based test case is planned and digitally submitted for each APBI technique to be offered at the facility. Once the site is credentialed, accrual may begin. The first case from each facility for any of the three APBI techniques to be offered is to be submitted for rapid review. The rapid review process allows the case to be evaluated prior to treatment initiation, assures that all of the parameters and guidelines have been followed, and assures that the patient will be treated according to the protocol. Immediate feedback to the site is important to correct any deviation from protocol that is seen. The subsequent four cases from that facility for that technique will be reviewed in a timely (5 days) fashion. After the first five cases are complete, all five cases are reviewed with recommendations to either proceed with continued enrollment or to repeat the review process. Once clearing the first five-case review process, additional review of completed cases is random. The process is efficient and allows immediate feedback to the treating facility in a timely manner that guarantees that each patient is treated according to protocol.

18.6 Conclusion

The management of early-stage breast cancer remains an area of active research. Standard breast-conservation therapy is now well established but the logistics of traditional whole-breast adjuvant irradiation limit the widespread use of breast conservation. A modern review of clinical and pathologic data suggests that adjuvant radiation of the entire breast is unnecessary and indicates that partial breast therapy may be appropriate, thus opening the possibilities of APBI. With more than 10 years experience, definitive data regarding the role of APBI have not yet been generated. The GEC-ESTRO multicenter phase III trial now underway in Europe and the NSABP B39/RTOG 0413 open in the United States are two, multi-institutional phase III trials constructed to deliver the answers to the many questions that remain. It is the role of these phase III trials to further define and potentially expand the patient selection criteria, elucidate which dosimetric parameters are critical to success and clarify which APBI technique is appropriate in which situation.

References

1. American Society of Breast Surgeons (2005) Consensus statement for accelerated partial breast irradiation. American Society of Breast Surgeons, Columbia, MD. http://www.breastsurgeons.org/apbi.shtml

2. Arthur D (2003) Accelerated partial breast irradiation: a change in treatment paradigm for early stage breast cancer. J Surg Oncol 84:185–191

3. Arthur DW, Vicini FA, Kuske RR, et al (2002) Accelerated partial breast irradiation: an updated report from the American Brachytherapy Society. Brachytherapy 1:184–190

4. Arthur DW, Koo D, Zwicker RD, et al (2003) Partial breast brachytherapy after lumpectomy: low-dose-rate and high-dose-rate experience. Int J Radiat Oncol Biol Phys 56:681–689

5. Edmundson GK, Vicini FA, Chen PY, et al (2002) Dosimetric characteristics of the MammoSite RTS, a new breast brachytherapy applicator. Int J Radiat Oncol Biol Phys 52:1132–1139

6. King TA, Bolton JS, Kuske RR, et al (2000) Long-term results of wide-field brachytherapy as the sole method of radiation therapy after segmental mastectomy for T(is,1,2) breast cancer. Am J Surg 180:299–304

7. Lawenda BD, Taghian AG, Kachnic LA, et al (2003) Dose-volume analysis of radiotherapy for T1N0 invasive breast cancer treated by local excision and partial breast irradiation by low-dose-rate interstitial implant. Int J Radiat Oncol Biol Phys 56:671–680

8. Polgar C, Sulyok Z, Fodor J, et al (2002) Sole brachytherapy of the tumor bed after conservative surgery for T1 breast cancer: five-year results of a phase I-II study and initial findings of a randomized phase III trial. J Surg Oncol 80:121–128; discussion 129

9. Silverstein MJ (2003) An argument against routine use of radiotherapy for ductal carcinoma in situ. Oncology (Huntingt) 17:1511–1533; discussion 1533–1514, 1539, 1542 passim

10. Strnad V, Polgar C (2004) Phase III multicenter trial – interstitial brachytherapy alone versus external beam radiation therapy after breast conserving surgery for low risk invasive carcinoma and low risk duct carcinoma in situ (DCIS) of the female breast. Study protocol. European Brachytherapy Breast Cancer GEC-ESTRO Working Group

11. Vicini FA, Kestin L, Chen P, et al (2003) Limited-field radiation therapy in the management of early-stage breast cancer. J Natl Cancer Inst 95:1205–1210

12. Vicini F, White J, Arthur D, et al (2004) NSABP protocol B39/RTOG protocol 0413: A randomized phase III study of conventional whole breast irradiation (WBI) versus partial breast irradiation (PBI) for women with stage 0, I, or II breast cancer

13. Wazer D, Berle L, Graham R, et al (2002) Preliminary results of a phase I/II study of HDR brachytherapy alone for T1/T2 breast cancer. Int J Radiat Oncol Biol Phys 53:889–897

Subject Index

Printing: Krips bv, Meppel
Binding: Stürtz, Würzburg